THE OFFICIAL PATIENT'S SOURCEBOOK

on

TINNITUS

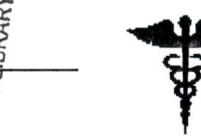

JAMES N. PARKER, M.D.
AND PHILIP M. PARKER, PH.D., EDITORS

ICON Health Publications
ICON Group International, Inc.
4370 La Jolla Village Drive, 4th Floor
San Diego, CA 92122 USA

Copyright ©2004 by ICON Group International, Inc.

Copyright ©2004 by ICON Group International, Inc. All rights reserved. This book is protected by copyright. No part of it may be reproduced, stored in a retrieval system, or transmitted in any form or by any means, electronic, mechanical, photocopying, recording or otherwise, without written permission from the publisher.

Printed in the United States of America.

Last digit indicates print number: 10 9 8 7 6 4 5 3 2 1

Publisher, Health Care: Philip Parker, Ph.D.
Editor(s): James Parker, M.D., Philip Parker, Ph.D.

Publisher's note: The ideas, procedures, and suggestions contained in this book are not intended as a substitute for consultation with your physician. All matters regarding your health require medical supervision. As new medical or scientific information becomes available from academic and clinical research, recommended treatments and drug therapies may undergo changes. The authors, editors, and publisher have attempted to make the information in this book up to date and accurate in accord with accepted standards at the time of publication. The authors, editors, and publisher are not responsible for errors or omissions or for consequences from application of the book, and make no warranty, expressed or implied, in regard to the contents of this book. Any practice described in this book should be applied by the reader in accordance with professional standards of care used in regard to the unique circumstances that may apply in each situation, in close consultation with a qualified physician. The reader is advised to always check product information (package inserts) for changes and new information regarding dose and contraindications before taking any drug or pharmacological product. Caution is especially urged when using new or infrequently ordered drugs, herbal remedies, vitamins and supplements, alternative therapies, complementary therapies and medicines, and integrative medical treatments.

Cataloging-in-Publication Data

Parker, James N., 1961-
Parker, Philip M., 1960-

The Official Patient's Sourcebook on Tinnitus: A Revised and Updated Directory for the Internet Age/James N. Parker and Philip M. Parker, editors
       p.   cm.
Includes bibliographical references, glossary and index.
ISBN: 0-597-84200-0
1. Tinnitus-Popular works.   I. Title.

Disclaimer

This publication is not intended to be used for the diagnosis or treatment of a health problem or as a substitute for consultation with licensed medical professionals. It is sold with the understanding that the publisher, editors, and authors are not engaging in the rendering of medical, psychological, financial, legal, or other professional services.

References to any entity, product, service, or source of information that may be contained in this publication should not be considered an endorsement, either direct or implied, by the publisher, editors or authors. ICON Group International, Inc., the editors, or the authors are not responsible for the content of any Web pages nor publications referenced in this publication.

Copyright Notice

If a physician wishes to copy limited passages from this sourcebook for patient use, this right is automatically granted without written permission from ICON Group International, Inc. (ICON Group). However, all of ICON Group publications are copyrighted. With exception to the above, copying our publications in whole or in part, for whatever reason, is a violation of copyright laws and can lead to penalties and fines. Should you want to copy tables, graphs or other materials, please contact us to request permission (E-mail: iconedit@san.rr.com). ICON Group often grants permission for very limited reproduction of our publications for internal use, press releases, and academic research. Such reproduction requires confirmed permission from ICON Group International, Inc. **The disclaimer above must accompany all reproductions, in whole or in part, of this sourcebook.**

Dedication

To the healthcare professionals dedicating their time and efforts to the study of tinnitus.

Acknowledgements

The collective knowledge generated from academic and applied research summarized in various references has been critical in the creation of this sourcebook which is best viewed as a comprehensive compilation and collection of information prepared by various official agencies which directly or indirectly are dedicated to tinnitus. All of the *Official Patient's Sourcebooks* draw from various agencies and institutions associated with the United States Department of Health and Human Services, and in particular, the Office of the Secretary of Health and Human Services (OS), the Administration for Children and Families (ACF), the Administration on Aging (AOA), the Agency for Healthcare Research and Quality (AHRQ), the Agency for Toxic Substances and Disease Registry (ATSDR), the Centers for Disease Control and Prevention (CDC), the Food and Drug Administration (FDA), the Healthcare Financing Administration (HCFA), the Health Resources and Services Administration (HRSA), the Indian Health Service (IHS), the institutions of the National Institutes of Health (NIH), the Program Support Center (PSC), and the Substance Abuse and Mental Health Services Administration (SAMHSA). In addition to these sources, information gathered from the National Library of Medicine, the United States Patent Office, the European Union, and their related organizations has been invaluable in the creation of this sourcebook. Some of the work represented was financially supported by the Research and Development Committee at INSEAD. This support is gratefully acknowledged. Finally, special thanks are owed to Tiffany Freeman for her excellent editorial support.

About the Editors

James N. Parker, M.D.

Dr. James N. Parker received his Bachelor of Science degree in Psychobiology from the University of California, Riverside and his M.D. from the University of California, San Diego. In addition to authoring numerous research publications, he has lectured at various academic institutions. Dr. Parker is the medical editor for the *Official Patient's Sourcebook* series published by ICON Health Publications.

Philip M. Parker, Ph.D.

Philip M. Parker is the Eli Lilly Chair Professor of Innovation, Business and Society at INSEAD (Fontainebleau, France and Singapore). Dr. Parker has also been Professor at the University of California, San Diego and has taught courses at Harvard University, the Hong Kong University of Science and Technology, the Massachusetts Institute of Technology, Stanford University, and UCLA. Dr. Parker is the associate editor for the *Official Patient's Sourcebook* series published by ICON Health Publications.

About ICON Health Publications

In addition to tinnitus, *Official Patient's Sourcebooks* are available for the following related topics:

- The Official Patient's Sourcebook on Acoustic Neurinoma
- The Official Patient's Sourcebook on Balance Disorders
- The Official Patient's Sourcebook on Cochlear Implants
- The Official Patient's Sourcebook on Hearing Loss
- The Official Patient's Sourcebook on Landau-kleffner Syndrome
- The Official Patient's Sourcebook on Ménière Disease
- The Official Patient's Sourcebook on Noise Induced Hearing Loss
- The Official Patient's Sourcebook on Otitis Media
- The Official Patient's Sourcebook on Otosclerosis
- The Official Patient's Sourcebook on Presbycusis
- The Official Patient's Sourcebook on Sudden Sensorineural Hearing Loss
- The Official Patient's Sourcebook on Usher Syndrome
- The Official Patient's Sourcebook on Waardenburg Syndrome

To discover more about ICON Health Publications, simply check with your preferred online booksellers, including Barnes&Noble.com and Amazon.com which currently carry all of our titles. Or, feel free to contact us directly for bulk purchases or institutional discounts:

ICON Group International, Inc.
4370 La Jolla Village Drive, Fourth Floor
San Diego, CA 92122 USA
Fax: 858-546-4341
Web site: **www.icongrouponline.com/health**

Table of Contents

INTRODUCTION 1
   Overview 1
   Organization 3
   Scope 3
   Moving Forward 4

PART I: THE ESSENTIALS 7

CHAPTER 1. THE ESSENTIALS ON TINNITUS: GUIDELINES 9
   Overview 9
   What Is Tinnitus? 10
   What Causes Tinnitus? 11
   What Should I Do If I Have Tinnitus? 11
   How Will Hearing Experts Treat My Tinnitus? 12
   What Can I Do to Help Myself? 12
   Where Can I Find More Information? 13
   More Guideline Sources 14
   Vocabulary Builder 36

CHAPTER 2. SEEKING GUIDANCE 39
   Overview 39
   Associations and Tinnitus 39
   Finding Associations 40
   Finding Doctors 42
   Finding an Otolaryngologist 43
   Selecting Your Doctor 44
   Working with Your Doctor 44
   Broader Health-Related Resources 46
   Vocabulary Builder 46

CHAPTER 3. CLINICAL TRIALS AND TINNITUS 47
   Overview 47
   Recent Trials on Tinnitus 50
   Benefits and Risks 51
   Keeping Current on Clinical Trials 54
   General References 55
   Vocabulary Builder 56

PART II: ADDITIONAL RESOURCES AND ADVANCED MATERIAL 57

CHAPTER 4. STUDIES ON TINNITUS 59
   Overview 59
   The Combined Health Information Database 59
   Federally Funded Research on Tinnitus 83

viii Contents

    E-Journals: PubMed Central 116
    The National Library of Medicine: PubMed 116
    Vocabulary Builder 170

CHAPTER 5. PATENTS ON TINNITUS 177
    Overview 177
    Patents on Tinnitus 178
    Patent Applications on Tinnitus 209
    Keeping Current 227
    Vocabulary Builder 227

CHAPTER 6. BOOKS ON TINNITUS 229
    Overview 229
    Book Summaries: Federal Agencies 229
    Book Summaries: Online Booksellers 233
    Chapters on Tinnitus 239
    Directories 266
    General Home References 267
    Vocabulary Builder 268

CHAPTER 7. MULTIMEDIA ON TINNITUS 271
    Overview 271
    Video Recordings 271

CHAPTER 8. PERIODICALS AND NEWS ON TINNITUS 273
    Overview 273
    News Services and Press Releases 273
    Newsletters on Tinnitus 276
    Newsletter Articles 277

CHAPTER 9. PHYSICIAN GUIDELINES AND DATABASES 279
    Overview 279
    NIH Guidelines 279
    NIH Databases 280
    Other Commercial Databases 293

CHAPTER 10. DISSERTATIONS ON TINNITUS 295
    Overview 295
    Dissertations on Tinnitus 295
    Keeping Current 296
    Vocabulary Builder 296

PART III. APPENDICES 297

APPENDIX A. RESEARCHING ALTERNATIVE MEDICINE 299
    Overview 299
    What Is CAM? 299
    What Are the Domains of Alternative Medicine? 300
    Can Alternatives Affect My Treatment? 303
    Additional Web Resources 339

General References 347
Vocabulary Builder 349
APPENDIX B. RESEARCHING NUTRITION 351
Overview 351
Food and Nutrition: General Principles 351
Finding Studies on Tinnitus 356
Federal Resources on Nutrition 361
Additional Web Resources 362
Vocabulary Builder 364
APPENDIX C. FINDING MEDICAL LIBRARIES 365
Overview 365
Preparation 365
Finding a Local Medical Library 366
Medical Libraries in the U.S. and Canada 366
APPENDIX D. NIH CONSENSUS STATEMENT ON NOISE AND HEARING LOSS 373
Overview 373
Abstract 374
Introduction 374
What Is Noise-Induced Hearing Loss? 376
What Sounds Can Damage Hearing? 379
What Factors, Including Age, Determine an Individual's Susceptibility to Noise-Induced Hearing Loss? 382
Differences among Individuals 382
Differences within Individuals 383
What Can Be Done to Prevent Noise-Induced Hearing Loss? 384
What Are the Directions for Future Research? 387
Conclusions and Recommendations 388
APPENDIX E. MORE ON NOISE-INDUCED HEARING LOSS 391
Overview 391
How Do We Hear? 391
What Sounds Cause NIHL? 392
What Are the Effects of NIHL? 393
What Are the Symptoms of NIHL? 393
Who Is Affected by NIHL? 393
Can NIHL Be Prevented? 394
What Research Is Being Done for NIHL? 394
Where Can I Get Additional Information? 395
APPENDIX F. PROTECT YOURSELF AND YOUR FAMILY FROM NOISE-INDUCED HEARING LOSS 397
Overview 397
How Much Noise Is Too Much? 398
Additional Resources 399

APPENDIX G. HOW LOUD IS TOO LOUD? 401
ONLINE GLOSSARIES 403
Online Dictionary Directories 404
TINNITUS GLOSSARY 405
General Dictionaries and Glossaries 414
INDEX 417

INTRODUCTION

Overview

Dr. C. Everett Koop, former U.S. Surgeon General, once said, "The best prescription is knowledge."[1] The Agency for Healthcare Research and Quality (AHRQ) of the National Institutes of Health (NIH) echoes this view and recommends that every patient incorporate education into the treatment process. According to the AHRQ:

> Finding out more about your condition is a good place to start. By contacting groups that support your condition, visiting your local library, and searching on the Internet, you can find good information to help guide your treatment decisions. Some information may be hard to find — especially if you don't know where to look.[2]

As the AHRQ mentions, finding the right information is not an obvious task. Though many physicians and public officials had thought that the emergence of the Internet would do much to assist patients in obtaining reliable information, in March 2001 the National Institutes of Health issued the following warning:

> The number of Web sites offering health-related resources grows every day. Many sites provide valuable information, while others may have information that is unreliable or misleading.[3]

---

[1] Quotation from **http://www.drkoop.com**.
[2] The Agency for Healthcare Research and Quality (AHRQ): **http://www.ahcpr.gov/consumer/diaginfo.htm**.
[3] From the NIH, National Cancer Institute (NCI): **http://cancertrials.nci.nih.gov/beyond/evaluating.html**.

Since the late 1990s, physicians have seen a general increase in patient Internet usage rates. Patients frequently enter their doctor's offices with printed Web pages of home remedies in the guise of latest medical research. This scenario is so common that doctors often spend more time dispelling misleading information than guiding patients through sound therapies. *The Official Patient's Sourcebook on Tinnitus* has been created for patients who have decided to make education and research an integral part of the treatment process. The pages that follow will tell you where and how to look for information covering virtually all topics related to tinnitus, from the essentials to the most advanced areas of research.

The title of this book includes the word "official." This reflects the fact that the sourcebook draws from public, academic, government, and peer-reviewed research. Selected readings from various agencies are reproduced to give you some of the latest official information available to date on tinnitus.

Given patients' increasing sophistication in using the Internet, abundant references to reliable Internet-based resources are provided throughout this sourcebook. Where possible, guidance is provided on how to obtain free-of-charge, primary research results as well as more detailed information via the Internet. E-book and electronic versions of this sourcebook are fully interactive with each of the Internet sites mentioned (clicking on a hyperlink automatically opens your browser to the site indicated). Hard copy users of this sourcebook can type cited Web addresses directly into their browsers to obtain access to the corresponding sites. Since we are working with ICON Health Publications, hard copy *Sourcebooks* are frequently updated and printed on demand to ensure that the information provided is current.

In addition to extensive references accessible via the Internet, every chapter presents a "Vocabulary Builder." Many health guides offer glossaries of technical or uncommon terms in an appendix. In editing this sourcebook, we have decided to place a smaller glossary within each chapter that covers terms used in that chapter. Given the technical nature of some chapters, you may need to revisit many sections. Building one's vocabulary of medical terms in such a gradual manner has been shown to improve the learning process.

We must emphasize that no sourcebook on tinnitus should affirm that a specific diagnostic procedure or treatment discussed in a research study, patent, or doctoral dissertation is "correct" or your best option. This sourcebook is no exception. Each patient is unique. Deciding on appropriate options is always up to the patient in consultation with their physician and healthcare providers.

Organization

This sourcebook is organized into three parts. Part I explores basic techniques to researching tinnitus (e.g. finding guidelines on diagnosis, treatments, and prognosis), followed by a number of topics, including information on how to get in touch with organizations, associations, or other patient networks dedicated to tinnitus. It also gives you sources of information that can help you find a doctor in your local area specializing in treating tinnitus. Collectively, the material presented in Part I is a complete primer on basic research topics for patients with tinnitus.

Part II moves on to advanced research dedicated to tinnitus. Part II is intended for those willing to invest many hours of hard work and study. It is here that we direct you to the latest scientific and applied research on tinnitus. When possible, contact names, links via the Internet, and summaries are provided. It is in Part II where the vocabulary process becomes important as authors publishing advanced research frequently use highly specialized language. In general, every attempt is made to recommend "free-to-use" options.

Part III provides appendices of useful background reading for all patients with tinnitus or related disorders. The appendices are dedicated to more pragmatic issues faced by many patients with tinnitus. Accessing materials via medical libraries may be the only option for some readers, so a guide is provided for finding local medical libraries which are open to the public. Part III, therefore, focuses on advice that goes beyond the biological and scientific issues facing patients with tinnitus.

Scope

While this sourcebook covers tinnitus, your doctor, research publications, and specialists may refer to your condition using a variety of terms. Therefore, you should understand that tinnitus is often considered a synonym or a condition closely related to the following:

- Subjective Tinnitus

In addition to synonyms and related conditions, physicians may refer to tinnitus using certain coding systems. The International Classification of Diseases, 9th Revision, Clinical Modification (ICD-9-CM) is the most commonly used system of classification for the world's illnesses. Your physician may use this coding system as an administrative or tracking tool. The following classification is commonly used for tinnitus:[4]

- 388.3 tinnitus
- 388.30 tinnitus, unspecified
- 388.31 subjective tinnitus
- 388.32 objective tinnitus

For the purposes of this sourcebook, we have attempted to be as inclusive as possible, looking for official information for all of the synonyms relevant to tinnitus. You may find it useful to refer to synonyms when accessing databases or interacting with healthcare professionals and medical librarians.

Moving Forward

Since the 1980s, the world has seen a proliferation of healthcare guides covering most illnesses. Some are written by patients or their family members. These generally take a layperson's approach to understanding and coping with an illness or disorder. They can be uplifting, encouraging, and highly supportive. Other guides are authored by physicians or other healthcare providers who have a more clinical outlook. Each of these two styles of guide has its purpose and can be quite useful.

As editors, we have chosen a third route. We have chosen to expose you to as many sources of official and peer-reviewed information as practical, for the purpose of educating you about basic and advanced knowledge as recognized by medical science today. You can think of this sourcebook as your personal Internet age reference librarian.

Why "Internet age"? All too often, patients diagnosed with tinnitus will log on to the Internet, type words into a search engine, and receive several Web site listings which are mostly irrelevant or redundant. These patients are left

---

[4] This list is based on the official version of the World Health Organization's 9th Revision, International Classification of Diseases (ICD-9). According to the National Technical Information Service, "ICD-9CM extensions, interpretations, modifications, addenda, or errata other than those approved by the U.S. Public Health Service and the Health Care Financing Administration are not to be considered official and should not be utilized. Continuous maintenance of the ICD-9-CM is the responsibility of the federal government."

to wonder where the relevant information is, and how to obtain it. Since only the smallest fraction of information dealing with tinnitus is even indexed in search engines, a non-systematic approach often leads to frustration and disappointment. With this sourcebook, we hope to direct you to the information you need that you would not likely find using popular Web directories. Beyond Web listings, in many cases we will reproduce brief summaries or abstracts of available reference materials. These abstracts often contain distilled information on topics of discussion.

While we focus on the more scientific aspects of tinnitus, there is, of course, the emotional side to consider. Later in the sourcebook, we provide a chapter dedicated to helping you find peer groups and associations that can provide additional support beyond research produced by medical science. We hope that the choices we have made give you the most options available in moving forward. In this way, we wish you the best in your efforts to incorporate this educational approach into your treatment plan.

The Editors

PART I: THE ESSENTIALS

ABOUT PART I

Part I has been edited to give you access to what we feel are "the essentials" on tinnitus. The essentials of a disease typically include the definition or description of the disease, a discussion of who it affects, the signs or symptoms associated with the disease, tests or diagnostic procedures that might be specific to the disease, and treatments for the disease. Your doctor or healthcare provider may have already explained the essentials of tinnitus to you or even given you a pamphlet or brochure describing tinnitus. Now you are searching for more in-depth information. As editors, we have decided, nevertheless, to include a discussion on where to find essential information that can complement what your doctor has already told you. In this section we recommend a process, not a particular Web site or reference book. The process ensures that, as you search the Web, you gain background information in such a way as to maximize your understanding.

CHAPTER 1. THE ESSENTIALS ON TINNITUS: GUIDELINES

Overview

Official agencies, as well as federally funded institutions supported by national grants, frequently publish a variety of guidelines on tinnitus. These are typically called "Fact Sheets" or "Guidelines." They can take the form of a brochure, information kit, pamphlet, or flyer. Often they are only a few pages in length. The great advantage of guidelines over other sources is that they are often written with the patient in mind. Since new guidelines on tinnitus can appear at any moment and be published by a number of sources, the best approach to finding guidelines is to systematically scan the Internet-based services that post them.

The National Institutes of Health (NIH)[5]

The National Institutes of Health (NIH) is the first place to search for relatively current patient guidelines and fact sheets on tinnitus. Originally founded in 1887, the NIH is one of the world's foremost medical research centers and the federal focal point for medical research in the United States. At any given time, the NIH supports some 35,000 research grants at universities, medical schools, and other research and training institutions, both nationally and internationally. The rosters of those who have conducted research or who have received NIH support over the years include the world's most illustrious scientists and physicians. Among them are 97 scientists who have won the Nobel Prize for achievement in medicine.

---

[5] Adapted from the NIH: **http://www.nih.gov/about/NIHoverview.html**.

There is no guarantee that any one Institute will have a guideline on a specific disease, though the National Institutes of Health collectively publish over 600 guidelines for both common and rare diseases. The best way to access NIH guidelines is via the Internet. Although the NIH is organized into many different Institutes and Offices, the following is a list of key Web sites where you are most likely to find NIH clinical guidelines and publications dealing with tinnitus and associated conditions:

- Office of the Director (OD); guidelines consolidated across agencies available at **http://www.nih.gov/health/consumer/conkey.htm**

- National Library of Medicine (NLM); extensive encyclopedia (A.D.A.M., Inc.) with guidelines available at **http://www.nlm.nih.gov/medlineplus/healthtopics.html**

- National Institute on Deafness and Other Communication Disorders (NIDCD); fact sheets and guidelines available at **http://www.nidcd.nih.gov/health/health.htm**

Among the above, the National Institute on Deafness and Other Communication Disorders (NIDCD) is particularly noteworthy. The mission of the NIDCD is to conduct and support biomedical and behavioral research and research training in the normal and disordered processes of hearing, balance, smell, taste, voice, speech, and language.[6] The Institute also conducts and supports research and research training related to disease prevention and health promotion; addresses special biomedical and behavioral problems associated with people who have communication impairments or disorders; and supports efforts to create devices which substitute for lost and impaired sensory and communication function.

The following patient guideline was recently published by the NIDCD on tinnitus.

What Is Tinnitus?[7]

Do you hear a ringing, roaring, clicking, or hissing sound in your ears? Do you hear this sound often or all the time? Does the sound bother you a lot? If you answer yes to these questions, you may have tinnitus (tin-NY-tus).

---

[6] This paragraph has been adapted from the NIDCD: **http://www.nidcd.nih.gov/about/about.htm**. "Adapted" signifies that a passage has been reproduced exactly or slightly edited for this book.
[7] Adapted from the National Institute on Deafness and Other Communication Disorders (NIDCD): **http://www.nidcd.nih.gov/health/pubs_hb/noiseinear.htm**.

Tinnitus is a symptom associated with many forms of hearing loss. It can also be a symptom of other health problems. According to estimates by the American Tinnitus Association, at least 12 million Americans have tinnitus. Of these, at least 1 million experience it so severely that it interferes with their daily activities. People with severe cases of tinnitus may find it difficult to hear, work, or even sleep.

What Causes Tinnitus?

- Hearing loss. Doctors and scientists have discovered that people with different kinds of hearing loss also have tinnitus.

- Loud noise. Too much exposure to loud noise can cause noise-induced hearing loss and tinnitus.

- Medicine. More than 200 medicines can cause tinnitus. If you have tinnitus and you take medicine, ask your doctor or pharmacist whether your medicine could be involved.

- Other health problems. Allergies, tumors, and problems in the heart and blood vessels, jaws, and neck can cause tinnitus.

What Should I Do If I Have Tinnitus?

The most important thing you can do is to go see your doctor. Your doctor can try to determine what is causing your tinnitus. He or she can check to see if it is related to blood pressure, kidney function, diet, or allergies. Your doctor can also determine whether your tinnitus is related to any medicine you are taking.

To learn more about what is causing your tinnitus, your doctor may refer you to an otolaryngologist (oh-toe-lair-in-GAH-luh-jist), an ear, nose, and throat doctor. He or she will examine your ears and your hearing to try to find out why you have tinnitus. Another hearing professional, an audiologist (aw-dee-AH-luh-jist), can measure your hearing. If you need a hearing aid, an audiologist can fit you with one that meets your needs.

How Will Hearing Experts Treat My Tinnitus?

Although there is no cure for tinnitus, scientists and doctors have discovered several treatments that may give you some relief. Not every treatment works for everyone, so you may need to try several to find the ones that help.

Treatments can include:

- Hearing aids. Many people with tinnitus also have a hearing loss. Wearing a hearing aid makes it easier for some people to hear the sounds they need to hear by making them louder. The better you hear other people talking or the music you like, the less you notice your tinnitus.

- Maskers. Maskers are small electronic devices that use sound to make tinnitus less noticeable. Maskers do not make tinnitus go away, but they make the ringing or roaring seem softer. For some people, maskers hide their tinnitus so well that they can barely hear it. Some people sleep better when they use maskers. Listening to static at a low volume on the radio or using bedside maskers can help. These are devices you can put by your bed instead of behind your ear. They can help you ignore your tinnitus and fall asleep.

- Medicine or drug therapy. Some medicines may ease tinnitus. If your doctor prescribes medicine to treat your tinnitus, he or she can tell you whether the medicine has any side effects.

- Tinnitus retraining therapy. This treatment uses a combination of counseling and maskers. Otolaryngologists and audiologists help you learn how to deal with your tinnitus better. You may also use maskers to make your tinnitus less noticeable. After a while, some people learn how to avoid thinking about their tinnitus. It takes time for this treatment to work, but it can be very helpful.

- Counseling. People with tinnitus may become depressed. Talking with a counselor or people in tinnitus support groups may be helpful.

- Relaxing. Learning how to relax is very helpful if the noise in your ears frustrates you. Stress makes tinnitus seem worse. By relaxing, you have a chance to rest and better deal with the sound.

What Can I Do to Help Myself?

Think about things that will help you cope. Many people find listening to music very helpful. Focusing on music might help you forget about your tinnitus for a while. It can also help mask the sound. Other people like to listen to recorded nature sounds, like ocean waves, the wind, or even crickets.

Avoid anything that can make your tinnitus worse. This includes smoking, alcohol, and loud noise. If you are a construction worker, an airport worker, or a hunter, or if you are regularly exposed to loud noise at home or at work, wear ear plugs or special earmuffs to protect your hearing and keep your tinnitus from getting worse.

If it is hard for you to hear over your tinnitus, ask your friends and family to face you when they talk so you can see their faces. Seeing their expressions may help you understand them better. Ask people to speak louder, but not shout. Also, tell them they do not have to talk slowly, just more clearly.

Where Can I Find More Information?

If you have any other questions, or if you need a large-print version of this fact sheet, call the NIDCD Information Clearinghouse. Here are several ways to contact us:

Toll-free: (800) 241-1044
Toll-free TTY: (800) 241-1055
Address: 1 Communication Avenue, Bethesda, MD 20892-3456
E-mail: nidcdinfo@nidcd.nih.gov
Internet: **www.nidcd.nih.gov**

You can contact other groups for more information on tinnitus as well:

American Tinnitus Association
P.O. Box 5
Portland, OR 97207
Voice: (503) 248-9985
Toll-free: (800) 634-8978
E-mail: tinnitus@ata.org
Internet: **www.ata.org**

American Academy of Otolaryngology-
Head and Neck Surgery
One Prince Street
Alexandria, VA 22314
Voice: (703) 836-4444
TTY: (703) 519-1585

E-mail: webmaster@ent.org
Internet: **www.entnet.org**

American Academy of Audiology
8300 Greensboro Drive, Suite 750
McLean, VA 22102
Voice: (703) 790-8466
Toll-free: (800) AAA-2336
TTY: (703) 790-8466
Internet: **www.audiology.org**

Self Help for Hard of Hearing People, Inc.
7910 Woodmont Avenue, Suite 1200
Bethesda, MD 20814
Voice: (301) 657-2248
TTY: (301) 657-2249
E-mail: national@shhh.org
Internet: **www.shhh.org**

American Speech-Language-Hearing Association
10801 Rockville Pike
Rockville, MD 20852
Voice: (301) 897-3279
Toll-free: (800) 638-8255
TTY: (301) 897-0157
E-mail: actioncenter@asha.org
Internet: **www.asha.org**

More Guideline Sources

The guideline above on tinnitus is only one example of the kind of material that you can find online and free of charge. The remainder of this chapter will direct you to other sources which either publish or can help you find additional guidelines on topics related to tinnitus. Many of the guidelines listed below address topics that may be of particular relevance to your specific situation or of special interest to only some patients with tinnitus. Due to space limitations these sources are listed in a concise manner. Do not hesitate to consult the following sources by either using the Internet hyperlink provided, or, in cases where the contact information is provided, contacting the publisher or author directly.

Topic Pages: MEDLINEplus

For patients wishing to go beyond guidelines published by specific Institutes of the NIH, the National Library of Medicine has created a vast and patient-oriented healthcare information portal called MEDLINEplus. Within this Internet-based system are "health topic pages." You can think of a health topic page as a guide to patient guides. To access this system, log on to **http://www.nlm.nih.gov/medlineplus/healthtopics.html**. From there you can either search using the alphabetical index or browse by broad topic areas. Recently, MEDLINEplus listed the following as being relevant to tinnitus:

- Other guides

    Dizziness and Vertigo
    http://www.nlm.nih.gov/medlineplus/dizzinessandvertigo.html

    Hearing Disorders and Deafness
    http://www.nlm.nih.gov/medlineplus/hearingdisordersanddeafness.html

    Hearing Problems in Children
    http://www.nlm.nih.gov/medlineplus/hearingproblemsinchildren.html

    Meniere's Disease
    http://www.nlm.nih.gov/medlineplus/menieresdisease.html

Within the health topic page dedicated to tinnitus, the following was recently recommended to patients:

- Treatment

    Tinnitus Management
    Source: American Speech-Language-Hearing Association
    http://www.asha.org/public/hearing/treatment/tinnitus_manage.htm

    Tinnitus Treatment Options
    Source: American Tinnitus Association
    http://www.ata.org/about_tinnitus/consumer/treatment.html

- Specific Conditions/Aspects

    Tinnitus: Questions to Ask Your Healthcare Provider
    Source: American Tinnitus Association
    http://www.ata.org/about_tinnitus/consumer/questions.html

- From the National Institutes of Health

    Noise in Your Ears: Facts about Tinnitus
    Source: National Institute on Deafness and Other Communication Disorders
    http://www.nidcd.nih.gov/health/hearing/noiseinear.asp

- Organizations

    American Academy of Otolaryngology--Head and Neck Surgery
    http://www.entnet.org/

    American Tinnitus Association
    http://www.ata.org/

    National Institute on Deafness and Other Communication Disorders
    http://www.nidcd.nih.gov/

- Pictures/Diagrams

    Inner Ear Anatomy
    Source: Vestibular Disorders Association
    http://www.vestibular.org/gallery.html

- Prevention/Screening

    Healthy Hearing
    Source: American Tinnitus Association
    http://www.ata.org/about_tinnitus/consumer/healthy_hearing1.html

- Research

    Tinnitus Research
    Source: National Institute on Deafness and Other Communication Disorders
    http://www.nidcd.nih.gov/health/hearing/tinnitus.asp

You may also choose to use the search utility provided by MEDLINEplus at the following Web address: **http://www.nlm.nih.gov/medlineplus/**. Simply type a keyword into the search box and click "Search." This utility is similar to the NIH search utility, with the exception that it only includes materials that are linked within the MEDLINEplus system (mostly patient-oriented information). It also has the disadvantage of generating unstructured results.

We recommend, therefore, that you use this method only if you have a very targeted search.

The Combined Health Information Database (CHID)

CHID Online is a reference tool that maintains a database directory of thousands of journal articles and patient education guidelines on tinnitus and related conditions. One of the advantages of CHID over other sources is that it offers summaries that describe the guidelines available, including contact information and pricing. CHID's general Web site is **http://chid.nih.gov/**. To search this database, go to **http://chid.nih.gov/detail/detail.html**. In particular, you can use the advanced search options to look up pamphlets, reports, brochures, and information kits. The following was recently posted in this archive:

- **Clinical Psychologists and Tinnitus**

    Source: London, England: Royal National Institute for Deaf People. 1998. 3 p.

    Contact: Available from RNID Helpline. P.O. Box 16464, London EC1Y 8TT, United Kingdom. 0870 60 50 123. Fax 0171-296 8199. E-mail: helpline@rnid.org.uk. Website: www.rnid.org.uk. Also available from RNID Tinnitus Helpline. Castle Cavendish Works, Norton Street, Radford, Nottingham NG7 5PN, United Kingdom. 0345 090210. Fax 0115-978 5012. E-mail: tinnitushelpline@btinternet.com. PRICE: Single copy free.

    Summary: Anxiety, depression, irritability, anger, tension, and insomnia are all common complaints of patients with tinnitus(ringing or other noises in the ear). These may be the effects of tinnitus itself, or they may have existed before it started and be made worse by the reaction to it. This fact sheet from the Royal National Institute for Deaf People (RNID) discusses the role of clinical psychologists in treating tinnitus. A clinical psychologist works within a clinical context, usually a hospital or medical setting, and deals primarily with alleviating people's psychological problems. The fact sheet reviews the strategies that clinical psychologists may offer to help people overcome or learn to deal better with the effects of tinnitus. A patient may see a clinical psychologist on a one to one basis or in group therapy sessions with other patients. The fact sheet describes the work of four different clinical psychologists, including their publications and concludes with information on the RNID Tinnitus Helpline (in Nottingham, UK), which is also accessible online at tinnitushelpline@btinternet.com. The RNID website is at www.rnid.org.uk.

- **Counselling for Tinnitus**

    Source: London, England: Royal National Institute for Deaf People. 1998. 3 p.

    Contact: Available from RNID Helpline. P.O. Box 16464, London EC1Y 8TT, United Kingdom. 0870 60 50 123. Fax 0171-296 8199. E-mail: helpline@rnid.org.uk. Website: www.rnid.org.uk. Also available from RNID Tinnitus Helpline. Castle Cavendish Works, Norton Street, Radford, Nottingham NG7 5PN, United Kingdom. 0345 090210. Fax 0115-978 5012. E-mail: tinnitushelpline@btinternet.com. PRICE: Single copy free.

    Summary: Counseling has been described as the most important single component in the management of tinnitus (ringing or other noises in the ears). Being able to talk to somebody who takes an interest and is prepared to listen can help a person understand tinnitus and learn to deal with it more effectively. This fact sheet from the Royal National Institute for Deaf People (RNID) discusses the use of counseling for patients with tinnitus. Topics include private, medical, and lay counseling (including support groups). The fact sheet reviews the strategies that counseling may offer to help people overcome or learn to deal better with the effects of tinnitus and concludes with information on the RNID Tinnitus Helpline (in Nottingham, UK), which is also accessible online at tinnitushelpline@btinternet.com. The RNID website is at www.rnid.org.uk. 8 references.

- **Underwater Diving and Tinnitus**

    Source: London, England: Royal National Institute for Deaf People. 2000. 4 p.

    Contact: Available from RNID Helpline. P.O. Box 16464, London EC1Y 8TT, United Kingdom. 0870 60 50 123. Fax 0171 296 8199. E-mail: helpline@rnid.org.uk. Website: www.rnid.org.uk. PRICE: Single copy free.

    Summary: Ear injuries and disorders are the most common occupational diseases of people who dive. This fact sheet offers information about underwater diving and tinnitus (ringing or other noises in the ears). The fact sheet, from the British based Royal National Institute for Deaf People (RNID), first discusses how pressure affects the ears when one dives, including middle ear squeeze, alternobaric vertigo (dizziness due to different pressures in the left and right middle ears), barotrauma, and decompression sickness (Caisson disease). The fact sheet then describes strategies that can be used to reduce the risks associated with diving. The fact sheet concludes with information about the British Sub Aqua Association (www.scubadiving.com) and about the RNID Tinnitus Helpline (www.rnid.org.uk). 6 references.

- **Diet and Tinnitus**

    Source: London, England: Royal National Institute for Deaf People. 1998. 2 p.

    Contact: Available from RNID Helpline. P.O. Box 16464, London EC1Y 8TT, United Kingdom. 0870 60 50 123. Fax 0171-296 8199. E-mail: helpline@rnid.org.uk. Website: www.rnid.org.uk. Also available from RNID Tinnitus Helpline. Castle Cavendish Works, Norton Street, Radford, Nottingham NG7 5PN, United Kingdom. 0345 090210. Fax 0115-978 5012. E-mail: tinnitushelpline@btinternet.com. PRICE: Single copy free.

    Summary: Many people have suggested that a wide variety of foods and drinks may cause or aggravate tinnitus (noise or ringing in the ears). This fact sheet from the Royal National Institute for Deaf People (RNID) discusses the relationship between diet and tinnitus by briefly examining the evidence for cheese and chocolate, coffee, tea, cola, salt, tonic water, alcohol, red wine, and spirits. Historical notes are provided for some of these categories. The fact sheet recommends that readers try keeping a detailed diary of their food and beverage intake and tinnitus levels for a few days, to see whether a particular food or drink is having any effect. If a suspicious food or drink becomes apparent, the fact sheet suggests no ingesting of that item for a few days to see whether the tinnitus improves but notes that, in general, the healthier and more balanced the diet, the better. The fact sheet concludes with information on the RNID Tinnitus Helpline (in Nottingham, UK), which is also accessible online at tinnitushelpline@btinternet.com. The RNID website is at www.rnid.org.uk.

- **Pulsatile Tinnitus**

    Source: London, England: Royal National Institute for Deaf People. 1999. 4 p.

    Contact: Available from RNID Helpline. P.O. Box 16464, London EC1Y 8TT, United Kingdom. 0870 60 50 123. Fax 0171-296 8199. E-mail: helpline@rnid.org.uk. Website: www.rnid.org.uk. Also available from RNID Tinnitus Helpline. Castle Cavendish Works, Norton Street, Radford, Nottingham NG7 5PN, United Kingdom. 0345 090210. Fax 0115-

978 5012. E-mail: tinnitushelpline@btinternet.com. PRICE: Single copy free.

Summary: Most people with tinnitus (ringing or noises in the ears) experience it as a constant or steady sound, a rushing, whistling, buzzing, or humming. However, up to 10 percent of those who hear tinnitus noises describe them as rhythmic, beating, pounding, throbbing, or swooshing, a condition know as pulsatile tinnitus. This fact sheet from the Royal National Institute for Deaf People (RNID) discusses the causes of pulsatile tinnitus, including benign intracranial hypertension, atherosclerotic carotid artery disease, and glomus tumors; the diagnosis of PT, including tests that may be used to confirm the condition; and the treatment options, including counseling, sound therapy (masking), cognitive therapy, or tinnitus retraining therapy. The fact sheet concludes with information on the RNID Tinnitus Helpline (in Nottingham, UK), which is also accessible online at tinnitushelpline@btinternet.com. The RNID website is at www.rnid.org.uk. 7 references.

- **Dental Drilling and Tinnitus**

Source: London, England: Royal National Institute for Deaf People. 1999. 3 p.

Contact: Available from RNID Helpline. P.O. Box 16464, London EC1Y 8TT, United Kingdom. 0870 60 50 123. Fax 0171 296 8199. E-mail: helpline@rnid.org.uk. Website: www.rnid.org.uk. PRICE: Single copy free.

Summary: People with tinnitus (ringing or other noises in the ear) have reason to be concerned about exposing themselves to any loud noise that may aggravate their tinnitus. Similarly, people who do not have tinnitus should take care to avoid too much loud noise, as it can cause hearing loss or tinnitus. This fact sheet from the Royal National Institute for Deaf People (RNID, London, England) reviews the problem of dental drilling and tinnitus. The author notes that research into the noise levels of dental drills and their potential for hearing damage has produced conflicting conclusions. Dentists themselves are at risk for noise induced hearing loss and or tinnitus. And although dental patients are exposed to dental drill noise for short periods of time, the noise is conducted directly to the ears through the bones of the jaw and skull, as well as through the air. The fact sheet reviews strategies that can reduce the risk of dental drill noise exacerbating tinnitus. The fact sheet concludes with information about the RNID tinnitus helpline, including the web site and email address of the organization. 7 references.

- **Malaria and Tinnitus**

  Source: London, England: Royal National Institute for Deaf People. 1998. 3 p.

  Contact: Available from RNID Helpline. P.O. Box 16464, London EC1Y 8TT, United Kingdom. 0870 60 50 123. Fax 0171-296 8199. E-mail: helpline@rnid.org.uk. Website: www.rnid.org.uk. Also available from RNID Tinnitus Helpline. Castle Cavendish Works, Norton Street, Radford, Nottingham NG7 5PN, United Kingdom. 0345 090210. Fax 0115-978 5012. E-mail: tinnitushelpline@btinternet.com. PRICE: Single copy free.

  Summary: Some antimalarial drugs have the potential to produce tinnitus or to aggravate existing tinnitus. This fact sheet from the Royal National Institute for Deaf People (RNID) discusses the fact some drugs used to prevent and treat malaria cause tinnitus (ringing or other noises in the ears). The fact sheet offers a chart that lists the main antimalarial drugs and the reporting of tinnitus as a possible side effect in two publications, the British National Formulary or Hearing and Medicines. These drugs are chloroquine, halofantrine hydrochloride, mefloquine, primaquine, proguanil hydrochloride, pyrimethamine, and quinine. The fact sheet notes that the risks of any side effect from antimalarials may be greater with the much higher doses given to treat the disease, than with the lower doses given for prevention before traveling. The overriding consideration is to balance the likely risks of experiencing a (probably temporary) generation of or increase in tinnitus against the chances of suffering from malaria. The fact sheet concludes with information on the RNID Tinnitus Helpline (in Nottingham, UK), which is also accessible online at tinnitushelpline@btinternet.com. The RNID website is at www.rnid.org.uk. 6 references.

- **Children and Tinnitus**

  Source: London, England: Royal National Institute for Deaf People. 200x. [2 p.].

  Contact: Available from RNID Helpline. P.O. Box 16464, London EC1Y 8TT, United Kingdom. 0870 60 50 123. Fax 0171 296 8199. E-mail: helpline@rnid.org.uk. Website: www.rnid.org.uk. PRICE: Single copy free.

  Summary: The incidence of tinnitus (a ringing or buzzing noise in the ears) may be greater among children than in adults, particularly among children with some degree of hearing loss. This fact sheet offers information about children and tinnitus. The fact sheet, from the British based Royal National Institute for Deaf People (RNID), first discusses the prevalence rates of tinnitus in children, the symptoms in children (which tend to be intermittent), risk factors for becoming aware of or bothered by the tinnitus, the need to reassure parents of children with tinnitus (children are often not bothered by their own tinnitus), and the association of tinnitus with otitis media with effusion (middle ear infection, called 'glue ear' in the British literature). The fact sheet then details the causes of tinnitus, including Meniere's disease, spontaneous emissions of tones, temporary conductive deafness, noise-induced tinnitus, and hearing loss with recruitment; and treatment options, including tinnitus maskers, hearing aids, and tinnitus retraining therapy (TRT). 1 reference.

- **15 Facts About Tinnitus**

  Source: Hearing Health. 17(1): 63. Spring 2001.

  Contact: Available from Voice International Publications, Inc. P.O. Drawer V, Ingleside, TX 78362-0500. Voice/TTY (361) 776-7240. Fax (361) 776-3278. Website: www.hearinghealthmag.com.

  Summary: This brief article provides 15 facts about tinnitus (ringing or other sounds in the ear or ears). Tinnitus is defined as the perception of head noise when none is present externally. Tinnitus can be intermittent or constant, with single or multiple tones and its perceived volume can range from subtle to shattering. Up to 90 percent of all people who seek treatment for tinnitus have some level of sensorineural hearing loss, usually noise induced. However, hearing loss and tinnitus have an unpredictable relationship. Exposure to loud noises is the primary cause of tinnitus; other causative factors can be aging, ototoxic drugs, stress and hypertension, wax buildup in the ear canal, ear or sinus infections, jaw misalignment, cardiovascular disease, tumors affecting the auditory system, thyroid disorders, and head and neck trauma. Hearing aids and ear level maskers are sometimes helpful in drowning out the sounds of tinnitus; stress reduction and relaxation therapy are often successful in tinnitus management strategies. The article includes the contact information for the American Tinnitus Association (800-634-8978 or www.ata.org).

- **'Doctor, What Causes the Noise in My Ears?': Ten Common Questions About Tinnitus**

  Source: Alexandria, VA: American Academy of Otolaryngology-Head and Neck Surgery Foundation, Inc. (AAO-HNS). 1993. 2 p.

  Contact: American Academy of Otolaryngology-Head and Neck Surgery Foundation, Inc. (AAO-HNS). One Prince Street, Alexandria, VA 22314.

(703) 836-4444. Fax (703) 683-5100. PRICE: Single copy free (send self-addressed, stamped envelope); $20.00 for members; $25.00 for non-members per 100. Item Number 4763020.

Summary: This brochure addresses ten common questions that patients often have about tinnitus. Topics covered include the causes of tinnitus; the difference between objective and subjective tinnitus; the epidemiology of tinnitus; the most common cause of tinnitus; treatment modalities; how to lessen tinnitus, even when the cause cannot be determined; biofeedback and its application in tinnitus; masking and tinnitus maskers; and the potential impact of hearing aids on tinnitus. The brochure concludes with a brief description of the specialty of otolaryngology-head and neck surgery.

- **American Speech-Language-Hearing Association Answers Questions About Tinnitus**

  Source: Rockville, MD: American Speech-Language-Hearing Association (ASHA). 199x. [2 p.].

  Contact: Available from American Speech-Language-Hearing Association (ASHA). Product Sales, 10801 Rockville Pike, Rockville, MD 20852. (888) 498-6699. TTY (301) 897-0157. Website: www.asha.org. PRICE: Single copy free; bulk orders available. Item Number 0210119.

  Summary: This brochure answers common questions about tinnitus, or hearing sounds coming from inside the head. Written in a question and answer format, the brochure addresses the incidence of tinnitus, the causes of tinnitus, tinnitus as a symptom rather than a disease entity, the interrelationship between tinnitus and hearing loss, diagnostic tests used to evaluate tinnitus, and treatment options, including the use of a tinnitus masker and hearing aids. The brochure briefly discusses resources for people who think they may have a hearing problem; the contact information for the American Speech Language Hearing Association (ASHA) is provided.

- **Tinnitus (Ringing in the Ears)**

  Source: Seattle, WA: University of Washington Virginia Merrill Bloedel Hearing Research Center. 199x. [4 p.].

  Contact: Available from Virginia Merrill Bloedel Hearing Research Center. University of Washington, Box 357923, Seattle, WA 98195-7923. (206) 616-4105. E-mail: bloedel@u.washington.edu. Website: weber.u.washington.edu/~hearing. PRICE: Single copy free.

  Summary: This brochure describes tinnitus (ringing in the ears). Tinnitus may be intermittent or constant in character, mild or severe in intensity, and vary from a low hiss to a high pitched tinkling or ringing type of sound. It may be subjective (audible only to the patient) or objective (audible to others). The brochure describes the anatomy of the ear and the physiology of normal hearing, the causes of tinnitus (by type: external, middle, or inner ear tinnitus), the pathology of the nerve pathways that may contribute to tinnitus or brain tinnitus, the presence of hearing impairment associated with tinnitus, and treatment options. The brochure concludes that treatment of tinnitus, while perhaps not curing the condition, is usually successful in helping people adapt and cope better. A thorough understanding of the problem helps patients to gain control over their reactions to the tinnitus. One illustration depicts the anatomy of the middle and inner ear. 1 figure.

- **Tinnitus, or Head Noises**

    Source: Washington, DC: Better Hearing Institute. 1998. [4 p.].

    Contact: Available from Better Hearing Institute (BHI). P.O. Box 1840, Washington, DC 20013. (800) EAR-WELL or (703) 684-3391. Fax (703) 750-9302. E-mail: mail@betterhearing.org. Website: www.betterhearing.org. PRICE: Single copy free; bulk orders available.

    Summary: This brochure describes tinnitus, sound heard in one or both ears that cannot be heard by others. Topics include a definition of tinnitus; its causes in the outer, middle, and inner ear; and treatment options, including correcting some causes of tinnitus (allergy, infection, syphilis) and masking. The brochure concludes that because tinnitus may be symptomatic of a more serious disorder, it is important to try to find the cause before treating the head noises with masking. 1 figure.

- **Discussion of Head Noise or Tinnitus**

    Source: Los Angeles, CA: House Ear Institute. 1996. 23 p.

    Contact: Available from House Ear Institute. 2100 West Third Street, Fifth Floor, Los Angeles, CA 90057. Voice (800) 552-HEAR; (213) 483-4431; TTY (213) 484-2642; Fax (213) 483-8789. PRICE: $1.00 per booklet. Order Number BR-5.

    Summary: This brochure discusses head noise or tinnitus. The booklet begins with a discussion of the five divisions of the hearing mechanism: the external ear, the middle ear, the inner ear, the nerve pathways, and the brain. Additional topics include objective tinnitus, including muscular tinnitus and vascular tinnitus; external ear tinnitus; middle and inner ear tinnitus; nerve pathway tinnitus; brain tinnitus; hearing impairment; the role of stress and depression; and treatment options, including general suggestions, noise maskers, hearing aids, biofeedback, and tinnitus maskers.

- **Ototoxic Medications: Drugs That Can Cause Hearing Loss and Tinnitus**

    Source: New York, NY: League for the Hard of Hearing. 2000. [4 p.].

    Contact: Available from League for the Hard of Hearing. 71 West 23rd Street, New York, NY 10010-4162. Voice (917) 305-7700. TTY (917) 305-7999. Fax (917) 305-7888. Website: www.lhh.org. PRICE: $2.00 plus shipping and handling.

    Summary: This brochure discusses which commonly used medications could potentially cause damage to one's hearing, or aggravate an already existing problem. Ototoxic medications are drugs that can cause hearing loss and tinnitus. The brochure notes that usually any hearing problem will only be caused by exceeding the recommended dosage of the medications. Often these problems are reversible upon discontinuation of the drug. Occasionally there are times when the change in hearing can be permanent. The bulk of the brochure includes lists and brief descriptions of drugs that can cause hearing loss, including salicylates, nonsteroidal antiinflammatory drugs (NSAIDs), antibiotics, diuretics, chemotherapeutic agents, quinine, mucosal protectant, and narcotic analgesics; and drugs that can cause tinnitus, including vapors, solvents, antibiotics, anti-neoplastics, diuretics, cardiac medications, psychopharmacologic agents, NSAIDs, glucocorticosteroids, anesthetics, antimalarials, and miscellaneous toxic substances. In the lists, the generic name of the drug is given first, with the trade name, if available, followed in parentheses and capitalized. Many times a particular generic drug is manufactured under several trade names. The brochure concludes with information about the activities of the League for the Hard of Hearing (www.lhh.org).

- **Information You Can Order: American Tinnitus Association (ATA)**

    Source: Portland, OR: American Tinnitus Association (ATA). 1998. [4 p.].

    Contact: Available from American Tinnitus Association (ATA). P.O. Box 5, Portland, OR 97207-0005. (800) 634-8978 or (503) 248-9985. Fax (503) 248-0024. E-mail: tinnitus@ata.org. Website: www.ata.org. PRICE: Single copy free.

    Summary: This brochure lists the publications available from the American Tinnitus Association (ATA). The brochure includes books, brochures, videos, and other information sources related to tinnitus and hearing loss. Also included are four items designed for professionals to use in educating their clients and patients. Books and brochures are described with a brief abstract; other items are only listed. The brochure includes pricing information and an order form.

- **Doctor, What Causes Tinnitus? Insight into Tinnitus, the Noise in Your Ears**

    Source: Alexandria, VA: American Academy of Otolaryngology-Head and Neck Surgery, Inc. 1997. 4 p.

    Contact: Available from American Academy of Otolaryngology-Head and Neck Surgery, Inc. 1 Prince Street, Alexandria, VA 22314-3357. (703) 836-4444. Fax (703) 683-5100. PRICE: Single copy free; bulk orders available.

    Summary: This brochure provides information about tinnitus, noises inside the head and ears that cannot be heard by other people. The brochure describes the many causes of tinnitus, including middle ear infection, eardrum perforation, fluid accumulation, otosclerosis of the middle ear, allergy, high or low blood pressure, diabetes, thyroid problems, injury to the head or neck, excessive noise, and drug side effects. The brochure lists seven suggestions to help lessen the severity of tinnitus: avoid exposure to loud sounds and noises; get blood pressure checked; decrease the intake of salt; avoid stimulants such as coffee, tea, cola and tobacco; exercise daily (to improve circulation); get adequate rest; and stop worrying about the noise. The brochure concludes with recommendations to help readers cope with the noise of tinnitus. These recommendations include concentration and relaxation exercises, masking, and the use of hearing aids. The brochure also includes a brief description of the specialty of otolaryngology-head and neck surgery. 2 figures.

- **American Tinnitus Association: Ringing in the Ears? There is Help and Hope**

    Source: Portland, OR: American Tinnitus Association (ATA). 1997. [2 p.].

    Contact: Available from American Tinnitus Association (ATA). P.O. Box 5, Portland, OR 97207-0005. (800) 634-8978 or (503) 248-9985. Fax (503) 248-0024. E-mail: tinnitus@ata.org. Website: www.ata.org. PRICE: Single copy free; bulk orders available.

    Summary: This brochure provides readers with information about tinnitus, or ringing in the ears, and the American Tinnitus Association (ATA). The brochure describes tinnitus and the steps readers can take to address the problem; the foundation of the ATA; medical research in the area of tinnitus; and the benefits of belonging to the ATA. The brochure includes a postage-paid postcard with which readers can join the ATA or request additional information. The brochure concludes with a list of the members of the ATA's Scientific Advisory Committee and Board of Directors.

- **Noise: Its Effects on Hearing and Tinnitus**

    Source: Portland, OR: American Tinnitus Association (ATA). 1999. [2 p].

    Contact: Available from American Tinnitus Association (ATA). P.O. Box 5, Portland, OR 97207-0005. (800) 634-8978 or (503) 248-9985. Fax (503) 248-0024. E-mail: tinnitus@ata.org. Website: www.ata.org. PRICE: $0.35 each for members; $1.00 each for nonmembers.

    Summary: This brochure reviews noise-induced hearing loss and noise-induced tinnitus. Topics covered include the importance of protecting one's ears from environmental sounds, an overview of noise-induced hearing loss, common noise sources and their approximate sound pressure levels, noise-induced tinnitus, symptoms, Hearing Conservation Programs and OSHA guidelines, how tinnitus can impact on one's social activities, and other health consequences of noise exposure. The brochure concludes with a list of three reminders for readers to help reduce noise-induced hearing loss and tinnitus. It is available in English or Spanish. 2 figures. 1 table.

- **Preventing Hearing Loss and Tinnitus**

    Source: Rockville, MD: American Speech-Language-Hearing Association (ASHA). 199x. [2 p.].

    Contact: Available from American Speech-Language-Hearing Association (ASHA). Product Sales, 10801 Rockville Pike, Rockville, MD 20852. (888) 498-6699. TTY (301) 897-0157. Website: www.asha.org. PRICE: $3.95 for 10 brochures plus shipping and handling.

    Summary: This brochure, from the American Speech-Language-Hearing Association (ASHA), describes the problem of hearing loss and the importance of lifestyle and health strategies to delay or prevent its occurrence. The brochure emphasizes that prevention and early identification of and intervention for hearing loss are crucial for developing, maintaining, or improving communication and quality of life. The brochure outlines three major factors that can cause hearing loss (noise, physical trauma, and disease, heredity and medications); in each category, the brochure describes the source of the problem and then outlines specific prevention strategies. A second section describes tinnitus (ringing or buzzing in the ears) and notes its causes and prevention strategies. The brochure concludes with a description of the work that audiologists perform in evaluating and treating hearing loss, the professional education that audiologists have completed, and how to find an ASHA certified audiologist. The brochure is illustrated with full color photographs of a variety of people engaged in activities of everyday life. 5 figures.

- **Aspirin and Tinnitus**

Source: London, England: Royal National Institute for Deaf People. 1999. 3 p.

Contact: Available from RNID Helpline. P.O. Box 16464, London EC1Y 8TT, United Kingdom. 0870 60 50 123. Fax 0171-296 8199. E-mail: helpline@rnid.org.uk. Website: www.rnid.org.uk. Also available from RNID Tinnitus Helpline. Castle Cavendish Works, Norton Street, Radford, Nottingham NG7 5PN, United Kingdom. 0345 090210. Fax 0115-978 5012. E-mail: tinnitushelpline@btinternet.com. PRICE: Single copy free.

Summary: This fact sheet from the Royal National Institute for Deaf People (RNID) considers the impact of aspirin on tinnitus (ringing or other noises in the ears). Aspirin has been used for over 80 years as an analgesic to relieve pain, reduce fever, and alleviate arthritis symptoms; it can also help prevent blood clots from forming. Aspirin contains salicylate which temporarily aggravates or causes tinnitus. This effect has been known for many years. Salicylate can cause reversible hearing loss and tinnitus, probably by its action on the outer hair cell system of the cochlea (inner ear). The fact sheet encourages readers to consult their health care providers about any concerns over the impact of aspirin on their tinnitus. The fact sheet discusses the use of aspirin as a treatment for a small number of people with tinnitus who have spontaneous otoacoustic emissions; aspirin may be useful in these cases. The fact sheet concludes with information on the RNID Tinnitus Helpline (in Nottingham, UK), which is also accessible online at tinnitushelpline@btinternet.com. The RIND website is at 5www.rnid.org.uk.

- **Noise in Your Ears: Facts About Tinnitus**

Source: Bethesda, MD: National Institute on Deafness and Other Communication Disorders (NIDCD), National Institutes of Health (NIH). February 2001. [3 p.].

Contact: Available from NIDCD Information Clearinghouse. 1 Communication Avenue, Bethesda, MD 20892-3456. Voice (800) 241-1044.

TTY (800) 241-1055. Fax (301) 907-8830. E-mail: nidcdinfo@nidcd.nih.gov. Website: www.nidcd.nih.gov. PRICE: Single copy free.

Summary: This fact sheet offers basic information about tinnitus, a ringing, buzzing, or roaring sound in the ears. Tinnitus is a symptom associated with many forms of hearing loss; it can also be a symptom of other health problems. The causes of tinnitus include hearing loss, loud noise, certain medications, and other health problems such as allergies, tumors, and problems in the heart and blood vessels, jaws, and neck. The fact sheet emphasizes the importance of having tinnitus diagnosed and reviews some of the treatments that may be used. Treatments can include hearing aids, maskers, medicine or drug therapy, tinnitus retraining therapy (TNT), counseling, and relaxation methods. Self care strategies are also outlined, including the importance of avoiding activities or behaviors that make the tinnitus worse (such as noise exposure or smoking or alcohol use). The fact sheet concludes with the contact information for a number of organizations including the National Institute on Deafness and Other Communication Disorders (NIDCD, 800-241-1044, www.nidcd.nih.gov), the American Tinnitus Association (800-634-8978, www.ata.org), the American Academy of Otolaryngology Head and Neck Surgery (www.entnet.org), the American Academy of Audiology (800-AAA-2336, www.audiology.org), Self Help for Hard of Hearing People (www.shhh.org), and the American Speech-Language-Hearing Association (800-638-8255, www.asha.org).

- **Tinnitus Retraining Therapy**

    Source: London, England: Royal National Institute for Deaf People. 2000. 4 p.

    Contact: Available from RNID Helpline. P.O. Box 16464, London EC1Y 8TT, United Kingdom. 0870 60 50 123. Fax 0171 296 8199. E-mail: helpline@rnid.org.uk. Website: www.rnid.org.uk. PRICE: Single copy free.

    Summary: This fact sheet offers information about the Tinnitus Retraining Therapy (TRT) methods developed by Jonathan Hazell and Pawel Jastreboff, and about the Neurophysiologically based Management (NBM) approach; both methods are used to manage tinnitus (a ringing or buzzing noise in the ears). The fact sheet, from the British based Royal National Institute for Deaf People (RNID), first discusses the development of TRT, including the natural process of habituation and how TRT attempts to speed up this natural process. TRT is based on a neurophysiological view of how the brain processes sound. This view suggests that tinnitus is more than just the passive sending of noise from the ear to the brain using the auditory system. This view says that two other systems come into play when tinnitus becomes troublesome: the limbic system (emotions and learning) and the autonomic nervous system. Hazell and Jastreboff's methods follow strict guidelines that first categorize patients according to the relative importance of tinnitus, hearing loss, and hyperacusis (sensitivity to noise), and then suggest different treatment programs. The fact sheet concludes with information about resources and programs that use TRT; most are based in Great Britain, but Jastreboff is also associated with Emory University in Atlanta, Georgia (in the United States).

- **Tinnitus: Fact Sheet**

   Source: St. Paul, MN: Sight and Hearing Association. 1997. 1 p.

   Contact: Available from Sight and Hearing Association. 674 Transfer Road, St. Paul, MN 55114. (800) 992-0424 or (612) 992-0424. Fax (612) 645-2742. E-mail: sha@mtn.org. Website: www.sightandhearing.org. PRICE: Single copy free; $20.00 per 100 copies.

   Summary: This fact sheet outlines tinnitus, the sensation of sound heard by one or both ears when no external physical sound is present. The sound varies from person to person, but may be described as a high-pitched ringing, whining, or hissing, or a low roaring noise. It can range from very mild (only heard in a quiet place) to a constant loud, annoying sound. The fact sheet reviews the causes of tinnitus, theories regarding the mechanisms responsible for tinnitus, treatment options, and statistics about tinnitus. Noise is by far the most probable cause of tinnitus. The fact sheet emphasizes that tinnitus does not cause hearing loss, and hearing loss does not cause tinnitus, although the two often exist together. One line drawing illustrates the anatomy of the ear. 1 figure.

- **Cochlear Implants and Tinnitus**

   Source: London, England: Royal National Institute for Deaf People. 1998. 5 p.

   Contact: Available from RNID Helpline. P.O. Box 16464, London EC1Y 8TT, United Kingdom. 0870 60 50 123. Fax 0171-296 8199. E-mail: helpline@rnid.org.uk. Website: www.rnid.org.uk. PRICE: Single copy free.

   Summary: This fact sheet, from the British Royal National Institute for Deaf People (RNID), describes the use of cochlear implants to help people with tinnitus (ringing or other sounds in the ears). A cochlear implant is an electronic device designed for people with profound or severe hearing loss who get little or no benefit from hearing aids. A small part of the cochlear implant is surgically implanted in the cochlea (inner ear), and an externally worn microphone and processor pick up sound and convert it into electrical signals which stimulate the auditory nerve. The fact sheet notes that a number of cochlear implant users have found that their tinnitus has been reduced or even abolished when their implants are switched on. The fact sheet briefly reviews research that supports these subjective impressions and then offers two lengthy quotations from personal experiences with cochlear implants and tinnitus. The fact sheet includes a list of resource organizations and references through which readers can obtain additional information.

- **Tinnitus Research**

    Source: Bethesda, MD: National Institute on Deafness and Other Communication Disorders (NIDCD). 1998. 2 p.

    Contact: Available from NIDCD Information Clearinghouse. National Institute on Deafness and Other Communications Disorders, National Institutes of Health, 1 Communication Avenue, Bethesda, MD 20892-3456. Voice (800) 241-1044. TTY (800) 241-1055. Fax (301) 907-8830. E-mail: nidcdinfo@nidcd.nih.gov. Website: www.nidcd.nih.gov. PRICE: Single copy free.

    Summary: This fact sheet, produced by the National Institute on Deafness and Other Communication Disorders (NIDCD), addresses tinnitus research. The fact sheet highlights tinnitus research conducted by Dr. Alan H. Lockwood of the University of New York at Buffalo and his colleagues. The research involved locating an area in the brain that is involved in the production of tinnitus. Researchers believe that the study, which included positron-emission tomography (PET) to map brain regions in individuals who had tinnitus in only one ear, will lead to further research and treatment options. The fact sheet notes that while tinnitus is a symptom that accompanies many kinds of hearing loss, the mechanisms that produce it are not fully understood. With its biomedical research projects and non-invasive imaging studies, the NIDCD hopes to provide data that will allow scientists to better understand tinnitus. The fact sheet concludes with a list of six organizations to contact for additional information. (AA-M).

- **Tinnitus Retraining Therapy (TRT) and Neurophysiologically-Based Management (NBM)**

    Source: London, England: Royal National Institute for Deaf People. 2000. 10 p.

    Contact: Available from RNID Helpline. P.O. Box 16464, London EC1Y 8TT, United Kingdom. 0870 60 50 123. Fax 0171 296 8199. E-mail:

helpline@rnid.org.uk. Website: www.rnid.org.uk. PRICE: Single copy free.

Summary: This lengthy fact sheet offers information about the Tinnitus Retraining Therapy (TRT) methods developed by Jonathan Hazell and Pawel Jastreboff, and about the Neurophysiologically based Management (NBM) approach; both methods are used to manage tinnitus (a ringing or buzzing noise in the ears). The fact sheet, from the British based Royal National Institute for Deaf People (RNID), first discusses the development of TRT, including the natural process of habituation and how TRT attempts to speed up this natural process. TRT is based on a neurophysiological view of how the brain processes sound. This view suggests that tinnitus is more than just the passive sending of noise from the ear to the brain using the auditory system. This view says that two other systems come into play when tinnitus becomes troublesome: the limbic system (emotions and learning) and the autonomic nervous system. Hazell and Jastreboff's methods follow strict guidelines that first categorize patients according to the relative importance of tinnitus, hearing loss, and hyperacusis (sensitivity to noise), and then suggest different treatment programs. The fact sheet describes some of the controversies over describing the role and value of TRT, including whether TRT works, or is that much better than counseling or other current mixes of therapies. 7 references.

- **Ear and Head Noises: Tinnitus**

    Source: San Bruno, CA: Krames Communications. 1993. 2 p.

    Contact: Available from Krames Communications. Order Department, 100 Grundy Lane, San Bruno, CA 94066-3030. (800) 333-3032; Fax (415) 244-4512. PRICE: Single copy free; $0.40 each for multiple copies; bulk discounts available. Order Number 1103.

    Summary: This patient education brochure discusses the problem of tinnitus (ear and head noises) in adults. After a description of the problem, the brochure discusses the anatomy of the ear and the etiology of tinnitus; the importance of a thorough patient history and examination; diagnostic tests conducted to confirm tinnitus, including hearing tests, balance tests, nerve conduction tests, and computed tomography (CT scan) or magnetic resonance imaging (MRI); and treatment options, including the use of masking. The brochure concludes that the key to successful treatment of tinnitus is getting the most accurate diagnosis possible.

- **Questions About Tinnitus**

    Source: London, England: Royal National Institute for Deaf People. 1998. 15 p.

    Contact: Available from RNID Helpline. P.O. Box 16464, London EC1Y 8TT, United Kingdom. 0870 60 50 123. Fax 0171-296 8199. E-mail: helpline@rnid.org.uk. Website: www.rnid.org.uk. PRICE: Single copy free.

    Summary: Tinnitus is the word for noises that some people hear 'in the ears' or 'in the head,' including buzzing, ringing, whistling, hissing, and other sounds that do not come from an external source. This brochure, from the British Royal National Institute for Deaf People (RNID), answers common questions about tinnitus. Topics include the causes of tinnitus, the types of tinnitus that are treatable, treatment options (counseling, hearing aids or maskers, Tinnitus Retraining Therapy, relaxation therapy, medication), self help strategies (including the importance of a positive attitude), activities or behaviors that can make tinnitus worse (including certain drugs, loud noise), and how to get additional information. The brochure includes a list of related materials available from RNID and a mail in form with which readers can request additional information. The inside back cover of the brochure summarizes the activities of the RNID. The brochure is illustrated with black and white photographs and line drawings.

- **Tinnitus**

    Source: American Academy of Audiology. Reston, VA. 2002.

    Contact: American Academy of Audiology. Publications, 11730 Plaza America Drive, Suite 300, Reston, VA 20190. Voice 800-AAA-2336; 703-790-8466. Fax: 703-790-8631. Web site: http://www.audiology.org/store. PRICE: Pkgs. of 100. Members: $40.00; Non-Members: $50.00.

    Summary: Tinnitus often is described by sufferers as a hissing, roaring, or ringing in the ears. This brochure includes detailed information on what causes tinnitus, who suffers from it, what treatments are currently available, and what one can do to minimize its effects. Geared toward patients and their families, the brochure encourages tinnitus sufferers to consult an audiologist who is knowledgeable about tinnitus to help develop a management program. 8-page fold-out.

Healthfinder™

Healthfinder™ is an additional source sponsored by the U.S. Department of Health and Human Services which offers links to hundreds of other sites that contain healthcare information. This Web site is located at **http://www.healthfinder.gov**. Again, keyword searches can be used to find guidelines. The following was recently found in this database:

- **FAQ - About Tinnitus**

    Summary: Answers to consumers' most commonly asked questions about this hearing impairment characterized by ringing in the ears and/or head noises. These noises can appear in a variety of forms...

    Source: American Tinnitus Association

    http://www.healthfinder.gov/scripts/recordpass.asp?RecordType=0&RecordID=2676

- **Tinnitus**

    Summary: This fact sheet provides information about the causes of and treatments for tinnitus.

    Source: National Institute on Deafness and Other Communication Disorders Information Clearinghouse

    http://www.healthfinder.gov/scripts/recordpass.asp?RecordType=0&RecordID=6696

- **Tinnitus Patient Information**

    Summary: This paitient education fact sheet contains basic information about tinnitus, its causes, diagnosis and treatment.

    Source: American Academy of Otolaryngology--Head and Neck Surgery

    http://www.healthfinder.gov/scripts/recordpass.asp?RecordType=0&RecordID=2675

- **Vestibular Schwannoma (Acoustic Neurinoma) and Neurofibromatosis**

    Summary: This fact sheet provides consumers with basic facts about acoustic neurinoma -- a benign tumor which often causes gradual hearing loss, tinnitus or ringing in the ears, and dizziness.

    Source: National Institute on Deafness and Other Communication Disorders Information Clearinghouse

    http://www.healthfinder.gov/scripts/recordpass.asp?RecordType=0&RecordID=2066

The NIH Search Utility

After browsing the references listed at the beginning of this chapter, you may want to explore the NIH search utility. This allows you to search for documents on over 100 selected Web sites that comprise the NIH-WEB-SPACE. Each of these servers is "crawled" and indexed on an ongoing basis. Your search will produce a list of various documents, all of which will relate in some way to tinnitus. The drawbacks of this approach are that the information is not organized by theme and that the references are often a mix of information for professionals and patients. Nevertheless, a large number of the listed Web sites provide useful background information. We can only recommend this route, therefore, for relatively rare or specific disorders, or when using highly targeted searches. To use the NIH search utility, visit the following Web page: **http://search.nih.gov/index.html**.

NORD (The National Organization of Rare Disorders, Inc.)

NORD provides an invaluable service to the public by publishing, for a nominal fee, short yet comprehensive guidelines on over 1,000 diseases. NORD primarily focuses on rare diseases that might not be covered by the previously listed sources. NORD's Web address is **www.rarediseases.org**. To see if a recent fact sheet has been published on tinnitus, simply go to the following hyperlink: **http://www.rarediseases.org/search/rdblist.html**. A complete guide on tinnitus can be purchased from NORD for a nominal fee.

Additional Web Sources

A number of Web sites that often link to government sites are available to the public. These can also point you in the direction of essential information. The following is a representative sample:

- AOL: **http://search.aol.com/cat.adp?id=168&layer=&from=subcats**
- Family Village: **http://www.familyvillage.wisc.edu/specific.htm**
- Google: **http://directory.google.com/Top/Health/Conditions_and_Diseases/**
- Med Help International: **http://www.medhelp.org/HealthTopics/A.html**
- Open Directory Project: **http://dmoz.org/Health/Conditions_and_Diseases/**
- Yahoo.com: **http://dir.yahoo.com/Health/Diseases_and_Conditions/**
- WebMD®Health: **http://my.webmd.com/health_topics**

Vocabulary Builder

The material in this chapter may have contained a number of unfamiliar words. The following Vocabulary Builder introduces you to terms used in this chapter that have not been covered in the previous chapter:

Antibiotic: A substance usually produced by vegetal micro-organisms capable of inhibiting the growth of or killing bacteria. [NIH]

Audiologist: Study of hearing including treatment of persons with hearing defects. [NIH]

Eardrum: A thin, tense membrane forming the greater part of the outer wall of the tympanic cavity and separating it from the external auditory meatus; it constitutes the boundary between the external and middle ear. [NIH]

Fold: A plication or doubling of various parts of the body. [NIH]

Formulary: A book containing a list of pharmaceutical products with their formulas and means of preparation. [NIH]

Habituation: Decline in response of an organism to environmental or other stimuli with repeated or maintained exposure. [NIH]

Impairment: In the context of health experience, an impairment is any loss or abnormality of psychological, physiological, or anatomical structure or function. [NIH]

Infections: The illnesses caused by an organism that usually does not cause disease in a person with a normal immune system. [NIH]

Insight: The capacity to understand one's own motives, to be aware of one's own psychodynamics, to appreciate the meaning of symbolic behavior. [NIH]

Need: A state of tension or dissatisfaction felt by an individual that impels him to action toward a goal he believes will satisfy the impulse. [NIH]

Nerve: A cordlike structure of nervous tissue that connects parts of the nervous system with other tissues of the body and conveys nervous impulses to, or away from, these tissues. [NIH]

Physiology: The science that deals with the life processes and functions of organismus, their cells, tissues, and organs. [NIH]

Refer: To send or direct for treatment, aid, information, de decision. [NIH]

Salicylate: Non-steroidal anti-inflammatory drugs. [NIH]

Stimulants: Any drug or agent which causes stimulation. [NIH]

CHAPTER 2. SEEKING GUIDANCE

Overview

Some patients are comforted by the knowledge that a number of organizations dedicate their resources to helping people with tinnitus. These associations can become invaluable sources of information and advice. Many associations offer aftercare support, financial assistance, and other important services. Furthermore, healthcare research has shown that support groups often help people to better cope with their conditions.[8] In addition to support groups, your physician can be a valuable source of guidance and support. Therefore, finding a physician that can work with your unique situation is a very important aspect of your care.

In this chapter, we direct you to resources that can help you find patient organizations and medical specialists. We begin by describing how to find associations and peer groups that can help you better understand and cope with tinnitus. The chapter ends with a discussion on how to find a doctor that is right for you.

Associations and Tinnitus

As mentioned by the Agency for Healthcare Research and Quality, sometimes the emotional side of an illness can be as taxing as the physical side.[9] You may have fears or feel overwhelmed by your situation. Everyone has different ways of dealing with disease or physical injury. Your attitude, your expectations, and how well you cope with your condition can all

---

[8] Churches, synagogues, and other houses of worship might also have groups that can offer you the social support you need.
[9] This section has been adapted from **http://www.ahcpr.gov/consumer/diaginf5.htm**.

influence your well-being. This is true for both minor conditions and serious illnesses. For example, a study on female breast cancer survivors revealed that women who participated in support groups lived longer and experienced better quality of life when compared with women who did not participate. In the support group, women learned coping skills and had the opportunity to share their feelings with other women in the same situation.

In addition to associations or groups that your doctor might recommend, we suggest that you consider the following list (if there is a fee for an association, you may want to check with your insurance provider to find out if the cost will be covered):

- **American Tinnitus Association**

    Telephone: (503) 248-9985 Toll-free: (800) 634-8978

    Fax: (503) 248-0024

    Email: tinnitus@ata.org

    Web Site: http://www.ata.org

    Background: The American **Tinnitus** Association is a national not-for-profit self-help organization dedicated to helping people with **tinnitus** and their health care providers. **Tinnitus** is a condition characterized by sensation of sound for which there is no external source. Such preceived sounds are often described as a buzzing, ringing, whistling, or clicking sensation. The Association's activities include research for a cure and management of the condition; production and distribution of public awareness materials; educational programs for the professional and lay communities; establishment of and guidance for self-help groups and their leaders; and promotion of community hearing protection programs. Founded in 1979, the organization maintains a bibliographic service and publishes a variety of informational brochures and a quarterly journal entitled 'Tinnitus Today.'.

    Relevant area(s) of interest: Tinnitus

Finding Associations

There are a several Internet directories that provide lists of medical associations with information on or resources relating to tinnitus. By consulting all of associations listed in this chapter, you will have nearly exhausted all sources for patient associations concerned with tinnitus.

The National Health Information Center (NHIC)

The National Health Information Center (NHIC) offers a free referral service to help people find organizations that provide information about tinnitus. For more information, see the NHIC's Web site at **http://www.health.gov/NHIC/** or contact an information specialist by calling 1-800-336-4797.

DIRLINE

A comprehensive source of information on associations is the DIRLINE database maintained by the National Library of Medicine. The database comprises some 10,000 records of organizations, research centers, and government institutes and associations which primarily focus on health and biomedicine. DIRLINE is available via the Internet at the following Web site: **http://dirline.nlm.nih.gov/**. Simply type in "tinnitus" (or a synonym) or the name of a topic, and the site will list information contained in the database on all relevant organizations.

The Combined Health Information Database

Another comprehensive source of information on healthcare associations is the Combined Health Information Database. Using the "Detailed Search" option, you will need to limit your search to "Organizations" and "tinnitus". Type the following hyperlink into your Web browser: **http://chid.nih.gov/detail/detail.html**. To find associations, use the drop boxes at the bottom of the search page where "You may refine your search by." For publication date, select "All Years." Then, select your preferred language and the format option "Organization Resource Sheet." By making these selections and typing in "tinnitus" (or synonyms) into the "For these words:" box, you will only receive results on organizations dealing with tinnitus. You should check back periodically with this database since it is updated every 3 months.

The National Organization for Rare Disorders, Inc.

The National Organization for Rare Disorders, Inc. has prepared a Web site that provides, at no charge, lists of associations organized by specific diseases. You can access this database at the following Web site:

http://www.rarediseases.org/search/orgsearch.html. Type "tinnitus" (or a synonym) in the search box, and click "Submit Query."

Online Support Groups

In addition to support groups, commercial Internet service providers offer forums and chat rooms for people with different illnesses and conditions. WebMD®, for example, offers such a service on its Web site: http://boards.webmd.com/roundtable. These online self-help communities can help you connect with a network of people whose concerns are similar to yours. Online support groups are places where people can talk informally. If you read about a novel approach, consult with your doctor or other healthcare providers, as the treatments or discoveries you hear about may not be scientifically proven to be safe and effective.

Finding Doctors

One of the most important aspects of your treatment will be the relationship between you and your doctor or specialist. All patients with tinnitus must go through the process of selecting a physician. While this process will vary from person to person, the Agency for Healthcare Research and Quality makes a number of suggestions, including the following:[10]

- If you are in a managed care plan, check the plan's list of doctors first.
- Ask doctors or other health professionals who work with doctors, such as hospital nurses, for referrals.
- Call a hospital's doctor referral service, but keep in mind that these services usually refer you to doctors on staff at that particular hospital. The services do not have information on the quality of care that these doctors provide.
- Some local medical societies offer lists of member doctors. Again, these lists do not have information on the quality of care that these doctors provide.

Additional steps you can take to locate doctors include the following:

- Check with the associations listed earlier in this chapter.

---

[10] This section has been adapted from the AHRQ: www.ahrq.gov/consumer/qntascii/qntdr.htm.

- Information on doctors in some states is available on the Internet at **http://www.docboard.org**. This Web site is run by "Administrators in Medicine," a group of state medical board directors.

- The American Board of Medical Specialties can tell you if your doctor is board certified. "Certified" means that the doctor has completed a training program in a specialty and has passed an exam, or "board," to assess his or her knowledge, skills, and experience to provide quality patient care in that specialty. Primary care doctors may also be certified as specialists. The AMBS Web site is located at **http://www.abms.org/newsearch.asp**.[11] You can also contact the ABMS by phone at 1-866-ASK-ABMS.

- You can call the American Medical Association (AMA) at 800-665-2882 for information on training, specialties, and board certification for many licensed doctors in the United States. This information also can be found in "Physician Select" at the AMA's Web site: **http://www.ama-assn.org/aps/amahg.htm**.

Finding an Otolaryngologist

An otolaryngologist is a medical doctor who specializes in the treatment of the ear, nose, throat, and related structures of the head and neck. The American Academy of Otolaryngology—Head and Neck Surgery (AAO-HNS) has created a "Find an Otolaryngologist" searchable database which contains information on the AAO-HNS's 9,300 members. To search the database, go to **http://www.entlink.net/aao-hns_otolaryngologist.cfm**. You will be given the option to search by the following criteria: doctor's name, city, state, zip code, country, or sub-specialty.

If the previous sources did not meet your needs, you may want to log on to the Web site of the National Organization for Rare Disorders (NORD) at **http://www.rarediseases.org/**. NORD maintains a database of doctors with expertise in various rare diseases. The Metabolic Information Network (MIN), 800-945-2188, also maintains a database of physicians with expertise in various metabolic diseases.

---

[11] While board certification is a good measure of a doctor's knowledge, it is possible to receive quality care from doctors who are not board certified.

Selecting Your Doctor[12]

When you have compiled a list of prospective doctors, call each of their offices. First, ask if the doctor accepts your health insurance plan and if he or she is taking new patients. If the doctor is not covered by your plan, ask yourself if you are prepared to pay the extra costs. The next step is to schedule a visit with your chosen physician. During the first visit you will have the opportunity to evaluate your doctor and to find out if you feel comfortable with him or her. Ask yourself, did the doctor:

- Give me a chance to ask questions about tinnitus?
- Really listen to my questions?
- Answer in terms I understood?
- Show respect for me?
- Ask me questions?
- Make me feel comfortable?
- Address the health problem(s) I came with?
- Ask me my preferences about different kinds of treatments for tinnitus?
- Spend enough time with me?

Trust your instincts when deciding if the doctor is right for you. But remember, it might take time for the relationship to develop. It takes more than one visit for you and your doctor to get to know each other.

Working with Your Doctor[13]

Research has shown that patients who have good relationships with their doctors tend to be more satisfied with their care and have better results. Here are some tips to help you and your doctor become partners:

- You know important things about your symptoms and your health history. Tell your doctor what you think he or she needs to know.

- It is important to tell your doctor personal information, even if it makes you feel embarrassed or uncomfortable.

---

[12] This section has been adapted from the AHRQ: **www.ahrq.gov/consumer/qntascii/qntdr.htm**.
[13] This section has been adapted from the AHRQ: **www.ahrq.gov/consumer/qntascii/qntdr.htm**.

- Bring a "health history" list with you (and keep it up to date).

- Always bring any medications you are currently taking with you to the appointment, or you can bring a list of your medications including dosage and frequency information. Talk about any allergies or reactions you have had to your medications.

- Tell your doctor about any natural or alternative medicines you are taking.

- Bring other medical information, such as x-ray films, test results, and medical records.

- Ask questions. If you don't, your doctor will assume that you understood everything that was said.

- Write down your questions before your visit. List the most important ones first to make sure that they are addressed.

- Consider bringing a friend with you to the appointment to help you ask questions. This person can also help you understand and/or remember the answers.

- Ask your doctor to draw pictures if you think that this would help you understand.

- Take notes. Some doctors do not mind if you bring a tape recorder to help you remember things, but always ask first.

- Let your doctor know if you need more time. If there is not time that day, perhaps you can speak to a nurse or physician assistant on staff or schedule a telephone appointment.

- Take information home. Ask for written instructions. Your doctor may also have brochures and audio and videotapes that can help you.

- After leaving the doctor's office, take responsibility for your care. If you have questions, call. If your symptoms get worse or if you have problems with your medication, call. If you had tests and do not hear from your doctor, call for your test results. If your doctor recommended that you have certain tests, schedule an appointment to get them done. If your doctor said you should see an additional specialist, make an appointment.

By following these steps, you will enhance the relationship you will have with your physician.

Broader Health-Related Resources

In addition to the references above, the NIH has set up guidance Web sites that can help patients find healthcare professionals. These include:[14]

- Caregivers:
  http://www.nlm.nih.gov/medlineplus/caregivers.html
- Choosing a Doctor or Healthcare Service:
  http://www.nlm.nih.gov/medlineplus/choosingadoctororhealthcareservice.html
- Hospitals and Health Facilities:
  http://www.nlm.nih.gov/medlineplus/healthfacilities.html

Vocabulary Builder

The following vocabulary builder provides definitions of words used in this chapter that have not been defined in previous chapters:

Specialist: In medicine, one who concentrates on 1 special branch of medical science. [NIH]

---

[14] You can access this information at http://www.nlm.nih.gov/medlineplus/healthsystem.html.

CHAPTER 3. CLINICAL TRIALS AND TINNITUS

Overview

Very few medical conditions have a single treatment. The basic treatment guidelines that your physician has discussed with you, or those that you have found using the techniques discussed in Chapter 1, may provide you with all that you will require. For some patients, current treatments can be enhanced with new or innovative techniques currently under investigation. In this chapter, we will describe how clinical trials work and show you how to keep informed of trials concerning tinnitus.

What Is a Clinical Trial?[15]

Clinical trials involve the participation of people in medical research. Most medical research begins with studies in test tubes and on animals. Treatments that show promise in these early studies may then be tried with people. The only sure way to find out whether a new treatment is safe, effective, and better than other treatments for tinnitus is to try it on patients in a clinical trial.

---

[15] The discussion in this chapter has been adapted from the NIH and the NEI: **http://www.nei.nih.gov/health/clinicaltrials%5Ffacts/index.htm**.

What Kinds of Clinical Trials Are There?

Clinical trials are carried out in three phases:

- **Phase I.** Researchers first conduct Phase I trials with small numbers of patients and healthy volunteers. If the new treatment is a medication, researchers also try to determine how much of it can be given safely.

- **Phase II.** Researchers conduct Phase II trials in small numbers of patients to find out the effect of a new treatment on tinnitus.

- **Phase III.** Finally, researchers conduct Phase III trials to find out how new treatments for tinnitus compare with standard treatments already being used. Phase III trials also help to determine if new treatments have any side effects. These trials--which may involve hundreds, perhaps thousands, of people--can also compare new treatments with no treatment.

How Is a Clinical Trial Conducted?

Various organizations support clinical trials at medical centers, hospitals, universities, and doctors' offices across the United States. The "principal investigator" is the researcher in charge of the study at each facility participating in the clinical trial. Most clinical trial researchers are medical doctors, academic researchers, and specialists. The "clinic coordinator" knows all about how the study works and makes all the arrangements for your visits.

All doctors and researchers who take part in the study on tinnitus carefully follow a detailed treatment plan called a protocol. This plan fully explains how the doctors will treat you in the study. The "protocol" ensures that all patients are treated in the same way, no matter where they receive care.

Clinical trials are controlled. This means that researchers compare the effects of the new treatment with those of the standard treatment. In some cases, when no standard treatment exists, the new treatment is compared with no treatment. Patients who receive the new treatment are in the treatment group. Patients who receive a standard treatment or no treatment are in the "control" group. In some clinical trials, patients in the treatment group get a new medication while those in the control group get a placebo. A placebo is a harmless substance, a "dummy" pill, that has no effect on tinnitus. In other clinical trials, where a new surgery or device (not a medicine) is being tested, patients in the control group may receive a "sham treatment." This treatment, like a placebo, has no effect on tinnitus and does not harm patients.

Researchers assign patients "randomly" to the treatment or control group. This is like flipping a coin to decide which patients are in each group. If you choose to participate in a clinical trial, you will not know which group you will be appointed to. The chance of any patient getting the new treatment is about 50 percent. You cannot request to receive the new treatment instead of the placebo or sham treatment. Often, you will not know until the study is over whether you have been in the treatment group or the control group. This is called a "masked" study. In some trials, neither doctors nor patients know who is getting which treatment. This is called a "double masked" study. These types of trials help to ensure that the perceptions of the patients or doctors will not affect the study results.

Natural History Studies

Unlike clinical trials in which patient volunteers may receive new treatments, natural history studies provide important information to researchers on how tinnitus develops over time. A natural history study follows patient volunteers to see how factors such as age, sex, race, or family history might make some people more or less at risk for tinnitus. A natural history study may also tell researchers if diet, lifestyle, or occupation affects how a disease or disorder develops and progresses. Results from these studies provide information that helps answer questions such as: How fast will a disease or disorder usually progress? How bad will the condition become? Will treatment be needed?

What Is Expected of Patients in a Clinical Trial?

Not everyone can take part in a clinical trial for a specific disease or disorder. Each study enrolls patients with certain features or eligibility criteria. These criteria may include the type and stage of disease or disorder, as well as, the age and previous treatment history of the patient. You or your doctor can contact the sponsoring organization to find out more about specific clinical trials and their eligibility criteria. If you are interested in joining a clinical trial, your doctor must contact one of the trial's investigators and provide details about your diagnosis and medical history.

If you participate in a clinical trial, you may be required to have a number of medical tests. You may also need to take medications and/or undergo surgery. Depending upon the treatment and the examination procedure, you may be required to receive inpatient hospital care. Or, you may have to return to the medical facility for follow-up examinations. These exams help find out how well the treatment is working. Follow-up studies can take months or years. However, the success of the clinical trial often depends on learning what happens to patients over a long period of time. Only patients who continue to return for follow-up examinations can provide this important long-term information.

Recent Trials on Tinnitus

The National Institutes of Health and other organizations sponsor trials on various diseases and disorders. Because funding for research goes to the medical areas that show promising research opportunities, it is not possible for the NIH or others to sponsor clinical trials for every disease and disorder at all times. The following lists recent trials dedicated to tinnitus.[16] If the trial listed by the NIH is still recruiting, you may be eligible. If it is no longer recruiting or has been completed, then you can contact the sponsors to learn more about the study and, if published, the results. Further information on the trial is available at the Web site indicated. Please note that some trials may no longer be recruiting patients or are otherwise closed. Before contacting sponsors of a clinical trial, consult with your physician who can help you determine if you might benefit from participation.

- **Epidemiology of Hearing Loss in Diabetic and Non-Diabetic Veterans**

    Condition(s): Diabetes; Tinnitus; Hearing Loss

    Study Status: This study is currently recruiting patients.

    Sponsor(s): Department of Veterans Affairs Medical Research Service

    Purpose - Excerpt: The purpose of this study is to determine if individuals with diabetes are at increased risk of hearing impairment or **tinnitus** (the perception of ringing or noises in the ears or head). An important goal of this research is also to obtain a better understanding of possible interactions between hearing disorders and other chronic conditions, such as diabetes. Participation in this research will be for a few hours only, to be scheduled at the participant's convenience and according to the testing schedules of the different clinics involved.

    Study Type: Observational

    Contact(s): see Web site below

    Web Site: http://clinicaltrials.gov/ct/show/NCT00018486

---

[16] These are listed at **www.ClinicalTrials.gov**.

- **Evaluation of Treatment Methods for Clinically Significant Tinnitus**

    Condition(s): Tinnitus

    Study Status: This study is no longer recruiting patients.

    Sponsor(s): Department of Veterans Affairs

    Purpose - Excerpt: The investigators propose to evaluate two different approaches to the alleviation of tinnitus symptoms by comparing changes from baseline performance on the Tinnitus Severity Index. They propose to provide an unbiased evaluation of competing methodologies. The design is one in which pairs of prospective subjects are randomly assigned to one of two treatment groups. Changes in group performance will be compared for selected measures.

    Phase(s): Phase II

    Study Type: Interventional

    Contact(s): see Web site below

    Web Site: http://clinicaltrials.gov/ct/show/NCT00013390

Benefits and Risks[17]

What Are the Benefits of Participating in a Clinical Trial?

If you are interested in a clinical trial, it is important to realize that your participation can bring many benefits to you and society at large:

- A new treatment could be more effective than the current treatment for tinnitus. Although only half of the participants in a clinical trial receive the experimental treatment, if the new treatment is proved to be more effective and safer than the current treatment, then those patients who did not receive the new treatment during the clinical trial may be among the first to benefit from it when the study is over.

- If the treatment is effective, then it may improve health or prevent diseases or disorders.

- Clinical trial patients receive the highest quality of medical care. Experts watch them closely during the study and may continue to follow them after the study is over.

- People who take part in trials contribute to scientific discoveries that may help other people with tinnitus. In cases where certain diseases or

---

[17] This section has been adapted from ClinicalTrials.gov, a service of the NIH: http://www.clinicaltrials.gov/ct/gui/c/a1r/info/whatis?JServSessionIdzone_ct=9jmun6f291.

disorders run in families, your participation may lead to better care or prevention for your family members.

The Informed Consent

Once you agree to take part in a clinical trial, you will be asked to sign an "informed consent." This document explains a clinical trial's risks and benefits, the researcher's expectations of you, and your rights as a patient.

What Are the Risks?

Clinical trials may involve risks as well as benefits. Whether or not a new treatment will work cannot be known ahead of time. There is always a chance that a new treatment may not work better than a standard treatment. There is also the possibility that it may be harmful. The treatment you receive may cause side effects that are serious enough to require medical attention.

How Is Patient Safety Protected?

Clinical trials can raise fears of the unknown. Understanding the safeguards that protect patients can ease some of these fears. Before a clinical trial begins, researchers must get approval from their hospital's Institutional Review Board (IRB), an advisory group that makes sure a clinical trial is designed to protect patient safety. During a clinical trial, doctors will closely watch you to see if the treatment is working and if you are experiencing any side effects. All the results are carefully recorded and reviewed. In many cases, experts from the Data and Safety Monitoring Committee carefully monitor each clinical trial and can recommend that a study be stopped at any time. You will only be asked to take part in a clinical trial as a volunteer giving informed consent.

What Are a Patient's Rights in a Clinical Trial?

If you are eligible for a clinical trial, you will be given information to help you decide whether or not you want to participate. As a patient, you have the right to:

- Information on all known risks and benefits of the treatments in the study.

- Know how the researchers plan to carry out the study, for how long, and where.
- Know what is expected of you.
- Know any costs involved for you or your insurance provider.
- Know before any of your medical or personal information is shared with other researchers involved in the clinical trial.
- Talk openly with doctors and ask any questions.

After you join a clinical trial, you have the right to:

- Leave the study at any time. Participation is strictly voluntary. However, you should not enroll if you do not plan to complete the study.
- Receive any new information about the new treatment.
- Continue to ask questions and get answers.
- Maintain your privacy. Your name will not appear in any reports based on the study.
- Know whether you participated in the treatment group or the control group (once the study has been completed).

What about Costs?

In some clinical trials, the research facility pays for treatment costs and other associated expenses. You or your insurance provider may have to pay for costs that are considered standard care. These things may include inpatient hospital care, laboratory and other tests, and medical procedures. You also may need to pay for travel between your home and the clinic. You should find out about costs before committing to participation in the trial. If you have health insurance, find out exactly what it will cover. If you don't have health insurance, or if your insurance company will not cover your costs, talk to the clinic staff about other options for covering the cost of your care.

What Questions Should You Ask before Deciding to Join a Clinical Trial?

Questions you should ask when thinking about joining a clinical trial include the following:

- What is the purpose of the clinical trial?

- What are the standard treatments for tinnitus? Why do researchers think the new treatment may be better? What is likely to happen to me with or without the new treatment?

- What tests and treatments will I need? Will I need surgery? Medication? Hospitalization?

- How long will the treatment last? How often will I have to come back for follow-up exams?

- What are the treatment's possible benefits to my condition? What are the short- and long-term risks? What are the possible side effects?

- Will the treatment be uncomfortable? Will it make me feel sick? If so, for how long?

- How will my health be monitored?

- Where will I need to go for the clinical trial? How will I get there?

- How much will it cost to be in the study? What costs are covered by the study? How much will my health insurance cover?

- Will I be able to see my own doctor? Who will be in charge of my care?

- Will taking part in the study affect my daily life? Do I have time to participate?

- How do I feel about taking part in a clinical trial? Are there family members or friends who may benefit from my contributions to new medical knowledge?

Keeping Current on Clinical Trials

Various government agencies maintain databases on trials. The U.S. National Institutes of Health, through the National Library of Medicine, has developed ClinicalTrials.gov to provide patients, family members, and physicians with current information about clinical research across the broadest number of diseases and conditions.

The site was launched in February 2000 and currently contains approximately 5,700 clinical studies in over 59,000 locations worldwide, with most studies being conducted in the United States. ClinicalTrials.gov receives about 2 million hits per month and hosts approximately 5,400 visitors daily. To access this database, simply go to their Web site (**www.clinicaltrials.gov**) and search by "tinnitus" (or synonyms).

While ClinicalTrials.gov is the most comprehensive listing of NIH-supported clinical trials available, not all trials are in the database. The database is updated regularly, so clinical trials are continually being added. The following is a list of specialty databases affiliated with the National Institutes of Health that offer additional information on trials:

- For clinical studies at the Warren Grant Magnuson Clinical Center located in Bethesda, Maryland, visit their Web site:
  http://clinicalstudies.info.nih.gov/

- For clinical studies conducted at the Bayview Campus in Baltimore, Maryland, visit their Web site:
  http://www.jhbmc.jhu.edu/studies/index.html

- For hearing-related trials, visit the National Institute on Deafness and Other Communication Disorders:
  http://www.nidcd.nih.gov/health/clinical/index.htm

General References

The following references describe clinical trials and experimental medical research. They have been selected to ensure that they are likely to be available from your local or online bookseller or university medical library. These references are usually written for healthcare professionals, so you may consider consulting with a librarian or bookseller who might recommend a particular reference. The following includes some of the most readily available references (sorted alphabetically by title; hyperlinks provide rankings, information and reviews at Amazon.com):

- **A Guide to Patient Recruitment : Today's Best Practices & Proven Strategies** by Diana L. Anderson; Paperback - 350 pages (2001), CenterWatch, Inc.; ISBN: 1930624115;
  http://www.amazon.com/exec/obidos/ASIN/1930624115/icongroupinterna

- **A Step-By-Step Guide to Clinical Trials** by Marilyn Mulay, R.N., M.S., OCN; Spiral-bound - 143 pages Spiral edition (2001), Jones & Bartlett Pub; ISBN: 0763715697;
  http://www.amazon.com/exec/obidos/ASIN/0763715697/icongroupinterna.

- **The CenterWatch Directory of Drugs in Clinical Trials** by CenterWatch; Paperback - 656 pages (2000), CenterWatch, Inc.; ISBN: 0967302935;
  http://www.amazon.com/exec/obidos/ASIN/0967302935/icongroupinterna

- **Extending Medicare Reimbursement in Clinical Trials** by Institute of Medicine Staff (Editor), et al; Paperback 1st edition (2000), National Academy Press; ISBN: 0309068886;
  http://www.amazon.com/exec/obidos/ASIN/0309068886/icongroupinterna

- **Handbook of Clinical Trials** by Marcus Flather (Editor); Paperback (2001), Remedica Pub Ltd; ISBN: 1901346293;
  http://www.amazon.com/exec/obidos/ASIN/1901346293/icongroupinterna

Vocabulary Builder

The following vocabulary builder gives definitions of words used in this chapter that have not been defined in previous chapters:

Consultation: A deliberation between two or more physicians concerning the diagnosis and the proper method of treatment in a case. [NIH]

Protocol: The detailed plan for a clinical trial that states the trial's rationale, purpose, drug or vaccine dosages, length of study, routes of administration, who may participate, and other aspects of trial design. [NIH]

Race: A population within a species which exhibits general similarities within itself, but is both discontinuous and distinct from other populations of that species, though not sufficiently so as to achieve the status of a taxon. [NIH]

PART II: ADDITIONAL RESOURCES AND ADVANCED MATERIAL

ABOUT PART II

In Part II, we introduce you to additional resources and advanced research on tinnitus. All too often, patients who conduct their own research are overwhelmed by the difficulty in finding and organizing information. The purpose of the following chapters is to provide you an organized and structured format to help you find additional information resources on tinnitus. In Part II, as in Part I, our objective is not to interpret the latest advances on tinnitus or render an opinion. Rather, our goal is to give you access to original research and to increase your awareness of sources you may not have already considered. In this way, you will come across the advanced materials often referred to in pamphlets, books, or other general works. Once again, some of this material is technical in nature, so consultation with a professional familiar with tinnitus is suggested.

CHAPTER 4. STUDIES ON TINNITUS

Overview

Every year, academic studies are published on tinnitus or related conditions. Broadly speaking, there are two types of studies. The first are peer reviewed. Generally, the content of these studies has been reviewed by scientists or physicians. Peer-reviewed studies are typically published in scientific journals and are usually available at medical libraries. The second type of studies is non-peer reviewed. These works include summary articles that do not use or report scientific results. These often appear in the popular press, newsletters, or similar periodicals.

In this chapter, we will show you how to locate peer-reviewed references and studies on tinnitus. We will begin by discussing research that has been summarized and is free to view by the public via the Internet. We then show you how to generate a bibliography on tinnitus and teach you how to keep current on new studies as they are published or undertaken by the scientific community.

The Combined Health Information Database

The Combined Health Information Database summarizes studies across numerous federal agencies. To limit your investigation to research studies and tinnitus, you will need to use the advanced search options. First, go to **http://chid.nih.gov/index.html**. From there, select the "Detailed Search" option (or go directly to that page with the following hyperlink: **http://chid.nih.gov/detail/detail.html**). The trick in extracting studies is found in the drop boxes at the bottom of the search page where "You may refine your search by." Select the dates and language you prefer, and the format option "Journal Article." At the top of the search form, select the number of records you would like to see (we recommend 100) and check the box to display "whole records." We recommend that you type in "tinnitus" (or synonyms) into the "For these words:" box. Consider using the option "anywhere in record" to make your search as broad as possible. If you want to limit the search to only a particular field, such as the title of the journal, then select this option in the "Search in these fields" drop box. The following is a sample of what you can expect from this type of search:

- **Masking Revisited: New Tinnitus Tools**

    Source: Hearing Health. 15(5): 34-38. September-October 1999.

    Contact: Available from Voice International Publications, Inc. P.O. Drawer V, Ingleside, TX 78362-0500. Voice/TTY (361) 776-7240. Fax (361) 776-3278. Website: www.hearinghealthmag.com.

    Summary: Although masking is not a cure for problem tinnitus, it offers a welcome respite from discomfort. This method traditionally uses devices worn at ear level to produce static white noise, a low level sound that is more acceptable to the listener than the intrusive noise of tinnitus. This article reviews advances in the use of masking for people with tinnitus. The authors offer a sampling of innovative treatment tools and therapeutic methods which display promise for treating tinnitus. Topics include dynamic tinnitus mitigation (DTM), the tinnitus relief system (TRS), the HiSonic bone conductor, Elite headphones, TRANQUIL (a broadband sound generator), Puretone products (16 different maskers), and tinnitus adaptation therapy (TAT), which teaches patients to focus away from the tinnitus. The authors note that for some individuals, the process of masking produces residual inhibition, a decreased awareness of tinnitus for a period of time after the masking sound is discontinued. One sidebar provides the addresses and telephone numbers of the product manufacturers and suppliers discussed.

- **The Costs of Tinnitus**

    Source: Tinnitus Today. The Journal of the American Tinnitus Association. 27(4): 18-19.

    Summary: An estimation of the costs of tinnitus is useful for assessing the effectiveness of treatments and justifying funding for research and education. Although the costs of tinnitus are difficult to calculate because of the wide range of treatments available, this article discusses the variables that should be considered when making those estimates. These include court awards; patient's age, gender, health, income, and employment history; number of treatments used; and perception of severity. The article also suggests ways to reduce the costs through prevention and management.

- **Tinnitus and Acoustic Neuroma**

    Source: ANA Notes. 2003;68.

    Contact: Available from Acoustic Neuroma Association. 600 Peachtree Parkway, Suite 108, Cumming, GA 30041. 770-205-8211; Fax:770-205-0239. Web site: http://www.ANAUSA.org. E-mail: ANAUSA@aol.com.

    Summary: Dr. John W. House discusses tinnitus, including diagnosis, treatment and prognosis, and its relationship to acoustic neuroma. Dr House describes tinnitus as a common symptom of hearing loss and a possible early sign of an acoustic neuroma.

- **Explosive Tinnitus: An Underrecognized Disorder**

    Source: Otolaryngology-Head and Neck Surgery. 118(1): 108-109. January 1998.

    Summary: Explosive tinnitus is a condition characterized by a frightening, loud, crashing or banging noise that occurs in association with sleep. Despite 60 case reports and typically dramatic auditory symptoms, a thorough MEDLINE review of the literature published since 1966 failed to identify mention of the disorder in the otologic literature. In this article, the body of information published to date is summarized, and two new cases are presented to illustrate the characteristics of this poorly understood phenomenon. Patients with the syndrome report a wide variety of medical and neurologic conditions, but in no cases have any significant associations been demonstrated. The condition is typically seen in the middle aged and elderly and is more common in women. The cause of the disorder remains speculative, and the condition is harmless. Patients typically have anxiety about their extreme symptoms, and reassurance can be offered if the condition is recognized. In some cases, sedative-hypnotic medications may significantly reduce symptoms by preventing periods of nighttime wakefulness, during which symptoms characteristically occur. 7 references.

- **Clinical Associations Between Tinnitus and Chronic Pain**

    Source: Otolaryngology-Head and Neck Surgery. 2003;128:706-10.

    Contact: Send requests to:.

    Summary: In this article the authors report on a prospective nonrandomized study in which a survey and the Tinnitus Handicap Inventory (THI) were distributed to 72 patients (50 women and 22 men) attending a tertiary chronic pain clinic, to determine the prevalence and severity of tinnitus inpatients with chronic pain. The research findings suggest a high incidence of tinnitus in people suffering with chronic pain.

- **Suicide in Tinnitus Sufferers**

    Source: Journal of Audiological Medicine. Volume 1: 30-37. 1992.

    Summary: In this article, the authors report six case histories of patients who died in violent circumstances (five suicides and one killed by his son). The authors discuss the role of tinnitus as a factor leading to their deaths, and also consider the potential risk factors for suicide, in terms of demographic features, associated mental illness, and tinnitus parameters. The patients in this group were mainly working class, male, lived alone, and had a history of psychiatric illness and previous suicide threats or attempts. Their tinnitus was generally of recent onset, pulsatile, and in their left ear. The number of cases quoted is small, so it is difficult to make firm conclusions, but the authors believe this represents the first published series on the subject. 1 table. 10 references. (AA-M).

- **Tinnitus Improvement Through TMD Therapy**

    Source: JADA. Journal of American Dental Association. 128(10): 1424-1432. October 1997.

    Summary: Many patients with temporomandibular disorder (TMD) and coexisting tinnitus find that therapy improves or resolves their tinnitus in conjunction with their TMD symptoms. This article reports on a study in which 93 patients with TMD who also reported having coexisting tinnitus were questioned and given clinical tests. These assessment instruments were then evaluated for their ability to suggest tinnitus improvement as a result of TMD therapy. The study suggests that asking targeted questions and performing a clinical test could be of significant value in helping practitioners decide which patients with TMD and coexisting tinnitus will experience improvement in, or resolution of, their tinnitus when TMD symptoms have improved significantly. Tables list characteristics of tinnitus, tinnitus-associated questions to ask patients, and specific clinical tests administered to subjects. 4 tables. 34 references. (AA-M).

- **Tinnitus Induced by Occupational and Leisure Noise**

    Source: Noise and Health. 8: 47-54. July-September 2000.

    Contact: Available from NRN Publications. Editorial Manager of Noise and Health, Institute of Laryngology and Otology, University College, London, 330 Gray's Inn Road, London WC1X 8EE, United Kingdom. 44 171 915 1575. Fax 44 171 278 8041. E-mail: m.patrick@ucl.ac.uk.

Summary: Noise exposure is the most common cause of tinnitus. Noise induced permanent tinnitus (NIPT) can derive from occupational noise exposure, leisure noise, or acoustic trauma. This article explores tinnitus induced by occupational and leisure noise. In general, NIPT is high pitched and tonal. The most common observed frequency of tinnitus on pitch matching is the same as the worst frequency for hearing. The sensation level of NIPT is usually low and sometimes negative. There is no correlation of significance between the discomfort caused by NIPT and audiometric findings. In occupational NIPT, the interval between the start of noisy work and the appearance of tinnitus is very long (many years) but with leisure noise and acoustic trauma, the interval between exposure and tinnitus is frequently very short (immediate). The incidence of musically induced tinnitus is increasingly more common. The authors contend that it is a much greater handicap for a young individual to suffer from tinnitus than from a small high tone hearing loss. The treatment of NIPT is not different from tinnitus treatment in general. 1 figure. 6 tables. 24 references.

- **Tinnitus and Vertigo in Patients with Temporomandibular Disorder**

    Source: Archives of Otolaryngology-Head and Neck Surgery. 118(8): 817-821. August 1992.

    Summary: The association of tinnitus and vertigo with temporomandibular disorder (TMD) has been debated for many years. This article reports on a study conducted to determine if tinnitus and vertigo are actually more prevalent in patients with TMD than in appropriate age-matched controls. One control group was recruited from patients seeking care for health maintenance and the other from patients seeking routine dental care. The authors surveyed 1032 patients: 338 had TMD and 694 served as two age-matched control groups. Tinnitus and vertigo symptoms were significantly more prevalent in the TMD group than in either of the control groups. The authors note that the mechanism of the association of TMD and otologic symptoms is unknown. 2 figures. 5 tables. 43 references. (AA-M).

- **Progressive Sensorineural Hearing Loss, Subjective Tinnitus and Vertigo Caused By Elevated Blood Lipids**

    Source: ENT. Ear, Nose, and Throat Journal. 76(10): 716-730. October 1997.

    Summary: The otologist frequently sees patients with progressive sensorineural hearing loss, subjective aural tinnitus, and vertigo with no apparent cause. Elevated blood lipids may be a cause of inner ear malfunction on a biochemical basis. This article reports on a study undertaken to establish the true incidence of this condition. All new patients (n = 4,251) seen during an eight-year period were evaluated; of these, 2,332 patients had complaints of inner ear disease. All the patients had a complete neurotologic examination, appropriate audiometric and vestibular studies and imaging, and blood tests including lipid phenotype studies. Hyperlipoproteinemia was found in 120 patients (5.1 percent). Most patients were found to be overweight and had additional coexisting conditions such as diabetes mellitus. Treatment with vasodilators and a 500 calorie, high-protein, low-carbohydrate diet yielded improvement of symptoms in 83 percent of patients within five months of initiation of treatment. The authors include three detailed case studies. The authors conclude that the cause-and-effect relationship between hyperlipoproteinemia and dysfunction of the inner ear is indisputable. 6 figures. 14 references. (AA-M).

- **Controlling Tinnitus**

    Source: Hearing Health. 13(4): 42-44. July-August 1997.

    Contact: Available from Voice International Publications, Inc. P.O. Drawer V, Ingleside, TX 78362-0500. Voice/TTY (361) 776-7240. Fax (361) 776-3278. Website: www.hearinghealthmag.com.

    Summary: This article addresses the therapeutic management of tinnitus. Tinnitus, noises that are heard by an individual but are not related to any external sound in the environment, is perceived as a variety of sounds. This article is the second in a series of three articles that focuses on a new neurophysiological model of tinnitus and a method of treatment called Tinnitus Retraining Therapy (TRT). In this article, the author describes TRT, a process which involves the habituation of the reactions evoked by tinnitus and one's perception of tinnitus. The author stresses that it is possible to achieve habituation only when tinnitus has no negative associations; therefore, it is necessary to include retraining counseling to de-mystify tinnitus. In addition, habituation occurs more quickly if the strength of tinnitus-related neuronal activity in the brain is decreased, which is achieved by sound therapy. The author describes the implementation of TRT, which consists of four steps: evaluation, consisting of initial interview, tinnitus oriented audiological evaluation, medical evaluation, and diagnosis, on the basis of which one of five major types of treatment is proposed; retraining counseling session; fitting of instruments, if needed; and follow up contacts. The author concludes that, while TRT is not a cure in the classical sense, it makes it possible to achieve a state where individuals are not aware of tinnitus for the majority of time. (AA-M).

- **Selective Cochlear Neurectomy for Debilitating Tinnitus**

  Source: Annals of Otology, Rhinology, and Laryngology. 106(7, Part 1): 568-570. July 1997.

  Summary: This article describes the use of selective cochlear neurectomy to treat debilitating tinnitus. Eight nerve sections have been performed for this purpose, with various success rates (45 to 76 percent). Patients with a unilateral, profound sensorineural hearing loss and disabling tinnitus are candidates for cochlear neurectomy. The authors introduce the use of a selective cochlear neurectomy with preservation of the vestibular nerve in two case presentations. The indications for surgery, surgical technique, and results are described. Advantages of preserving the vestibular nerve fibers include the lack of postoperative vertigo and disequilibrium and a short length of hospital stay. Another advantage is the conservation of a symmetric vestibular input, obviating the lengthy compensation process that might otherwise be needed, particularly in the elderly. A selective cochlear neurectomy for the control of debilitating tinnitus has proven to be successful in controlling tinnitus in the two patients presented, with the added advantage of preservation of their vestibular function. The authors call for further studies to confirm the advantages and effectiveness of this technique. 11 references. (AA).

- **Tinnitus: An Obscure Symptom**

  Source: Hearing Health. 10(2): 17-19. February-March 1994.

  Contact: Available from Voice International Publications, Inc. P.O. Drawer V, Ingleside, TX 78362-0500. Voice/TTY (361) 776-7240. Fax (361) 776-3278. Website: www.hearinghealthmag.com.

  Summary: This article discusses the etiological factors accounting for tinnitus, including those of the external ear, the middle ear, the inner ear, and the central nervous system. The article includes a case study used to show the obscure nature of tinnitus and how unconventional treatments sometimes help. The article concludes with the contact information for two resource organizations. The author stresses that varied etiologic factors make it important that every patient have a thorough medical examination, preferably by an otologist who works closely with an audiologist experienced with tinnitus. 1 figure. 1 table.

- **Tinnitus and Craniomandibular Disorders: Is There A Link?**

  Source: Swedish Dental Journal Supplement. Volume 95: 1-46. 1993.

  Summary: This article discusses the relationship between tinnitus and craniomandibular disorder (CMD) symptoms. Craniomandibular disorders consist of musculoskeletal discomfort or dysfunction in the stomatognathic system, which is aggravated by mandibular function. The author reviews the literature in an attempt to find parameters which could define a CMD-related tinnitus, and to identify predictors of stomatognathic and biofeedback treatment outcome in this group of patients. The author concludes that several findings in the studies reviewed indicate an association between signs and symptoms of CMD and tinnitus. The relationship between tinnitus complains and several symptoms of CMD, including frequent headaches, seems to be independent of the degree of hearing loss, occupational noise exposure, general morbidity, medication, and socioeconomic status. 2 figures. 1 table. 334 references.

- **Tinnitus Management in the Dispensing Practice**

  Source: Audecibel. 42(4): 7-10. October-November-December 1993.

  Summary: This article discusses tinnitus management in the dispensing practice. The author first defines aspects of tinnitus which may apply to the dispensing practice and then sets forth a basic tinnitus analysis screening protocol as it applies to the hearing aid evaluation process. Topics covered include personal descriptions of tinnitus; Residual Inhibition (RI); masking with hearing aids, including pitch matching and intensity matching; auditory reattention and stress relief; adjustment of tinnitus instruments; and the protocol. 1 figure. 23 references.

- **Counseling the Tinnitus Patient: Often It's What We Say That Counts**

  Source: Hearing Journal. 52(3): 36-37. March 1999.

  Contact: Available from Lippincott Williams and Wilkins. Customer Service, P.O. Box 1175, Lowell, MA 01853.

  Summary: This article encourages hearing health care professionals to make a concerted effort to offer proper education and unwavering compassion and understanding to their patients with tinnitus. The author describes the typical encounter with a patient with tinnitus and the often failed treatment that can result. The author notes that tinnitus patients typically develop a heightened sense of awareness of everything about themselves and their bodies. As a result, every word uttered by their audiologist or their physician takes on increased significance. Misinformation, misrepresentation, or miscommunication can send a patient with tinnitus into complete despair. The author stresses that one does not have to have tinnitus in order to be an advocate for tinnitus patients or to demonstrate compassion and understanding. Information about tinnitus is plentiful and is easily accessible through audiology journals, books, conferences, and the Internet.

- **Clinical Management of Tinnitus and Hyperacusis**

    Source: The ASHA Leader. 8(20): 4-5, 24. November 4, 2003.

    Contact: Available from American Speech-Language-Hearing Association (ASHA). Product Sales, 10801 Rockville Pike, Rockville, MD 20852. (888) 498-6699. TTY (301) 897-0157. Website: www.asha.org.

    Summary: This article is presented as an introduction to Tinnitus Retraining Therapy (TRT), defined by the author as an individualized, noninvasive treatment that is effective for patients with intrusive tinnitus. The topics covered include habituation to the tinnitus signal and assessment of sound sensitivity; the implementation process; options for sound therapy; and efficacy.

- **Learning to Control Tinnitus. Part IV of IV**

    Source: Hearing Health. 14(4): 40-42. July-August 1998.

    Contact: Available from Voice International Publications, Inc. P.O. Drawer V, Ingleside, TX 78362-0500. Voice/TTY (361) 776-7240. Fax (361) 776-3278. Website: www.hearinghealthmag.com.

    Summary: This article is the final installment in a four-part series on an integrated treatment approach for tinnitus. The author reports that tinnitus is the most frustrating symptom presented to him by patients. Many people with tinnitus first consult with their primary care physician, internist, or neurologist before reaching an otologist or neurotologist such as the author. By then, besides being frustrated by their condition, these prospective patients generally report discontent with their previous medical experience. The author discusses strategies used to pinpoint the source of the tinnitus. No matter what treatment plan is ultimately established, an accurate diagnosis is the first step in evaluation and management. Once a diagnosis is reached, therapy is tailored so that all the treatable causes of tinnitus can be addressed. For patients who continue to have chronic tinnitus, many techniques and treatment plans can either reduce the severity of the problem or enable the patient to establish and maintain some control. These techniques include masking, cognitive therapy, and a combination of both which is called tinnitus retraining therapy. The author concludes that management of chronic tinnitus is very complex, requiring commitment and dedication from the patient, treating physician, and other healthcare professionals involved. (AA-M).

- **Contribution of Social Noise to Tinnitus in Young People: A Preliminary Report**

    Source: Noise and Health. Volume 1: 40-46. September-December 1998.

    Contact: Available from Noise and Health. Institute of Laryngology and Otology, University College London, 330 Gray's Inn Road, London WC1X 8EE, United Kingdom. +44 171 915 1575. Fax +44 171 278 8041.

    Summary: This article offers a preliminary report on a study of the contribution of social noise to tinnitus in young people. In the authors' original study of the Hearing in Young Adults (HIYA) aged 18 to 25 years, there appeared to be little effect of social noise (primarily amplified music) on hearing thresholds. There was however, a threefold increase in the reports of tinnitus in those subjects with significant social noise exposure. No other hearing function abnormality was found for those who were exposed to social noise. The authors invited a subsample of those tested in the earlier phase of the study, resulting in three groups: those in the most social noise group who reported tinnitus (n = 15) and those who did not (n = 15), plus a group of people who had no social noise exposure but who reported tinnitus (n = 8). All groups were retested for their hearing thresholds, using standard audiometry and also the Audioscan technique to look for notches in the audiogram. Speech tests were carried out using an adaptive FAAF test. Transient evoked otoacoustic emissions were measured and also suppressed with a contralateral broad band noise. Some evidence has been found to suggest that those young people who reported tinnitus are affected by social noise exposure, in terms of pure tone thresholds, speech tests, otoacoustic emissions, and reported hearing problems. The authors share some of the lessons to be learned from their attempt to follow up this interesting population. The population is highly mobile and follow up is difficult; and the presumed noise exposure was often not appropriate because even after a year it was possible for several individuals with insignificant social noise to move into the group with significant social noise exposure. The authors conclude with a call for a larger multi center study to look at the effect of social noise in more detail, using a common protocol. 14 references. (AA-M).

- **Tinnitus Thru the Ages**

    Source: Hearing Health. 16(1): 90-93. January-February 2000.

    Contact: Available from Voice International Publications, Inc. P.O. Drawer V, Ingleside, TX 78362-0500. Voice/TTY (361) 776-7240. Fax (361) 776-3278. Website: www.hearinghealthmag.com.

Summary: This article offers a summary of tinnitus (ringing or other sounds in the ears) and its treatments. The authors present a brief overview of the progression of methods for treating tinnitus, including only those clinical protocols that seem to have a certain degree of acceptance among the majority of qualified tinnitus therapists. The authors stress that a number of theories exist about the causes of tinnitus onset, yet there is no agreement as to the neurophysiologic mechanisms of tinnitus. In addition, there is no common consensus of the best treatment or management strategy. Treatments discussed include medical intervention (drug therapy), masking (using another sound to cover up the tinnitus sounds), and other nonmedical therapies, including Tinnitus Retraining Therapy (TRT) which involves a combination of directive counseling coupled with the use of a noise generator in each ear (for masking), and Cognitive Therapy, a psychologically based behavioral modification approach to treatment.

- **Neurophysiological Approach to Tinnitus Patients**

    Source: American Journal of Otology. 17(2): 236-240. March 1996.

    Summary: This article outlines a neurophysiologic model of tinnitus and an approach to tinnitus management. The model is based on the concept that all levels of the auditory pathways and several nonauditory systems play essential roles in tinnitus. The nonauditory systems may be dominant in determining the level of annoyance caused by the tinnitus. The authors propose to treat tinnitus by inducing and facilitating habituation to the tinnitus signal. The goal is to reach the stage at which patients are unaware of tinnitus unless they focus on it. Even when perceived, tinnitus should not evoke annoyance. Habituation is achieved by directive counseling combined with low-level, broad-band noise generated by wearable generators, and environmental sounds, according to a specific protocol. The authors briefly report on their experiences using this model to treat patients with tinnitus. 2 figures. 38 references. (AA-M).

- **Update on Tinnitus from the NIDCD**

    Source: Tinnitus Today. 19(1): 18-20. March 1994.

    Contact: Available from American Tinnitus Association (ATA). P.O. Box 5, Portland, OR 97207-0005. (800) 634-8978 or (503) 248-9985. Fax (503) 248-0024. E-mail: tinnitus@ata.org. Website: www.ata.org.

    Summary: This article presents an update on current research activities on tinnitus. Written by the director of the National Institute on Deafness and Other Communication Disorders (NIDCD), Dr. James B. Snow, Jr., the article discusses the mechanisms of tinnitus; the etiology of tinnitus; ototoxicity; side effects of aminoglycoside antibiotics; the prevention of noise-induced hearing loss; the diseases and disorders with which tinnitus is associated; therapeutic modalities, including surgery; the mission of the NIDCD; present research supported by the NIDCD; a planned NIDCD workshop on tinnitus in 1995; the infrastructure of the NIDCD; temporal bone donation; research funding; and research goals for the future.

- **Modulation of Tinnitus by Voluntary Jaw Movements**

    Source: American Journal of Otology. 19(6): 785-789. November 1998.

    Contact: Available from Lippincott Williams and Wilkins. 12107 Insurance Way, Hagerstown, MD 21740. (800) 638-3030 or (301) 714-2300. Fax (301) 824-7390.

    Summary: This article reports on a study in which the authors describe symptoms and population characteristics in patients with tinnitus who report the ability to control the loudness of their tinnitus by performing voluntary movements. The authors used a questionnaire, administered at a tertiary care center, to investigate respondents with the self-reported ability to control the loudness of their tinnitus by using voluntary jaw movements. The authors describe 93 patients with tinnitus (83 percent men, 17 percent women); 85 percent of these patients report jaw movements and 9 percent report eye movements that affect their tinnitus. In the jaw movement group, tinnitus loudness increased in 90 percent. Jaw movement affected the pitch in 51 percent, with an increase in pitch reported by 90 percent of those. Other maneuvers, such as pressure applied to the head, affected tinnitus in many subjects. Tinnitus had a major impact on the lives of the authors respondents: 27 percent registered mild to moderate depression and 8 percent moderate to severe depression as shown by the Beck Depression Inventory. The authors conclude that the ability to modulate tinnitus by performing voluntary somatosensory or motor acts is likely the result of plastic changes in the brains of these patients with the development of aberrant connections between the auditory and sensory motor systems. The strong predominance of men in the sample suggests the presence of a gender specific factor that mediates these changes. 2 tables. 20 references. (AA-M).

- **Computer-Automated Clinical Technique for Tinnitus Quantification**

    Source: American Journal of Audiology. 9(1): 36-49. June 2000.

Contact: Available from American Speech-Language-Hearing Association (ASHA). Product Sales, 10801 Rockville Pike, Rockville, MD 20852. (888) 498-6699. TTY (301) 897-0157. Website: www.asha.org.

Summary: This article reports on a study that addressed the need for uniformity in techniques for clinical quantification of tinnitus (ringing or other sounds in the ear). The authors' laboratory is developing techniques to perform computer automated tinnitus testing. A computer controlled psychoacoustical system was developed to quantify tinnitus loudness and pitch using a tone matching technique. Hearing thresholds were also obtained as part of the procedure. The system generated test stimuli and simultaneously controlled a notebook computer positioned in the sound chamber facing the patient. The notebook computer displayed instructions for responding and relayed response choices through on screen 'buttons' that the patient touched with a pen device. Twenty individuals with tinnitus were evaluated with the technique over two sessions, and responses were analyzed for test retest reliability. Analyses revealed good reliability of thresholds, loudness matches, and pitch matches. The authors conclude that these results demonstrate that use of a fully automated system to obtain reliable measurements of tinnitus loudness and pitch is feasible for clinical application. 5 figures. 5 tables. 62 references.

- **Longitudinal Follow-Up of Tinnitus Complaints**

    Source: Archives of Otolaryngology-Head and Neck Surgery. 127(2): 175-179. February 2001.

    Contact: Available from American Medical Association. Subscriber Services, P.O. 10946, Chicago, IL 60610-0946. (800) 262-3250 or (312) 670-7827. Fax (312) 464-5831. E-mail: ama-subs@ama-assn.org. Website: www.ama-assn.org/oto.

    Summary: This article reports on a study undertaken to investigate the long term outcome of patients with tinnitus (ringing or other sounds in the ears), the long term effects of cognitive behavior therapy for their tinnitus, and what characteristics of tinnitus predict distress at follow up. The study consisted of longitudinal follow up of a consecutive sample of patients with tinnitus initially seen by a clinical psychologist at the Department of Audiology, University Hospital in Uppsala, Sweden. The consecutive series of 189 patients with tinnitus treated between January 1988 and March 1995 were sent a mailed questionnaire. One hundred forty six (77 women and 69 men) provided usable responses, in all yielding a 77 percent response rate. Questionnaire data showed that many patients with tinnitus still experienced distress an average of 4.9 years after admission. Tolerance of tinnitus increased over time overall.

For patients who had received cognitive behavior therapy (59 percent), there was a reduction in tinnitus related distress. Further, an open ended question showed that the benefits from treatment outweighed the deficits. Analysis showed that tinnitus maskability at admission was a significant predictor of distress at follow up. The authors conclude that severe tinnitus shows some signs of improvement over time, especially when psychological treatment has been given. Tinnitus maskability is an important prognostic factor of future tinnitus annoyance. 3 figures. 22 references.

- **Tinnitus: In the Eyes of the Law**

    Source: Tinnitus Today. 21(1): 9-14. March 1996.

    Contact: Available from American Tinnitus Association (ATA). P.O. Box 5, Portland, OR 97207-0005. (800) 634-8978 or (503) 248-9985. Fax (503) 248-0024. E-mail: tinnitus@ata.org. Website: www.ata.org.

    Summary: This article reports on legal issues specific to tinnitus, particularly as tinnitus is recognized as a compensable disability. Topics covered include Social Security, how disability claims are processed, pitch and loudness matching, Worker's Compensation laws, the Department of Veteran's Affairs, the Americans With Disabilities Act, and actual courtroom experiences. The article concludes with a list of technical and legal consultants on tinnitus and other hearing issues and a brief list of lawyers who represented successful tinnitus cases. 17 references.

- **Tinnitus: Keeping Up to Date**

    Source: Hearing Health. 12(6): 40-42. November-December 1996.

    Contact: Available from Voice International Publications, Inc. P.O. Drawer V, Ingleside, TX 78362-0500. Voice/TTY (361) 776-7240. Fax (361) 776-3278. Website: www.hearinghealthmag.com.

    Summary: This article reviews some recent research on tinnitus and its management. Topics include tinnitus in children, benefits or detriments of alcohol use in people with tinnitus, drug treatment and tinnitus, psychological factors, and future research, particularly that on children with tinnitus. Drugs discussed include carbamazepine, betahistine hydrochloride, benzodiazepines, propranol, pitzotifen, and antidepressants. The author notes that most children with tinnitus believe it is normal, a regular aspect of every day life. The author stresses that children must be educated about avoiding loud noise.

- **Tinnitus: Among Many Uncertainties, A Message of Hope is One Constant**

    Source: SHHH Journal. 17(1): 16-20, 22-23. January-February 1996.

    Contact: Available from Self Help for Hard of Hearing People, Inc. (SHHH). 7910 Woodmont Avenue, Suite 1200, Bethesda, MD 20814. (301) 657-2248; TTY (301) 657-2249; Fax (301) 913-9413.

    Summary: This article reviews the controversies surrounding tinnitus and its treatment. Topics covered include the connections between tinnitus and hearing loss, the hidden nature of tinnitus, medical referrals, the need to provide tinnitus patients with information and reassurance, the American Tinnitus Association, the role of counseling for tinnitus patients, diagnostic considerations, lifestyle factors, psychoacoustic testing, treatment options, the use of amplification, masking devices, drug therapy, habituation, support groups, cognitive behavioral therapy, other treatments that may be of some use, and research on tinnitus and its treatments. The author includes the address and telephone number of the American Tinnitus Association at the end of the article.

- **Tinnitus: Etiology and Management**

    Source: Clinics in Geriatric Medicine. 15(1): 193-204. February 1999.

    Contact: Available from W.B. Saunders. Periodicals Fulfillment, 6277 Sea Harbor Drive, Orlando, FL 32887-4800. (800) 654-2452. Website: www.wbsaunders.com.

    Summary: This article reviews the etiology and management of tinnitus, defined as the perceived sensation of sound in the absence of an acoustic stimulus. The authors contend that because tinnitus has the potential to drastically affect a person's life (particularly older adults), it is important for physicians to take the time to closely evaluate this complaint. The authors review the causes of objective and subjective tinnitus, patient evaluation strategies, and the management of tinnitus. The authors include information about the American Tinnitus Association, cited as a source for excellent information on tinnitus. The authors reiterate that a caring physician can make a significant difference in the tinnitus patient's quality of life by properly evaluating the patient to rule out significant underlying disease and explaining the commonality of their condition. Many times, these patients will show much improvement with reassurance and some basic guidance. 27 references.

- **Managing Tinnitus: What You Can Do!**

    Source: Hearing Health. 16(1): 93-96. January-February 2000.

Contact: Available from Voice International Publications, Inc. P.O. Drawer V, Ingleside, TX 78362-0500. Voice/TTY (361) 776-7240. Fax (361) 776-3278. Website: www.hearinghealthmag.com.

Summary: This article reviews the impact that tinnitus (ringing or other noises in the ear) can have on a person's quality of life, focusing on the ways that an individual's perspective and approach can make their tinnitus problem greater or less. The author stresses the importance of continuing to do activities that one enjoys, even when there are some things that might need to be limited. The author outlines six basic guidelines: excessively loud noise for any appreciable amount of time should be avoided; medication which is known to potentially cause damage to the auditory system should never be taken, unless the situation is life threatening and no acceptable alternative can be found; exposure to all kinds of sounds that are not excessively loud should be incorporated as a way of life; medically indicated drugs and medications should be used (not avoided); in moderation, one can and should feel comfortable about participating prudently in life's activities; and look forward to a future that might bring about more understanding or even a cure for tinnitus. The author uses the story of one of his patients to explain how these guidelines can be used to cope with tinnitus. The author stresses that even though there is not a cure for tinnitus, there are treatment and approach methods that can ease suffering.

- **Drug-Induced Tinnitus and Other Hearing Disorders**

   Source: Drug Safety. 14(3): 198-212. March 1996.

   Summary: This article reviews the pharmacoepidemiology of drug-induced tinnitus and other hearing disorders. Tinnitus and hearing loss, both reversible and irreversible, are associated both with acute intoxication and long term administration of a large range of drugs. The mechanism causing drug-induced ototoxicity is unclear, but may involve biochemical and consequent electrophysiological changes in the inner ear and eighth cranial nerve impulse transmission. Over 130 drugs and chemicals have been reported to be potentially ototoxic. The major classes are the aminoglycosides and other antimicrobials, anti-inflammatory agents, diuretics, antimalarial drugs, antineoplastic agents, and some topically administered agents. Prevention of drug-induced ototoxicity is generally based upon consideration and avoidance of appropriate risk factors, as well as on monitoring of renal function, serum drug concentrations, and cochlear and auditory functions before and during drug therapy. Ototoxicity, although not life-threatening, may cause considerable discomfort to patients taking ototoxic drugs, and in some cases, drug discontinuation may be necessary to prevent permanent damage. Drug categories discussed include antimicrobials, salicylates and other nonsteroidal anti-inflammatory drugs, loop diuretics, antimalarial drugs, antineoplastic drugs, topically and regionally applied drugs, and miscellaneous drugs. 2 tables. 168 references. (AA).

- **New Look at Tinnitus**

    Source: Hearing Health. 13(3): 16-17. May-June 1997.

    Contact: Available from Voice International Publications, Inc. P.O. Drawer V, Ingleside, TX 78362-0500. Voice/TTY (361) 776-7240. Fax (361) 776-3278. Website: www.hearinghealthmag.com.

    Summary: This article reviews the problem of tinnitus, including a brief discussion of hyeracusis (extremely sensitive hearing). Tinnitus, noises that are heard by an individual but are not related to any external sound in the environment, is perceived as a variety of sounds. This article is the first in a series of three articles that focuses on a new neurophysiological model of tinnitus and a method of treatment called Tinnitus Retraining Therapy (TRT). In this first article, the author describes the symptoms and effects of tinnitus, the interrelationship of tinnitus and hearing loss, brain function, and habituation (of the reactions and of tinnitus perception). The author concludes that, once the habituation of reaction is achieved, patients are no longer annoyed by tinnitus, disregarding the fact that their tinnitus has the same loudness and pitch as before treatment. (AA-M).

- **Meeting of the Minds: What's Up with Tinnitus?**

    Source: Hearing Health. 15(2): 27-29. March-April 1999.

    Contact: Available from Voice International Publications, Inc. P.O. Drawer V, Ingleside, TX 78362-0500. Voice/TTY (361) 776-7240. Fax (361) 776-3278. Website: www.hearinghealthmag.com.

    Summary: This article summarizes the activities of the 1998 Sixth Annual Conference on Management of the Tinnitus Patient (Iowa City, Iowa), including an overview of the event's origins and a sneak preview of the 1999 workshop. The conference was initially intended for professionals (otologists, audiologists, psychologists, nurses) who provide clinical services, but in 1997 it was opened to people who have tinnitus. The conference is intended to disseminate the current thinking on evaluation and treatment strategies for tinnitus. The article briefly reviews the psychological approaches covered in the conference, the use of cognitive therapy, Tinnitus Retraining Therapy (TRT), the role of psychological factors in tinnitus, social activity (coffeehouses) as a treatment strategy, tinnitus and sleep, and tinnitus in children. The author concludes the article by briefly introducing the topics and speakers who will be presenting in October 1999, at the next conference. One sidebar summarizes present tinnitus research activities. 2 figures.

- **Update on Tinnitus**

    Source: Otolaryngologic Clinics of North America. 29(3): 455-465. June 1996.

    Summary: This article updates readers on tinnitus, the perception of sound or noise without any external stimulation. The authors discuss attempts to objectify tinnitus. They describe the relationship between active cochlear processes and tinnitus, eighth nerve and brain stem considerations, the cerebral cortex, and evaluation of patients with tinnitus. The author also addresses the management of tinnitus, medicolegal concerns, the need for an international tinnitus classification system, and other philosophical issues. The authors conclude that the problems of managing tinnitus are compounded by the several different mechanisms that contribute to the persistent sensation of tinnitus. They conclude that it is naive to conceptualize tinnitus as a disease with a single origin and treatment. 3 tables. 28 references.

- **Tinnitus: Research Highlights, Treatment Options**

    Source: Advance for Speech-Language Pathologists and Audiologists. 6(28): 6-7. July 15, 1996.

    Contact: Available from Merion Publications, Inc. 650 Park Avenue, Box 61556, King of Prussia, PA 19406-0956. (800) 355-1088 or (610) 265-7812.

    Summary: This article, from a professional newsletter for speech language pathologists and audiologists, describes research and treatment in the area of tinnitus. The author describes recent research that has revealed new information about the disorder and paved the way for new treatment options, including habituation, medication, hearing aids, and maskers. Topics include tinnitus in children and in elderly people, audiological evaluation and habituation therapy, therapeutic results using habituation therapy, a comparison of maskers and habituation therapy, and a brief discussion of drug therapy for tinnitus. The article concludes with the addresses and telephone numbers of the researchers interviewed in the article.

- **Tinnitus: From Symptom to Management**

    Source: Hearing Health. 14(3): 30-32. May-June 1998.

Contact: Available from Voice International Publications, Inc. P.O. Drawer V, Ingleside, TX 78362-0500. Voice/TTY (361) 776-7240. Fax (361) 776-3278. Website: www.hearinghealthmag.com.

Summary: This article, the third in a four-part series on tinnitus, outlines treatment and management options. The author first stresses that an accurate diagnosis underlies all successful attempts to manage tinnitus. The author notes that tinnitus is a symptom, not a disease unto itself. It can be an early signal of a hearing loss in progress or an auditory condition in a period of change, either for the better or the worse. Tinnitus can be caused by impacted cerumen (earwax), foreign bodies, otosclerosis, auditory nerve tumor, sensorineural hearing loss, ototoxicity (drugs that damage the ear), or noise exposure. A complete evaluation by an audiologist experienced in tinnitus treatment is recommended. The maskability of the sound and the presence or absence of residual inhibitions should be assessed. Residual inhibition occurs after exposure to a narrow band of noise surrounding the frequency of the person's tinnitus. Maskable tinnitus is a good predictor of success with maskers or hearing aids, which are among the most effective forms of instrumentation for this type of problem. The author includes a section discussing the emotional component of chronic tinnitus. In addition, a major aspect to be evaluated in the success of tinnitus management is how long the improvement is maintained. Only when a person with severe tinnitus experiences significant relief which is maintained over time can it be considered that this symptom is truly managed. One sidebar lists the steps to successful treatment for tinnitus and notes the addresses of four resource and support organizations (in the United States, Canada, England, and Germany).

- **New Finding in Tinnitus Research**

    Source: Hearing Health. 14(3): 52. May-June 1998.

    Contact: Available from Voice International Publications, Inc. P.O. Drawer V, Ingleside, TX 78362-0500. Voice/TTY (361) 776-7240. Fax (361) 776-3278. Website: www.hearinghealthmag.com.

    Summary: This brief article provides readers with new information about identifying and treating tinnitus. The article reports on a study in that used positron emission tomography (PET) scans to determine neural activity in the brains of four tinnitus patients and six control subjects. PET is an imaging technique that can show functional activity in the body as opposed to only showing the anatomy of the organ. Neural activity is determined by the amount of cerebral (brain) blood flow, which increases as neural activity in a certain region of the brain rises. This increase shows up on the PET scans. The tinnitus patients in the study all had cochlear hearing loss, and were able to control the loudness of their tinnitus through oral facial movements, such as clenching the jaws. Although loudness and pitch of tinnitus are subjective measures, changes in cerebral blood flow (as shown on the PET scans) indicated that the patients were indeed changing something. Researchers used an injection of a liquid tracer to measure cerebral blood flow in all test subjects at rest, and tinnitus patients were also scanned while they manipulated their symptoms through facial movements. Study of images taken from each patient pinpointed the origin of the tinnitus activity to sites in the temporal lobe opposite the affected ear. In other words, if a patient reported tinnitus in the right ear, the origin of the activity was in the left temporal lobe. The remainder of the article describes ongoing and planned research in this area. 1 figure.

- **Tinnitus: Its Causes, Diagnosis, and Treatment**

  Source: British Medical Journal. Volume 326: 1490-1491. April-June 1993.

  Summary: This brief article reviews the causes, diagnosis of, and treatment for tinnitus. After a discussion of the pathophysiology and diagnosis of tinnitus, the author summarizes management issues. The main management of tinnitus is medical and comprises psychological, pharmacological, and prosthetic considerations. The author stresses that surgery must be reserved for rare cases. She notes that it is much better for patients with troublesome tinnitus to be investigated for a cause and managed by someone with a positive attitude towards the condition, prepared to give an informed explanation and appropriate psychological or psychiatric support. 11 references.

- **Tinnitus Caused By Sudden, Intense Changes in Air Pressure**

  Source: Tinnitus Today. 25(1): 17. March 2000.

  Contact: Available from American Tinnitus Association. P.O. Box 5, Portland, OR 97207. (800) 634-8978 or (503) 248-9985. E-mail: tinnitus@ata.org. Website: www.ata.org.

  Summary: This brief article reviews the problem of tinnitus (ringing or other sounds in the ear) caused by sudden, intense changes in air trauma (barotrauma). Normally the air pressure within the middle ear (the space enclosed by the ear drum) is equalized to the outside air pressure whenever the Eustachian tube opens. But sometimes equalization cannot occur, causing pain, feeling of intense pressure, and sometimes bleeding or rupture of the eardrum. Hearing damage or tinnitus may then result. The authors report on their findings of tinnitus caused by barotrauma, as demonstrated by data from the Tinnitus Data Registry (collected at the

Tinnitus Clinic of the Oregon Health Sciences University in Portland, Oregon). The authors note that a total of 17 patients in the database reported barotrauma as the cause of their tinnitus (about seven-tenths of 1 percent of the database). The authors report on the characteristics of this subgroup, noting similarities and differences between this group and the overall Clinic group.

- **Tinnitus with Calcium-Channel Blockers (Letter)**

   Source: Lancet. 343(8907): 1229-1230. May 14, 1994.

   Summary: This brief letter to the editor discusses the problem of tinnitus associated with calcium-channel blockers (CCB); the authors stress that this side-effect has only been reported with nicardipine. They report information on eight patients who developed tinnitus while being treated with CCBs. Five of these patients were being treated only with a CCB, while three were also receiving other well-known ototoxic drugs. The induction period was 1 day or less in all 5 cases; all patients completely recovered after drug withdrawal. The authors conclude that the close temporal relation between drug exposure and tinnitus in the five patients who had been exposed only to a CCB suggests a possible causal relation. 3 references.

- **Tinnitus: Tuning Out the Noises in Your Head**

   Source: One in Seven. Supplement: 1-27. February-March 1999.

   Contact: Available from RNID Helpline. P.O. Box 16464, London EC1Y 8TT, United Kingdom. 0870 60 50 123. Fax 0171-296 8199. E-mail: helpline@rnid.org.uk. Website: www.rnid.org.uk. PRICE: 1.99 pounds.

   Summary: This issue focusing on tinnitus is a special supplement to 'One in Seven,' a magazine published by the British Royal National Institute for Deaf People (RNID). Tinnitus is the word for noises that some people hear in their ears or in their head, including buzzing, ringing, whistling, hissing, and other sounds that do not come from any external source. Most people have experienced tinnitus on occasion, but it can become a problem when it persists. The issue offers eight articles that cover the causes and effects of tinnitus; treatment options after receiving a diagnosis of tinnitus; self help strategies for diet and lifestyle; recommendations for managing tinnitus; products available to help with relaxation and stress reduction; the latest developments in the treatment of tinnitus; research studies on tinnitus; and facts about tinnitus. The magazine features interviews with people who have tinnitus and who explain their own coping and management strategies. The magazine contains numerous full color photographs and graphics. The inside back cover of the magazine lists the patient education leaflets available from RNID.

- **Elderly People and Tinnitus**

   Source: Tinnitus Today. 22(2): 9-10. June 1997.

   Contact: Available from American Tinnitus Association (ATA). P.O. Box 5, Portland, OR 97207-0005. (800) 634-8978 or (503) 248-9985. Fax (503) 248-0024. E-mail: tinnitus@ata.org. Website: www.ata.org.

   Summary: This newsletter article reviews the issue of tinnitus in elderly people. The author discusses hearing loss, health and mobility problems, depression, polypharmacy (taking multiple medications), isolation and loneliness, and attitudes (of health care providers and of the patients themselves). The author cautions that the increasing loss of hearing that often accompanies aging can accentuate the internal sounds of tinnitus and make the intervention of low noise therapy or masking techniques more problematic and less effective. In addition, mobility difficulties that can interfere with a range of everyday activities can also make it hard to get to a doctor, hospital, or local tinnitus group, or to simply get out of the house and away from tinnitus. Debilitating conditions can lower confidence and self-esteem, and the motivation to seek help. However, the author encourages readers to think optimistically about managing tinnitus problems in the elderly. 8 references. (AA-M).

- **Unique Case of Pulsatile Tinnitus**

   Source: Annals of Otology, Rhinology and Laryngology. 109(12, Part 1): 1103-1106. December 2000.

   Contact: Available from Annals Publishing Company. 4507 Laclede Avenue, St. Louis, MO 63108.

   Summary: Tinnitus (noise or ringing in the ears) is a common symptom encountered by otolaryngologists (ear, nose and throat specialists). However, pulsatile tinnitus (where the symptom of sound is perceived in pulses or beats, like a heart beat) is rare and can present a diagnostic challenge. Establishing a diagnosis is important because pulsatile tinnitus may indicate serious intracranial (inside the skull) or extracranial (outside the skull) disease. This article presents a case of pulsatile tinnitus caused by cervical artery dissection; the authors discuss the differential diagnosis and treatment. The case subject, a 32 year old woman driving a car, was involved in a head on motor vehicle accident in December 1993. She was wearing a combination shoulder lap belt at the time of the accident. She had no loss of consciousness, head injury, or external signs of trauma other than a fractured clavicle (shoulder blade). Three days after the accident, she noted a right sided aural (ear) pressure and pulsatile tinnitus. There was no associated earache, otorrhea (drainage from the ear), hearing loss, headache, or visual changes. Because of the high suspicion for possible vascular injury, the patient was sent for magnetic resonance imaging (MRI) which demonstrated a right vertebral (neck) artery dissection. The authors discuss the therapy (hospitalization and anticoagulation therapy) and her follow up, which was uneventful. The authors reiterate the importance of accurate and speedy diagnosis: in dissections of the internal carotid artery (ICA), stroke usually occurs in the first few days. 2 figures. 37 references.

- **Tinnitus in Childhood**

    Source: International Journal of Pediatric Otorhinolaryngology. 49(2): 99-105. August 5, 1999.

    Contact: Available from Elsevier Science. P.O. Box 945, New York, NY 10159-0945. (888) 437-4636. Fax (212) 633-3680. E-mail: usinfo-f@elsevier.com.

    Summary: Tinnitus (ringing or other sounds in the ears) is a common symptom in adults and there is a wealth of published information on the pathogenesis and management of the condition. Tinnitus in childhood is likewise quite common when children are directly asked about the symptom. This article reviews the literature regarding the prevalence and nature of pediatric tinnitus and suggests a logical and practical approach to managing this symptom. The authors caution that children rarely spontaneously complain of tinnitus. Little is known about effective management strategies for pediatric tinnitus. The authors recommend an initial appointment with a pediatric otologist to exclude significant, potentially treatable, pathology and to introduce the concept that tinnitus is a treatable condition. Therapy should then focus on the reduction of tinnitus associated distress and reduction of tinnitus awareness. Counseling, and the use of white noise generators (maskers) or hearing aids should then be considered. Care should also be taken to address the concerns and anxieties of the parent. 1 table. 26 references.

- **Tinnitus: Current Evaluation and Management**

    Source: Medical Clinics of North America. 83(1): 125-137. January 1999.

    Contact: Available from W.B. Saunders. Periodicals Fulfillment, 6277 Sea Harbor Drive, Orlando, FL 32887-4800. (800) 654-2452. Website: www.wbsaunders.com.

    Summary: Tinnitus is defined as any abnormal noise perceived by the patient when no external acoustic stimulus exists. Tinnitus may be described as low pitched or high pitched, loud or soft, buzzing or ringing, paroxysmal or constant. This article reviews the current evaluation and management of tinnitus. The authors give the primary care physician a basis of understanding of the various types of tinnitus, the diseases that are commonly associated with tinnitus, the current options available for treatment of the disease, and criteria for referral to an otolaryngologist and audiologist for evaluation of tinnitus. The authors also review recent research data on tinnitus. The causes of subjective tinnitus are categorized in six groups: dental factors, metabolic dysfunction, neurologic abnormalities, otologic, pharmacologic factors, and psychological factors. The authors note that separating patients into two groups, either objective or subjective tinnitus, will assist with evaluation and treatment regimens. In certain situations, multidisciplinary care is required for tinnitus patients (e.g., glomus tumors, benign intracranial hypertension). Patients with objective tinnitus do well over time with treatment. Subjective tinnitus responds well to management of the primary systemic disorder when one can be identified. The article includes the contact information for the American Tinnitus Association, cited as a good source of current information on tinnitus and management options. 2 tables. 17 references.

- **Tinnitus: Current Concepts in Diagnosis and Management**

Source: Volta Review. 9(5): 119-127. November 1999.

Contact: Available from Alexander Graham Bell Association for the Deaf and Hard of Hearing. Subscription Department, 3417 Volta Place, NW, Washington, DC 20007-2778. Voice/TTY (202) 337-5220. Website: www.agbell.org. Also available as individual copies from Publication Sales Department, 3417 Volta Place, NW, Washington, DC 20007-2778. Voice/TTY (202) 337-5220. Website: www.agbell.org. PRICE: $22.95 plus shipping and handling.

Summary: Tinnitus is defined as the perception of sound or noise in the ears or head without any external stimulation. It can present itself in many forms, such as a ringing, a hissing, a jetstream, crickets chirping, or even the sound of the ocean. This chapter on tinnitus is from a monograph that was written by assembling the leading experts from all over the country to present to both the consumer and the professional the latest information on the diagnosis and management of hearing loss in children and adults. The author notes that a pulsating type of tinnitus is unique in the sense that it may represent a muscle spasm or an abnormality of the blood vessels within the ear or head and neck area. Tinnitus can be continuous or intermittent, and may be aggravated by loud noises, certain medications, stress, and changing positions of the head and neck. It is usually more noticeable to people in a relatively quiet environment. Although tinnitus in one ear is less common than complaints of tinnitus in both ears, it may be suggestive of an inner ear tumor, vascular abnormality, or spasm of palatal, face, or neck muscles. Subjective tinnitus is heard by the affected person only and is usually related to some form of hearing loss. Objective tinnitus is heard by both the affected person and the examiner and is generally caused by a blood vessel abnormality, muscle spasm, or joint clicking within the head or neck area. The author reviews treatment options, including reassurance of the patient, diet, avoidance of certain medication, reduction of exposure to loud music and noise, the use of amplification and masking, medications, surgery, and habituation or Tinnitus Retraining Therapy (TRT).

- **A Primer on Tinnitus**

    Source: Tinnitus Today. The Journal of the American Tinnitus Association. 27(4):5-7.

    Summary: Until there is a cure for tinnitus, people who have the condition can use several strategies to manage or relieve their symptoms. This journal article provides an overview of tinnitus and some of the available treatment methods, including the use of maskers, background sounds that help cover up the ringing; vitamin B3, or niacin; music therapy; homeopathy; and positioning. In addition, readers are provided with suggestions for locating additional information on tinnitus and its possible treatment.

Federally Funded Research on Tinnitus

The U.S. Government supports a variety of research studies relating to tinnitus and associated conditions. These studies are tracked by the Office of Extramural Research at the National Institutes of Health.[18] CRISP (Computerized Retrieval of Information on Scientific Projects) is a searchable database of federally funded biomedical research projects conducted at universities, hospitals, and other institutions. Visit CRISP at **http://crisp.cit.nih.gov/crisp/crisp_query.generate_screen**. You can perform targeted searches by various criteria including geography, date, as well as topics related to tinnitus and related conditions.

---

[18] Healthcare projects are funded by the National Institutes of Health (NIH), Substance Abuse and Mental Health Services (SAMHSA), Health Resources and Services Administration (HRSA), Food and Drug Administration (FDA), Centers for Disease Control and Prevention (CDCP), Agency for Healthcare Research and Quality (AHRQ), and Office of Assistant Secretary of Health (OASH).

For most of the studies, the agencies reporting into CRISP provide summaries or abstracts. As opposed to clinical trial research using patients, many federally funded studies use animals or simulated models to explore tinnitus and related conditions. In some cases, therefore, it may be difficult to understand how some basic or fundamental research could eventually translate into medical practice. The following sample is typical of the type of information found when searching the CRISP database for tinnitus:

- **Project Title: ACTIVE AND NONLINEAR MODELS FOR COCHLEAR MECHANICS**

  Principal Investigator & Institution: Grosh, Karl; Mechanical Engineering; University of Michigan at Ann Arbor 3003 South State, Room 1040 Ann Arbor, Mi 481091274

  Timing: Fiscal Year 2002; Project Start 01-MAY-1999; Project End 30-APR-2004

  Summary: In order to better understand the hearing process, numerous efforts in cochlear modeling and physiological measurement have been undertaken. Understanding the process of normal auditory function holds the significant promise of assisting in the determination of the causes of hearing loss and **tinnitus.** Understanding the morphology and function of each component can lead the way to the development of better cochlear prostheses and diagnostic processes for noninvasive determination of disease. Biologically inspired designs for speech recognition and signal processing of non--auditory systems are also possible and could have a significant impact for applications other than hearing. Current research in cochlear mechanics is focussed on determining the source of the enhanced filtering and nonlinear compression seen in in vivo measurements. The hypothesis that an active amplification process is the source of the enhanced filtering has been studied widely since first proposed in 1948. In this grant a comprehensive, efficient numerical strategy for nonlinear and active macroscopic cochlear mechanics is proposed. Through this capability, a virtual laboratory for model testing will be developed capable of incorporating the most general nonlinear models for activity and geometric nonuniformity. Using a hybrid analytic and numeric approach the micromechanics of the Organ of Corti, especially the outer hair cells and their connecting structures, will be included in the global response modeling. These predictions will be compared to in vivo data obtained from physiological experiments. Experimental validation is a central focus of this modeling effort. Close ties to the physiological measurements is important to validate modeling parameters, most importantly the relation of the hypothesized transductions models to the endocochlear potential (or current). Controlled experiments will be used to both identify transducer model parameters (e.g., gains) and to validate/invalidate the hypothesis.

Website: http://crisp.cit.nih.gov/crisp/Crisp_Query.Generate_Screen

- **Project Title: ADENYLYL CYCLASE SIGNALING IN EAR SENSORY EPITHELIA**

    Principal Investigator & Institution: Drescher, Marian J.; Otolaryngology; Wayne State University 656 W. Kirby Detroit, Mi 48202

    Timing: Fiscal Year 2002; Project Start 01-MAY-1999; Project End 30-APR-2004

    Summary: Adenylyl cyclase isoform expression in hair cells and their neural contacts, both efferent axons and afferent dendrites, will determine the pharmacology of cAMP-mediated signal transduction at the specified cellular sites, hypothesized to modulate receptoneural transmission and adaptation of mechanosensory transduction. (1) A goal is to ascertain this expression, utilizing RT-PCR applied to the organ of Corti and spiral ganglion tissue fractions and PCR with nested primers applied to lambdaZAP cDNA libraries of inner hair cells and outer hair cells and in a teleost hair cell preparation. (2) Gprotein coupling to adenylyl cyclase enzymatic activity will be determined at an ultrastructural level with pertussis/cholera toxins, and if evidence of Galphas is absent, the effect of calcium ionophores will be examined as a putative mechanism for activating adenylyl cyclase isoforms, specifically, in hair cells. Inhibition of adenylyl cyclase enyzmatic activity by glutamate metabotropic agonists will be analyzed. (3) Protein targets of adenylyl cyclase action in hair cells will be identified including those proteins that are substrates for protein kinase A phosphorylation and cyclic nucleotide gated ion channels. (4) Dopaminergic efferent regulation via D2L receptor coupling of Galphai2 to adenylyl cyclase will be ascertained with agonist-elicited modulation of intracellular cAMP in the intact rat organ of Corti compared to the intact sensory epithelia and separately, hair cells, of the teleost saccular macula. Proteins specifically targeted by D2L receptor occupation for PKA-driven phosphorylation (or inhibition of PKA-driven phosphorylation) will be identified. A consequential presynaptic modulation of dopamine synthesis and content in the lateral efferents will be determined with radioactive precursors and electrochemical detection of dopamine chromatographically resolved by HPLC. The elucidation of adenylyl cyclase-mediated signal transduction in inner-ear sensory epithelia through dopaminergic innervation may allow eventual pharmacological amelioration of sensorineural deafness and **tinnitus.**

Website: http://crisp.cit.nih.gov/crisp/Crisp_Query.Generate_Screen

- **Project Title: ANATOMY OF THE AUDITORY SYSTEM**

Principal Investigator & Institution: Morest, D Kent.; Professor of Anatomy; Anatomy; University of Connecticut Sch of Med/Dnt Bb20, Mc 2806 Farmington, Ct 060302806

Timing: Fiscal Year 2002; Project Start 01-JUL-1979; Project End 30-JUN-2004

Summary: The focus of this research is the synaptic nests of the mammalian cochlear nucleus. The unifying hypothesis is that the nests are structured so as to mediate plastic changes in response to acoustic overstimulation and damage to the auditory system. These newly discovered nests consist of aggregations of closely packed synaptic endings which are unusual in not being separated from each other by glial processes. The nests occur throughout the cochlear nucleus and may reach their greatest development in the human. Their fine structure and lack of astrocytic processes having high-affinity glutamate transporters may endow the nests with an unusual potential for producing plastic changes to ongoing stimulation and to damaging levels of noise. A specific hypothesis is that overstimulation produces structural and histochemical changes, including chronic degeneration and new growth of synaptic endings in the nests and the regions associated with them. To see if the balance of excitatory and inhibitory input is thereby disturbed, the analysis will focus on the relative proportions of the different types of synaptic ending in the nests, the transmitter-related molecules associated with them, their origins, and the plastic changes they undergo in response to noise damage. Electron microcopy will be used to characterize the fine structure and quantify the types of synaptic endings in the nests of the chinchilla and mouse cochlear nucleus. The origins of the major inputs for each type of ending will be determined with anterograde-labeling and silver-degeneration methods. Immunocytochemistry and in situ hybridization will be used to identify the transmitter-related molecules associated with each type of ending. These normative data will be used as a basis for determining changes in the relative proportions of ending types in the nests following exposure to noise. These findings will suggest ways of perturbing the degenerative and regenerative changes of these endings, including the insertion of small lesions, cells or latex microspheres for delivery of growth factors, and single gene deletions or overexpression. These changes may account for some of the auditory dysfunction in human nerve deafness caused by noise, including **tinnitus** and loudness recruitment. The perturbation experiments should lead directly to proposals for new therapies in this disorder.

Website: http://crisp.cit.nih.gov/crisp/Crisp_Query.Generate_Screen

- **Project Title: AUDITORY SIGNALING, THE FUNCTIONAL ROLE OF KV CHANNELS**

Principal Investigator & Institution: Tempel, Bruce L.; Professor of Otolaryngology-Hns and Pha; Otolaryn & Head & Neck Surgery; University of Washington Grant & Contract Services Seattle, Wa 98105

Timing: Fiscal Year 2002; Project Start 01-AUG-1999; Project End 31-JUL-2004

Summary: from applicant's summary) A major challenge confronting neurobiology is to define how specific voltage-gated potassium (Kv) channel genes influence the timing, duration and frequency of the neuronal signals that encode and transmit information. Neurons in the auditory system have the unique advantages of relatively simple circuitry, well defined functional roles (involving precise signal fidelity) and strong expression of Kv currents. The goal of this proposal is to examine the functional roles of Kv channel genes in three types of auditory neuron-bushy neurons and octopus cells of the cochlear nucleus. and neurons of the medial nucleus of the trapezoid body -each performing related but distinct information processing tasks. Using molecular and irnmunocytochemical techniques, the applicant will determine the complement of Kv channel subunits expressed in these neurons and examine their subcellular localizations. Using electrophysiological techniques, the applicant will characterize Kv currents in these auditory neurons in brainstem slices from wildtype mice and from hearing impaired mice that lack the Kv1.1 channel subunit gene (i.e. Kvl.l knockout mice). These data should reveal rules governing Kv channel assembly and localization in parts of the neuron specialized for either encoding or transmission of information, and elucidate specialized roles in auditory information processing for different subunits, or subsets of subunits within a subfamily. Our thorough characterization of the functional role of Kv channels at the cellular level will also help to explain at the organismal level the hearing loss, movement abnormalities and seizures observed in Kvl.1 knockout mice. Using both anatomical and electrophysiological data, the applicant will develop computer models to assess the relevance of Kv channels/currents in auditory information processing. The model will be used to predict the effects of removing other Kv genes strongly expressed in auditory neurons, such as Kv 1.2 for which the applicant's predictions will be tested directly by examining

Kv1.2 knockout mice. Episodic ataxia myokymia is caused by mutations in the Kv1.1 (KCNA1) gene in humans. Clinical reports on these patients often include **tinnitus,** vertigo and sometimes profound hearing loss. The proposed studies and models based on the Kv1.1 knockout mouse mutants should also be informative regarding the neuronal dysfunction that underlies this human disease.

Website: http://crisp.cit.nih.gov/crisp/Crisp_Query.Generate_Screen

- **Project Title: CENTRAL MECHANISMS RELATED TO TINNITUS**

Principal Investigator & Institution: Kaltenbach, James A.; Professor; Otolaryngology; Wayne State University 656 W. Kirby Detroit, Mi 48202

Timing: Fiscal Year 2002; Project Start 01-JAN-1997; Project End 30-JUN-2004

Summary: The main objective of this study is to further develop our animal model of **tinnitus** with the goal of defining physiological and chemical correlates of this hearing disorder at the level of the cochlear nucleus. This project builds on our recent studies showing that intense sound exposure at levels sufficient to induce **tinnitus** in humans leads to increases in spontaneous neural activity (hyperactivity) in the dorsal cochlear nucleus. The specific aims of this project are as follows: 1) Two-choice behavioral tests will be employed to characterize the pitch and loudness of sound-induced **tinnitus** in hamsters. The relationship of these measures to altered activity in the cochlear nucleus will be investigated by quantifying the magnitude and spatial distribution patterns of hyperactivity in the same animals. 2) The laminar distribution of the hyperactive cells will be determined by marking sites where activity is highest with horseraddish peroxidase,HRP. Further clarification of the cellular substrates underlying hyperactivity will be sought by immunolabeling hyperactive cells with antibodies to the c-fos gene product in cochlear nucleus sections. 3) The cochlear nuclei will then be analyzed chemically to determine whether increases in spontaneous activity are correlated with chemical changes. The concentrations of selected neurotransmitter candidates, neurotransmitter-associated enzymes, and neurotransmitter receptors will be assayed using high performance liquid chromatography and autoradiography. Changes in these elements will be mapped along the tonotopic axis. Chemically altered areas will be identified and correlated with regions showing hyperactivity. 4) The possible role of cochlear outer hair cell loss as a trigger of hyperactivity and **tinnitus** will be investigated by testing whether animals treated with cisplatin, an agent known to induce **tinnitus** in humans and to cause selective outer hair cell loss in humans and animals, show evidence of behavioral **tinnitus** and hyperactivity in the cochlear nucleus. Findings from these experiments are expected to contribute to an understanding of central mechanisms of **tinnitus** and pave the way toward the development of anti-tinnitus therapies.

Website: http://crisp.cit.nih.gov/crisp/Crisp_Query.Generate_Screen

- **Project Title: CHARACTERIZATION OF THE HUMAN HAIR CELL RECEPTOR ALPHA-9**

Principal Investigator & Institution: Lustig, Lawerence R.; Professor; Otolaryn & Head & Neck Surgery; Johns Hopkins University 3400 N Charles St Baltimore, Md 21218

Timing: Fiscal Year 2002; Project Start 01-AUG-2000; Project End 31-JUL-2005

Summary: The family of nicotinic acetylcholine receptors supports chemical synaptic transmission throughout the nervous system, including efferent, or centrifugal regulation of the inner ear. While cholinergic innervation of the inner-ear has been studied in several animal models, our understanding of cholinergic transmission within the human inner ear is quite limited. We propose here to undertake molecular, electrophysiological and histological studies of a putative nicotinic receptor, alpha-9, in the human inner ear. This work will provide not only a molecular basis for the cholinergic modulation of human hair cells, but also will establish targets of novel therapies for diseases such as vertigo and **tinnitus.** Furthermore, mutations and disorders of nicotinic receptor function have been implicated in such diverse diseases as myasthenia gravis, nocturnal frontal lobe epilepsy and schizophrenia. Thus, the present work may also have wider implications for understanding otologic diseases without a known etiology, including autoimmune inner ear disorders or M ni re's syndrome. Recent work in our lab has led to the identification of the human ortholgue of alpha-9, included a complete elucidation of its cDNA and genomic sequence. The goal of the current research proposal is to fully characterize this newly identified receptor, which is a likely mediator of the efferent cholinergic response in the human inner-ear. Ongoing work during the initial characterization will include the search for splice variants within human tissue, as well as further genomic analysis of its regulatory elements. The second phase of the project will include the cellular localization of the alpha-9 gene product within surgically-derived hair populations and other tissue types. The third phase of the project will include functional expression of human alpha-9 to evaluate its physiologic response to acetylcholine and its antagonists. The final phase of the project will employ these same techniques in an effort to identify additional cholinergic receptor types that may be involved in efferent cholinergic transmission within the inner-ear.

Website: http://crisp.cit.nih.gov/crisp/Crisp_Query.Generate_Screen

- **Project Title: CLINICAL TRIAL FOR TINNITUS RETRAINING THERAPY(TRT)**

Principal Investigator & Institution: Formby, C C.; Surgery; University of Maryland Balt Prof School Baltimore, Md 21201

Timing: Fiscal Year 2002; Project Start 01-FEB-2002; Project End 31-JAN-2004

Summary: (provided by applicant): The purpose of this Planning Grant is to develop operations and procedures as part of the planning process for conducting a large-scale, multi-center trial of **Tinnitus** Retraining Therapy (TRT). TRT is a habituation-based intervention that uses directive counseling and low-level sound therapy to facilitate habituation of the awareness of **tinnitus,** its annoyance, and impact on the patient's life. Millions of Americans experience **tinnitus,** but for about 2.5 million individuals it is severely disabling. With no other proven or more successful intervention, TRT has become the therapeutic intervention "of this decade" for disabling **tinnitus.** TRT, however, remains highly controversial despite many reported successes in this country and abroad. It now lacks and requires validation in a controlled clinical trial. In light of a real need for a rigorous controlled study of TRT, we will develop, organize, and plan a formal randomized, double-blind, placebo-controlled, longitudinal clinical trial of TRT. The trial will be conducted at flagship Army, Air Force, and Navy Medical Centers with active duty and retired military personnel and their dependents. The likely higher incidence of noise-induced **tinnitus** (than in the general population) and the great diversity of this study population make the U.S. Armed Forces an ideal study group for a clinical trial of TRT. The 3x2 trial design will incorporate six treatment arms to control for the treatment effects of directive counseling and sound therapy, including a double-blind placebo sound therapy and a "no treatment" control arm to establish the natural history of **tinnitus.** The trial will use a repeated-measures questionnaire, psychoacoustic, and audiologic data as outcome measures to evaluate the validity and efficacy of TRT and its component parts in habituating the perceived **tinnitus** sensation, awareness, annoyance, and overall impact on life (Aim 1); characterize and monitor the temporal courses of the habituation effects over the course of TRT in relation to the non-treatment control arm and those arms receiving alternative placebo and partial treatments (lacking either the counseling or sound therapy components) (Aim 2); establish the permanence and sustained benefits of

TRT and the alternative interventions, post-treatment (Aim 3); and develop statistical models and methods to establish and predict the success of TRT, the treatment effects from directive counseling and sound therapy, the mechanisms by which each works, and the target population for TRT (Aim 4).

Website: http://crisp.cit.nih.gov/crisp/Crisp_Query.Generate_Screen

- **Project Title: COCHLEAR BLOOD FLOW AND NEUROPEPTIDES**

Principal Investigator & Institution: Nuttall, Alfred L.; Professor; Otolaryngology Head & Neck Surgery; Oregon Health & Science University Portland, or 972393098

Timing: Fiscal Year 2002; Project Start 30-SEP-1995; Project End 31-JUL-2004

Summary: The migraine related inner ear symptoms for phonopobia, **tinnitus,** hearing fluctuation, hearing loss, and increased noise sensitivity provide evidence for a possible neurological substrate connecting basilar artery migraine and cochlear pathophysiological mechanisms. Recently we have identified a previously unreported sensory innervation of the cochlear blood vessels originating from the trigeminal ganglia. We have shown that this sensory innervation has a significant effect on cochlear blood flow (CBF) in both normal and pathological conditions (e.g., in the animal model of endolymphatic hydrops, one of the symptoms of Meniere's disease). This proposal seeks to further define the anatomical basis and mechanisms of the trigemino-sensory network around the vertebrovasilar and cochlear vascular system. The proposal offers the hypothesis that the trigemino-sensory system and its related neuropeptide system are important factors contributing to basilar migraine and vascular homeostasis of the cochlea. The study has three specific aims. Aim 1. To establish if there is a physiological basis for the cochlear symptoms in basilar artery migraine headache. Positive results will confirm a common functional basis for basilar migraine and cochlear symptoms, the basis could be neurogenic inflammation. Aim 2. To demonstrate if vanilloid receptor (VR1) and substance P (SP) are co-localized around cochlear blood vessels, the basilar artery and its related branches. Positive immunocytochemical results will demonstrate: (a) network of the VR1 and (b) SP co-labeled primary sensory neurons around the basilar artery; anterior inferior cerebellar artery (AICA), spiral modiolar artery (SMA) and radial artery; (c), Capsaicin will cause a significant reduction in the density of labeled sensory fibers. Aim 3. To determine the vasoregulatory disturbance of the trigemino-sensory neurons in endolymphatic hydrops. In this study positive results will demonstrate that endolymphatic hydrops causes a reduction in the stimulated trigeminal ganglion induced CBF change. The studies of the proposal will help clarify how trigemino-sensory neurons regulate the vertebro-basilar vascular system and cochlear fluid balance under normal and pathological conditions.

Website: http://crisp.cit.nih.gov/crisp/Crisp_Query.Generate_Screen

- **Project Title: CORTICAL PLASTICITY AND PROCESSING OF COMPLEX STIMULI**

Principal Investigator & Institution: Kilgard, Michael P.; Assistant Professor; Neuroscience; University of Texas Dallas Richardson, Tx 75080

Timing: Fiscal Year 2002; Project Start 01-JAN-2000; Project End 31-DEC-2003

Summary: The insights derived from neuroscience studies of cortical plasticity have been indispensable in the development of treatment strategies for a number of neurological disorders, including dyslexia, **tinnitus,** and stroke. However, because most of these studies were focused on relatively simple sensory stimuli, our understanding of the plasticity principles that shape the cortical representation of more complex stimuli, such as speech, remains rudimentary. The proposed experiments document how experience-dependent plasticity improves the auditory cortex representation of spectro temporally complex stimuli and, by advancing our understanding of brain mechanisms involved in the learning of language, will aid in the treatment of communicative disorders. Using simple stimuli, we have demonstrated that electrical stimulation of the cholinergic nucleus basalis (NB) generates robust cortical plasticity that parallels natural learning. The proposed experiments will extend this series by pairing NB stimulation with complex spectrotemporal stimuli. Two different coding strategies, which have demonstrated stimulation of the cholinergic nucleus basis (NB) generates robust cortical plasticity that parallels natural learning. The proposed experiments will extend this series by pairing NB stimulation with complex spectrotemporal stimuli. Two different strategies, which have been proposed to represent the neural basis of memory, emerge with natural learning of behaviorally important complexes stimuli. In the first, complex features are represented by the distributed activity of neurons (coarse coding); while in the second, complex stimuli are represented with specialized filters tuned to specific spectrotemporal transitions (sparse coding). Our preliminary evidences indicates that NB-stimulation leads to representational plasticity that combines both coding strategies. In addition to sharpening spectral and temporal responses generally, NB activation paired with a spectrotemporal sequence created combination selective neural responses that do not exist in naive cortex.

These results demonstrate that combination selectivity is not limited to species/specific vocalizations, and representations of the acoustic environment. Our continuing studies will examine several other acoustic stimuli to determine precisely what stimulus features are required to generate each element of representational plasticity observed in our preliminary results.

Website: http://crisp.cit.nih.gov/crisp/Crisp_Query.Generate_Screen

- **Project Title: DANGEROUS DECIBELS--PARTNERSHIPS IN PUBLIC HEALTH**

    Principal Investigator & Institution: Jackman, Andrew M.; Vp of Education; Oregon Museum of Sciences and Industry and Industry Portland, or 97214

    Timing: Fiscal Year 2002; Project Start 30-SEP-2000; Project End 31-AUG-2005

    Summary: (Adapted from the applicants abstract): A consortium of innovative basic science researchers, museum educators, civic leaders and volunteers propose a unique partnership to reduce the incidence and prevalence of Noise Induced Hearing Loss (NIHL), a growing problem among children and adults. To address this critical public health concern, a unique public/private partnership, including the Oregon Museum of Science and Industry (OMSI), the Oregon Hearing Research Center at the Oregon Health Sciences University (OHSU), the Portland Veterans Administration Medical Center National Center for Rehabilitative Auditory Research (NCRAR), the American **Tinnitus** Association (ATA), and Oregon and Southwest Washington elementary and secondary schools, propose a regional campaign to significantly reduce the prevalence of preventable hearing loss and **tinnitus.** The project is comprised of three freestanding, but interlocking components that create a strong public health campaign against Noise Induced Hearing Loss. These components are: (1) exhibitry; (2) curriculum; and (3) research. We propose a three phase, five-year program, directly targeting school-age youth, using established volunteer and volunteer training programs among each of the participating institutions: Phase 1: Prototype exhibit development and full production of one exhibit incorporating education, entertainment and pre-post knowledge evaluation; test-ready curriculum; draft evaluation tools and hearing screening capabilities for data acquisition. Phase 11: Classroom presentations with exhibitry and data acquisition in six Oregon and Southwest Washington for pilot testing. Phase III: Regional model program and implementation strategy for hearing science education and hearing loss prevention. Program evaluation analysis will include research results regarding subject factors and noise induced hearing loss in children.

Website: http://crisp.cit.nih.gov/crisp/Crisp_Query.Generate_Screen

- **Project Title: EXPRESSION OF ION CHANNELS IN THE AUDITORY SYSTEM**

Principal Investigator & Institution: Kaczmarek, Leonard K.; Professor; Pharmacology; Yale University 47 College Street, Suite 203 New Haven, Ct 065208047

Timing: Fiscal Year 2002; Project Start 01-APR-1993; Project End 31-MAR-2006

Summary: The firing patterns of neurons in central auditory pathways encode specific features of sound stimuli, such as frequency, intensity and localization in space. The generation of the appropriate pattern depends, to a major extent, on the properties of the voltage-dependent potassium channels in these neurons. The Shaw-family Kv3.1 and Kv3.3 channels and the two-pore family rTWIK channel are expressed at high levels in neurons that are capable to firing at very rapid rates and that lock their action potentials to specific phases of auditory stimuli. We plan to determine the mechanisms that regulate these channels in the presynaptic terminals of cochlear nucleus neurons and their postsynaptic targets, neurons of the medial nucleus of the trapezoid body. To test the roles of these channels in timing and regulation of transmitter release, we shall record the responses of neuronal terminals and somata in which the genes for these channels have been eliminated by homologous recombination. We shall test the hypothesis that phosphorylation of the channel proteins alters the transmission of information through this synaptic pathway. Using transgenic animals in which the promoters for the channels are coupled to a fluorescent reporter gene, we shall test whether the naturally occurring differences in the level of expression of the Kv3.l channel along tonotopic axes can be induced by changes in the pattern of activity to which the neurons are exposed. An understanding of how ion channels are regulated in central auditory neurons is likely to lead to therapies for certain forms of deafness, as well as for **tinnitus,** disorders in the interpretation of auditory stimuli, and states of hyperexcitability such as audiogenic seizures.

Website: http://crisp.cit.nih.gov/crisp/Crisp_Query.Generate_Screen

- **Project Title: FUNCTION OF THE TRIGEMINAL GANGLION-COCHLEAR NUCLEUS**

  Principal Investigator & Institution: Shore, Susan E.; Otolaryngology; University of Michigan at Ann Arbor 3003 South State, Room 1040 Ann Arbor, Mi 481091274

  Timing: Fiscal Year 2002; Project Start 01-APR-2001; Project End 31-MAR-2006

  Summary: (Adapted from applicant's abstract): We have demonstrated that the trigeminal ganglion sends a projection to the auditory brain stem and to the cochlear vasculature. The terminations in the brainstem end in granular and magnocellular regions of the ventral cochlear nucleus (VCN) and at the locations of olivocochlear neurons in the superior olivary complex. The cochlear portion of the innervation modulates blood flow within the cochlea. However, the function of the brainstem projection is unknown. Preliminary findings suggest that the projection to the VCN is excitatory. The axons of granule' cells (parallel fibers) project to the dorsal cochlear nucleus (DCN). Therefore, excitation by the trigeminal innervation could affect most of the output neurons of the cochlear nucleus (CN). A series of studies is designed to elucidate the function of the CN portion of this new projection and define its neurotransmitters: The trigeminal ganglion will be electrically stimulated while observing the responses of single units in the CN. The candidate neurotransmitters, Substance P and Nitric Oxide, will be evaluated using immunocytochemistry and neuropharmacology. A role for the trigeminal ganglion in the generation and modulation of **tinnitus** will be explored: As many as two thirds of **tinnitus** patients are able modulate their **tinnitus** by clenching the jaw or touching the skin on the face, areas innervated by the trigeminal ganglion. Others can attribute the onset of **tinnitus** to a somatic insult in the head and neck region ("somatic tinnitus"). On the assumption that increased spontaneous rate is a manifestation of **tinnitus,** its modulation by somatosensory input to the CN could play a role in the generation and modulation of **tinnitus.** The hypothesis wifi be tested by electrically stimulating the trigeminal ganglion while recording spontaneous activity in single units of the CN. Identifying the neurotransmitter used in this pathway could then set the stage for later drug treatments.

  Website: http://crisp.cit.nih.gov/crisp/Crisp_Query.Generate_Screen

- **Project Title: FUNCTIONAL IMAGING OF TINNITUS AND HEARING LOSS**

  Principal Investigator & Institution: Lockwood, Alan H.; Professor of Neurology and Nuclear Medic; Neurology; State University of New York at Buffalo Suite 211 Ub Commons Amherst, Ny 14228

  Timing: Fiscal Year 2002; Project Start 01-JAN-1998; Project End 31-DEC-2002

  Summary: The overall goal of this project is to develop a better understanding of the functional neuroanatomy of the auditory system and how this is affected by **tinnitus,** sensorineural hearing loss (SNHL) and phenomena associated with SNHL such as loudness recruitment. In preliminary studies, using positron emission tomography (PET) to measure cerebral blood flow (CBF), we have identified spontaneous neural activity in the central auditory system associated with **tinnitus,** evidence for plastic reorganization of central auditory systems, and links between sensory-motor systems and limbic and frontal brain regions that may mediate the emotional disability associated with **tinnitus.** We will broaden our successful preliminary approach by using statistical parametric mapping (SPM) to map CBF to focus on 5 specific aims: 1) What is the relationship between the intensity of an external tone and the degree of activation in the auditory cortex for subjects who have: (A) normal hearing, (B) loudness recruitment and (C) loudness recruitment plus tinnitus? 2) What effects do **tinnitus** and SNHL have on resting neural activity and what are the effects of high-frequency SNHL and **tinnitus** on the cortical frequency-place map? 3) What regions of the cerebral cortex are activated in patients who can modulate the loudness or pitch of their **tinnitus** with an oral-facial movement or eye movements? 4) Do lidocaine and residual inhibition reduce activity in regions of the brain activated by tinnitus? 5) What is the anatomical link between **tinnitus** and depression? This application of advanced imaging technology to study patients with communication disorders to investigate perception, and plasticity in the central auditory system should elucidate normal sensory processing of auditory information and how this is disturbed by **tinnitus** and SNHL. We expect to identify neural systems mediating **tinnitus** and related phenomena that will lead to the development of rational therapy targeted at affected neural areas.

  Website: http://crisp.cit.nih.gov/crisp/Crisp_Query.Generate_Screen

- **Project Title: FUNCTIONS OF CORTICOFUGAL AUDITORY SYSTEMS**

  Principal Investigator & Institution: Suga, Nobuo; Biology; Washington University Lindell and Skinker Blvd St. Louis, Mo 63130

Timing: Fiscal Year 2002; Project Start 01-JUL-1981; Project End 30-JUN-2005

Summary: Our ultimate goal is the complete understanding of neural mechanisms for both species-specific (biosonar) and common (communication) auditory functions. Unlike the auditory periphery, the central auditory system contains many different types of neurons. Some neurons are tuned to particular acoustic parameters characterizing sounds other than frequency. Some of these, called "combination-sensitive" neurons, are tuned to specific parameters characterizing combinations of signal elements in complex sounds. Different types of neurons are clustered in different cortical areas. It has been explained that all these neurons result from the divergent and convergent projections within the ascending auditory system. However, the descending (corticofugal) system plays a very important role in signal processing. Response properties of subcortical neurons, and accordingly those of cortical neurons, are shaped by both the ascending and descending systems. The organization of the subcortical nucleus can be changed by the corticofugal system according to auditory experience, including associative learning. Our aims for the proposed research are to explore the functions of the corticofugal system and to test our hypotheses: (1) that the auditory cortex has an intrinsic mechanism which works together with the corticofugal system to adjust and improve auditory signal processing according to auditory experience, (2) that this mechanism is augmented if the acoustic signals become behaviorally relevant to the animal, e.g., through associative learning, and (3) that such augmentation is mediated by the cholinergic basal forebrain. Our proposed research will contribute further toward our understanding of the neural mechanisms for processing behaviorally relevant sounds and the functional organization of the central auditory system. We will be able to propose possible neural mechanisms for hearing disorders such as neural **tinnitus.** We will study the response properties of cortical and subcortical neurons to acoustic stimuli. We will then study how their response properties are changed by focal electrical stimulation of the auditory cortex, somatosensory cortex and/or basal forebrain or classical conditioning and also by focal applications of different types of drugs to the auditory cortex and subcortical nuclei. All the data which will be obtained will be evaluated in relation to our hypotheses.

Website: http://crisp.cit.nih.gov/crisp/Crisp_Query.Generate_Screen

- **Project Title: GABAPENTIN FOR RELIEF OF IDIOPATHIC SUBJECTIVE TINNITUS**

Principal Investigator & Institution: Piccirillo, Jay F.; Associate Professor; Otolaryngology; Washington University Lindell and Skinker Blvd St. Louis, Mo 63130

Timing: Fiscal Year 2004; Project Start 01-APR-2004; Project End 31-MAR-2006

Summary: (provided by applicant): **Tinnitus** is the perceived sensation of sound without actual acoustic stimulation. Approximately, 40 million people in the United States experience chronic **tinnitus** and 10 million of these people consider their **tinnitus** to be a significant problem. There are many different treatments for **tinnitus**. However, no one treatment or combinations of treatments have been found to be significantly effective and consequently the FDA has not approved any drugs for **tinnitus**. Many investigators have noted similarities between **tinnitus** and chronic naturopathic pain. This has lead to the chronic pain model for **tinnitus**. Gabapentin is a drug that is widely used for naturopathic pain because it is generally well tolerated, easily triturated, has few drug interactions, and does not require laboratory monitoring. We recently completed an open-label pilot study of gabapentin for troublesome **tinnitus**. Between November 2001 and April 2002, 19 patients were placed on 900 mg per day of gabapentin. The range of scores on the **Tinnitus** Handicap Inventory (THI) at baseline was 10 to 94 and the average (+/- 95% CI) score was 44 (32-55). At the end of Week 4, the average (+ 95% CI) score for the 16 (84%) patients who remained in the study was 28 (18-38). The difference in average THI score between Week 0, 2, and 4 was statistically significant (F test =10.31, p=0004). Gabapentin was well tolerated by most patients. The primary specific aim of this study is to evaluate the effect of gabapentin on **tinnitus** as measured by the change in the THI. The null hypothesis is that gabapentin is no more effective than placebo in the treatment of **tinnitus**. The alternative hypothesis is that gabapentin is different than placebo in the treatment of **tinnitus**. There will be four secondary aims of the study. The secondary aims will focus on interesting subgroup responses or interaction between treatment response and important covariates. The results of these secondary aims are likely to generate new and interesting hypotheses. We will employ a double-blind placebo-controlled randomized clinical trial design to assess the efficacy of gabapentin. Adults, between the ages of 18 and 70 with idiopathic, subjective, troublesome, unilateral or bilateral, non-pulsate **tinnitus** (ICD-9 --388.31) of 6 month's duration or greater and score of 38 or greater on the THI will be eligible. We plan to enroll a total of 160 patients and expect to be able to detect a 30% change in score on the THI Enrollment will begin May 2004 and continue until 160 valuable patients have been enrolled (anticipated end date: January, 2006). The significance of this research is that troublesome **tinnitus** is a very common health problem and treatment options for these patients are quite limited. The findings from this research could have significant health impact for a large number of Americans.

Website: http://crisp.cit.nih.gov/crisp/Crisp_Query.Generate_Screen

- **Project Title: GENE REGULATION OF RAT DENTIN SIALOPROTEIN**

    Principal Investigator & Institution: Ritchie, Helena H.; Cariology/Restor Sci/Endod; University of Michigan at Ann Arbor 3003 South State, Room 1040 Ann Arbor, Mi 481091274

    Timing: Fiscal Year 2003; Project Start 30-SEP-1995; Project End 30-JUN-2007

    Summary: (provided by applicant): During tooth development, odontoblasts modulate dentin formation by producing a predentin matrix into which additional NCPs are subsequently secreted to initiate the mineralization process so necessary for healthy tooth formation. Abnormalities in dentin mineralization due to genetic diseases such as dentinogenesis imperfecta II (DGI-II; affecting 1 in 7,000 newborns) leave these children few choices other than placement of crowns on the teeth or a complete denture. A nonsense mutation, located in the coding sequence for dentin sialoprotein (DSP) is likely responsible for blocking both DSP and phosphophoryn (PP) expression in these individuals because these two NCPs are located on a single DSP-PP transcript. Importantly, some DGI patients also experience **tinnitus** as well as balancing problems making it necessary to consider problems in DSP-PP transcript and protein expression as an important public health concern. This application proposes a series of studies to better define DSP-PP transcript expression and DSP/PP protein function in dentin mineralization. The specific aims of this proposal are 1) to test the hypothesis that odontoblast-specific factors acting on the DSP-PP gene promoter, regulate DSP-PP expression, 2) to test the hypothesis that multiple DSP-PP transcripts generate functionally distinct PP isoforms with distinct calcium binding capacity and hydroxyapatite forming ability which are required for orderly dentin mineralization, 3) to correlate DSP-PP transcript and DSP-only transcript expression patterns with dentin mineralization, and 4) to validate Aims 2 and 3 by examining mineral formation as a function of DSP and PP isoform expression in cell culture. These ongoing studies, which combine gene regulation and protein function approaches, will reveal underlying mechanisms of dentin mineralization and will later be applicable to reparative dentistry.

Website: http://crisp.cit.nih.gov/crisp/Crisp_Query.Generate_Screen

- **Project Title: HEALTH COMMUNICATION: NIHL AND TINNITUS PREVENTION**

Principal Investigator & Institution: Martin, William H.; Otolaryngology Head & Neck Surgery; Oregon Health & Science University Portland, or 972393098

Timing: Fiscal Year 2004; Project Start 01-DEC-2003; Project End 30-NOV-2006

Summary: (provided by applicant): Noise-induced hearing loss (NIHL) and related **tinnitus** pose significant health risks to millions of Americans. Educational interventions, based upon health communication theory, have yet to be systematically applied to NIHL and **tinnitus** prevention. The purpose of this project is to design, implement and evaluate intervention strategies applying current health communication and behavior theory, to increase knowledge, change attitude and behavioral intention consistent with hearing loss prevention. The target population will be 4th grade school students in Oregon and SW Washington. Four single educational interventions (some established and some new innovations) will be compared to a non-intervention, control group. Also, health communication theory predicts that certain intervention strategies will be more effective than others. Health communication research demonstrates that paired-interventions, especially in the form of a "booster" separated in time from the initial program, will be more effective than a single-intervention approach. Once evaluation of the four interventions is complete, a second evaluation will be conducted using paired combinations of the most effective educational interventions. Subjects will receive pre- and post-intervention and follow-up questionnaires. Intervention 1: Classroom Presentation by Older-Peer Educators. High school students will present an NIHL and **tinnitus** prevention program. Intervention 2: Classroom Presentation by Health Professional Educators. School nurses will present an NIHL and **tinnitus** prevention program. Intervention 3: On-site Museum Experience. Students will visit a 12-component exhibition of noise-induced hearing loss and **tinnitus** prevention. The exhibit provides a novel and innovative method of communicating information to visitors, young and old. Intervention 4: Web-based Museum Experience. A web-based version of the above museum exhibit will be the vehicle to communicate information about noise-induced hearing loss and **tinnitus** prevention to fourth-grade students. Non-Intervention: Control groups matched for age, gender, socioeconomic and geographic (rural/ urban) factors will receive pre- and post-evaluation questionnaires without receiving an educational intervention. Results from the comparison of these interventions will be used to enhance delivery methods and vehicles for public education to increase awareness, change attitudes and behavioral intentions about the dangers of noise-induced hearing loss and **tinnitus.** The goal is to decrease the number of cases of preventable noise induced hearing loss and **tinnitus,** and to promote healthy hearing and good aural communication in the population.

Website: http://crisp.cit.nih.gov/crisp/Crisp_Query.Generate_Screen

- **Project Title: IDENTIFICATION OF ACOUSTICO-LATERALIS TRANSMITTERS**

  Principal Investigator & Institution: Drescher, Dennis G.; Professor and Director of Molecular Rese; Otolaryngology; Wayne State University 656 W. Kirby Detroit, Mi 48202

  Timing: Fiscal Year 2002; Project Start 01-MAY-1980; Project End 30-JUN-2003

  Summary: (from the Applicant's abstract). The major objective of the present proposal is to identify peripheral neurotransmitters/neuromodulators and associated biochemical systems of hair-cell organs. Peripheral neurotransmitters voltage-gated calcium channels, and neurotransmitter receptors will be examined for mammalian and fish model systems. The main hypotheses address the existence and function of non-glutamate hair cell transmitter(s), non-L-type voltage- gated calcium channel(s), and recently-described efferent neurotransmitter receptors for acetylcholine and dopamine. Methods include: 1) high- resolution, high-performance liquid chromatography (HPLC) with detection by electrochemistry, fluorescence, radioactivity, and radioimmunoassay, 2) analysis of tissue content, and depolarization-induced release in vitro of presumptive neurotransmitters and neuromodulators from a saccular hair cell sheet for which the hair cell is the only intact cell type, and sound-induced release in vivo into cochlear perilymph, 3) biological assay of compounds utilizing Xenopus laevis lateral line, 4) morphological localization of molecular entities by immunochemical and in situ hybridization methods, 5) sequence analysis as to molecular function after RT-PC (reverse transcription polymerase chain reaction) of voltage-gated calcium channels associated with transmitter release of haircells, and 6) functional sequence analysis after RT-PCR of efferent neurotransmitter receptors for acetylcholine and dopamine. Using these methods, it is planned to identify chemically and determine the biological activity of compounds release from saccular sensory cells in a calcium-dependent manner by low level potassium depolarization and released into perilymph by sound stimulation. Biosynthesis of neuroactive monoamines and related molecules will be studied utilizing radioactive precursors and HPLC. We will demonstrate molecular characteristics and localization of a hair cell-associated, non-L-type voltage-gated calcium channel and efferent- related a. nicotinic receptor and dopamine D2(ing) and D, receptors. This approach, utilizing methods of micro-biochemistry, should result in continued, detailed elucidation of structure and molecular function of peripheral neurotransmitter systems of hearing and balance, pointing the way to development of therapies for transmitter-related hearing loss, vertigo, and **tinnitus.**

Website: http://crisp.cit.nih.gov/crisp/Crisp_Query.Generate_Screen

- **Project Title: MEMBRANE PROPERTIES OF CELLS COMPRISING THE OUTER HAIR C**

Principal Investigator & Institution: Santos-Sacchi, Joseph R.; Professor; Surgery; Yale University 47 College Street, Suite 203 New Haven, Ct 065208047

Timing: Fiscal Year 2002; Project Start 01-FEB-1984; Project End 31-MAR-2005

Summary: The organ of Corti is composed of a variety of cell types including sensory, supporting and neural elements. Taken together, these cells comprise a functionally intricate and cohesive electrical unit that initiates the analysis of acoustic information within our environment. This electrical unit is extremely complex and nearly anatomically inaccessible, making an analysis of the whole quite a challenge. Fortunately, during the last several years the in vitro approach, including the isolated cochlea and cell preparations, has aided in the elucidation of cell function; the strategy is to understand the cells first on an individual basis, and finally to integrate this knowledge into a complete understanding of the organ of Corti. The overall aim of this project is to analyze the membrane properties of the outer hair cell (OHC), one of the major players in auditory function, principally using variations on the whole cell voltage clamp technique. Three areas of investigation are proposed. Specifically, we intend to 1) analyze the mobility OHC sensor/motors in the lateral plasma membrane, 2) study in detail and make modifications to the electrical correlate of OHC motility, its nonlinear capacitance and analyze what such modifications will do to the high frequency mechanical activity of the OHC, and 3) study the mechanical coupling among OHCs that we have just discovered. These results will lead to a deeper understanding of inner ear function and aid in understanding auditory pathologies which may result from OHC insult and homeostatic imbalance, including sensorineural hearing loss and **tinnitus.**

Website: http://crisp.cit.nih.gov/crisp/Crisp_Query.Generate_Screen

- **Project Title: MODULATION OF COCHLEAR MECHANICS**

Principal Investigator & Institution: Oghalai, John S.; Otolaryngology; University of California San Francisco 500 Parnassus Ave San Francisco, Ca 941222747

Timing: Fiscal Year 2002; Project Start 01-AUG-2001; Project End 31-MAY-2003

Summary: (provided by applicant): The long-term goal of these studies is to understand how drugs modulate the cochlear amplifier. The mammalian cochlea is a mechanical structure that is tuned along its length tonotopically. Outer hair cells (OHCs) within the cochlea undergo high-speed length changes in sync with sound vibrations, adding energy via a positive feedback loop. This is called the cochlear amplifier and provides exquisite hearing sensitivity and frequency selectivity. OHC motility is based upon the highly organized biomechanical structure of the cell's lateral wall, which contains a plasma membrane, a cytoskeleton, and motor proteins. The specific objective of this project is to determine whether drugs that change OHC lateral wall biomechanics in vitro will modulate cochlear mechanics in vivo. There are three categories of drugs that will be tested: amphipathic drugs which change membrane tension by causing cell membranes to bend, drugs that affect the actin-spectrin cytoskeleton and change cell stiffness, and drugs that directly block the electromotility motor. The compound action potential (CAP), distortion product otoacoustic emissions (DPOAEs), and the medial olivocochlear (MOC) reflex will be monitored to assess cochlear function in anesthetized guinea pigs before and during the administration of these drugs. Because OHCs are the most sensitive cell in the cochlea to noise exposure, drugs that change OHC biomechanics may also modulate noise-induced hearing loss. This will be tested in the guinea pig model. Finally, the effect of these drugs on sound conditioning will be assessed. This is a protective process whereby long-term exposure to moderate-level sound can reduce permanent threshold shifts from subsequent high-level noise exposure. Overall, these studies are designed to understand how OHCs transmit forces within the cochlea and the mechanisms behind sound conditioning. Clinically, they will improve our comprehension of the generation of otoacoustic emissions, as well as the role of the efferent nerves on the cochlear amplifier in health and disease.

Additionally, these studies may lead to therapeutic interventions for noise-induced hearing loss and **tinnitus.**

Website: http://crisp.cit.nih.gov/crisp/Crisp_Query.Generate_Screen

- **Project Title: MOLECULAR DEVELOPMENT OF THE ENDOLYMPHATIC DUCT AND SAC**

Principal Investigator & Institution: Choo, Daniel I.; Assistant Professor; Children's Hospital Med Ctr (Cincinnati) 3333 Burnet Ave Cincinnati, Oh 45229

Timing: Fiscal Year 2002; Project Start 02-APR-2001; Project End 31-MAR-2006

Summary: (from applicant's abstract): Homeostasis of inner ear endolymph is critical to sensory transduction in the inner ear. Failure to maintain endolymph homeostasis is thought to result in deafness, vestibular dysfunction and **tinnitus** in pathologies such as Meniere's disease or certain forms of hereditary hearing impairment. The endolymphatic duct and sac (ELDS) are key structures in maintaining this fluid homeostasis. Therefore, data on the molecular development of the ELDS are very relevant. By focusing on a mouse mutant (kreisler) with an ELDS phenotype, this application seeks to define the molecular pathways involved in induction and differentiation of the ELDS. To determine early targets of kr signaling, this application will test the hypothesis that expression of early molecular markers of the ELDS anlage is down-regulated in homozygote kr embryos at embryonic day 10-11 compared to controls. The effects of kr mutation on cellular differentiation within the developing ELDS will be studied by testing the hypothesis that expression of a battery of genes specific for cells in the embryonic day 12 to 18 ELDS is down-regulated in kreisler homozygotes compared to controls. To facilitate direct experimental manipulation of the developing ELDS, this application will develop an in vitro model of the developing kreisler otocyst and ELDS. Experiments will first test the hypothesis that cultured kreisler otocysts developmentally mimic the in vivo system morphologically and functionally. This model will then be used to test the hypothesis that virally mediated expression of kr can rescue the ELDS phenotype in vitro. To test the hypothesis that hindbrain sources of kr induce ELDS differentiation, we will culture kreisler otocysts with wild-type hindbrain explants. Such data will provide insights into the molecular pathways involved in kr signaling and in development of the ELDS. The PI's obvious commitment to medicine and science has been demonstrated by his extensive pursuit of training in the clinical and basic science facets of inner ear biology. The success of these efforts are reflected in his publications which also demonstrate his ability to accomplish quality basic science investigation. In combination with the outstanding academic environment at Children's Hospital Research Foundation, the RCA will allow the PI to continue a rigorous scientific training and successfully address the specific aims outlined in the application. The proposed program of study and the science generated will undoubtedly advance the PI toward his goals of successfully competing for a future R01, and in the long term, becoming a successful independent Clinician scientist. Significantly, this proposal includes challenging but achievable goals that will provide important knowledge to the field of inner ear development.

Website: http://crisp.cit.nih.gov/crisp/Crisp_Query.Generate_Screen

- **Project Title: MOLECULAR MECHANISMS IN CENTRAL AUDITORY FUNCTION,**

Principal Investigator & Institution: Altschuler, Richard A.; Professor; Otolaryngology; University of Michigan at Ann Arbor 3003 South State, Room 1040 Ann Arbor, Mi 481091274

Timing: Fiscal Year 2003; Project Start 01-JUL-2003; Project End 30-JUN-2004

Summary: (provided by applicant): This proposal is for a third Symposium on "Molecular Mechanisms in Central Auditory Function, Plasticity and Disorders" at the Snow King Resort in Jackson Hole, Wyoming to be held in late June 2004. The central focus of the conference is the "molecular mechanisms" regulating neurotransmission. The premise of the conference is that these molecular features regulate auditory activity, shape auditory neuronal response properties, influence development and provide for central auditory plasticity. Furthermore, changes in these molecular mechanisms can underlie genetic disorders or acquired central auditory disorders such as age related hearing loss, seizures and **tinnitus**. The topic remains important and timely, with new and exciting results being generated from an increasing number of laboratories, generating new insights. The Symposium will present and highlight new developments and to provide a forum where they can be synthesized, integrated and correlated. This will be a three day meeting, under a similar format to our 1999 meeting, with platform presentations, posters and time for formal and informal discussions. The goals are: 1) To provide an understanding of molecular mechanisms underlying functional diversity in central auditory neurons; 2) To develop correlation between molecular mechanisms and the shaping of cell specific response characteristics; 3) To examine molecular mechanisms underlying central auditory plasticity; 4) To examine molecular mechanisms underlying disorders such as **tinnitus**, seizures and age related hearing loss; 5) To explore the role of genetics in central auditory system function and dysfunction; 6) To provide interaction between molecular and systems researchers The conference will consist of platform presentations by approximately 50 invited speakers from the auditory system and two additional speakers from outside the auditory field as well as a Poster Session open to contributions from all participants. Based on our previous experience and the attraction of the location, we expect to draw another 30 - 50 additional participants (including recipients of two minority fellowships) from other scientists and students interested in this topic.

Website: http://crisp.cit.nih.gov/crisp/Crisp_Query.Generate_Screen

- **Project Title: NEURITE DENSITY IN SKIN AS A MARKER FOR NEUROPATHIC PAIN**

Principal Investigator & Institution: Oaklander, Anne L.;; Massachusetts General Hospital 55 Fruit St Boston, Ma 02114

Timing: Fiscal Year 2002; Project Start 01-SEP-2002; Project End 31-AUG-2006

Summary: (provided by applicant): Chronic pain has been recognized as an underserved area of medicine. Clinical care and research are hampered by the lack of objective correlates for the subjective complaint of pain. This is especially a problem for neuropathic pain patients, where the pain is caused by malfunction of the pain-sensing neurons, rather than injury to the area where the pain is felt. In this translational project we will evaluate two types of objective evidence of neural damage to see whether they correlate with the complaint of pain. We will investigate the usefulness of these methods in adults with one of two common neuropathic pain conditions, postherpetic neuralgia (PHN) after shingles (herpes zoster), or painful neuropathy in the lower legs from diabetes mellitus, and in rat models of these conditions. Data from individuals with and without pain will be compared. We will evaluate the usefulness of tests of specific sensory functions, using standardized quantitative sensory stimuli, for predicting who does or does not have pain from shingles or diabetes. We will also evaluate the usefulness of a new technique, counting the density of pain-sensing (nociceptive) nerve endings within the epiderrnal layer of small skin punch biopsies. Surprisingly, work by our group and others show that neuropathic pain patients usually have fewer nociceptive nerve endings in painful skin. When the amount of signal coming in from the periphery decreases, pain-processing neurons in the brain and spinal cord become hyperactive. The result can be pain in the absence of tissue injury. This is similar to the development of **tinnitus** (ringing in the ears) when people lose hearing.

Our data suggests that after shingles, PEN pain is felt by only those patients whose density of nociceptive nerve endings has been reduced below a threshold value (650 neurites/mm2 skin surface area). In Specific Aim I, we will study patients about 6 weeks after onset of shingles with quantitative sensory testing and skin biopsies, and repeat them 6 months later. We will evaluate whether data from the first set of tests, or changes between the two test sessions, can provide a marker for those who recover from pain or not. In Specific Aim II we will compare sensory testing and skin biopsy data from normal people and diabetics with and without pain to see whether there is evidence for a threshold value separating individuals with and without pain, and whether we can identify a presymptomatic state. In Specific Aim III, we plan to evaluate sensory function of the paw in rat models of pain after sciatic nerve injury. At sacrifice, biopsies will be taken from the bottom of the rat's paws as well as from the injured nerves to see whether changes in the density of nociceptive nerve endings in the foot correlate with severity of damage in the nerve and with the rat's behavior during sensory testing. The goal of this research is to improve medical care for patients with chronic neuropathic pain, and facilitate research by identifying "biomarkers" that can be used as surrogate measures for the presence of neuropathic pain.

Website: http://crisp.cit.nih.gov/crisp/Crisp_Query.Generate_Screen

- **Project Title: NEUROGENIC CONTROL OF COCHLEAR BLOOD FLOW**

Principal Investigator & Institution: Wangemann, a P.;; Father Flanagan's Boys' Home Boys Town, Ne 68010

Timing: Fiscal Year 2002

Summary: This project will focus on the neurogenic regulation of cochlear blood flow and on the interactions between neurogenic and endothelium-mediated mechanisms. Receptors controlling vascular diameter of the spiral modiolar artery and the identity of locally released vasoactive substances will be determined. Locally-released vasoactive substances will include those from neuronal elements innervating the spiral modiolar artery and those from endothelial cells lining the lumen of this vessel. The spiral modiolar artery is the main blood supply of the cochlea. Aberrations in the regulation of cochlear blood flow have been suspected to play a major part in the etiology of a variety of inner ear disorders including sudden and fluctuating hearing loss, Meniere's disease, **tinnitus** and autoimmune-related hearing loss. Fundamental to these etiologies are the receptors present on the cochlear blood vessels and their function in the regulation of cochlear blood flow. Hypotheses pertaining to the presence of receptors and to the identity of released vasoactive substances will be tested with a functional assay based on newly-developed in vitro preparations of the isolated spiral modiolar artery. The vascular diameter and the release of vasoactive substance from neuronal elements and from the endothelium will be measured. The measurement of the vascular diameter is the most physiologically-relevant parameter since change in the vascular diameter is the single most effective means of regulating blood flow. Receptors will be determined pharmacologically utilizing selective agonists and antagonists. Release of neurotransmitter from neuronal elements which remain with the isolated spiral modiolar artery will be triggered by electric field stimultation. The identity of the released neurotransmitters will be determined by their functional effect on their respective target receptors and by a highly specific bioluminescence assay. All techniques are well established in this laboratory. This project evolved out of the previous one on isolated medial efferent nerve terminals. Common to both projects is the focus on the function of isolated nerve terminals. Whereas the experimental access was previously limited to prejunctional processes, the proposed studies include both pre- and post junctional mechanisms and their complex interactions leading to the regulation of cochlear blood flow. The completion of the proposed studies are expected to provide a foundation for the pharmacologic management of inner ear disorders.

Website: http://crisp.cit.nih.gov/crisp/Crisp_Query.Generate_Screen

- **Project Title: NEUROTRANSMITTERS IN THE AUDITORY SYSTEM**

Principal Investigator & Institution: Potashner, Steven J.; Professor; Anatomy; University of Connecticut Sch of Med/Dnt Bb20, Mc 2806 Farmington, Ct 060302806

Timing: Fiscal Year 2002; Project Start 01-DEC-1990; Project End 30-JUN-2005

Summary: Our long-term goal is to understand the changes in the brain after an injury to the adult auditory system consisting of the ablation of one cochlea and sensorineural hearing loss. This injury initially destroyed the cochlear nerve, which carried cochlear excitation into the brain. Subsequently, the injury induced growth of new synapses, changes of synaptic strengths, and axonal and synaptic pruning in brain stem auditory nuclei. Since these plasticities may produce pathologic symptoms, such as **tinnitus,** rehabilitating the system after injury could depend on control of the mechanisms underlying plasticity. Because plastic changes and the mechanisms which generate them are poorly understood, we wish to identify more plastic changes, the signals that induce them, and the biochemical transduction pathways that link the signals to the plasticities. First, we will study synaptic rearrangements in the young adult guinea pig superior olive after cochlear ablation, using histological methods. Next, using neurochemical methods, we will study the auditory brain stem nuclei of adult guinea pigs, including the subdivisions of the cochlear nucleus, the nuclei of the superior olive, and the inferior colliculus. We will evaluate candidate signals, such as altered synaptic excitation, altered, neurotrophic support, and injury, each transduced through distinct second messenger pathways. We will determine if protein kinases, employed by second messenger pathways that transduce synaptic excitation and neuronal depolarization, can regulate synaptic activities in the brain stem auditory nuclei. We will also determine if protein kinases are involved in changes of synaptic strength after cochlear ablation. We will determine if neurotrophic support is available and can regulate synaptic activities in the brain stem auditory nuclei, if it is altered after cochlear ablation, and if it is involved in postlesion changes of synaptic strength. We will determine if transduction of altered neuronal excitation and neurotrophic support regulate nuclear factors that may induce plasticity through regulation of gene expression. Finally, we will determine if cochlear ablation activates second messenger pathways that transduce signals of injury to regulate nuclear factors that may change gene expression and induce degenerative pruning.

Website: http://crisp.cit.nih.gov/crisp/Crisp_Query.Generate_Screen

- **Project Title: NOVEL INNER EAR DRUG DELIVERY SYSTEM**

  Principal Investigator & Institution: Petelenz, Tomasz J.;; Sarcos Research Corporation 360 Wakara Wy Salt Lake City, Ut 84108

  Timing: Fiscal Year 2002; Project Start 01-SEP-2002; Project End 31-AUG-2004

  Summary: (provided by applicant): Sarcos Research Corporation proposes a novel microinfusion system for administration of medications for treatment of middle ear and cochlear diseases, such as sudden hearing loss, Menieres disease, instances of **tinnitus,** and for providing pharmacological hearing protection in chemotherapy. Methods that are currently in use cause systemic toxicity, do not provide suffient dose control (injections, wicks) or are impractical (waist-mounted pumps) and expensive. The proposed system will be small size, light-weight, will fit safely and comfortably behind the patient's ear, and will deliver medications into the middle ear in precise, controlled programmable and convenient manner, increasing effectiveness, reducing side effects and improving compliance with the therapy. In the future, the system will evove into totally implantable unit for treatment of chronic and/or recurrent conditions. In addition to improving the existing treatment regimens, the system will enable application of chronotherapy and other temporal dose patterns to increase effectiveness and reduce side effects, and will allow administration of medications in the head-and-neck area for treament of cancer in both hospital and at-home settings. For this application, Sarcos will adapt its microinfusion pump and microcatheter technologies to create a system that will consist of a micropump, a programmer with a wireless data link, and a drug delivery catheter. Due to the significant advancement of the already developed technology base that is available at Sarcos for this project, and in order to accelerate the development of the commercial product, Sarcos proposes a joint Phase I/II (Fast Track) effort that will result in a validated system ready for commercialization and clinical implementation. Phase I of this project will result in a definitive feasibiility prototype, wherease the projected Phase II will end with a commercial product and completed regulatory submission to the FDA. The proposed system will have significant health and economic impact as it it is estimated that more than 28 millions Americans suffer from preventable hearing loss, at least 3 million are affected by Menieres disease, and 40 to 45 million have life-impairing **tinnitus,** resulting in an estimated cost of lost productivity that exceeds 30 billion dollars per year.

Website: http://crisp.cit.nih.gov/crisp/Crisp_Query.Generate_Screen

- **Project Title: PERIPHERIAL AND CENTRAL MECHANISMS OF TINNITUS GENERAT**

Principal Investigator & Institution: Bauer, Carol A.; Associate Professor; Surgery; Southern Illinois University Sch of Med Box 19616, 801 Rutledge St Springfield, Il 62794

Timing: Fiscal Year 2002; Project Start 25-APR-2002; Project End 31-MAR-2007

Summary: This study is designed to investigate the aspects of peripheral and central auditory pathology that are necessary for the development of **tinnitus. Tinnitus** is considered to be a serious, often debilitating handicap. Chronic **tinnitus** is a symptom experienced by 35% of the U.S. population and 10% of people with chronic **tinnitus** consider the problem to be severe and to significantly interfere with activities of daily life. Although there has been increased interest in studying **tinnitus** over the last decade, understanding the pathophysiology of chronic **tinnitus** remains rudimentary. Consequently there are no uniformly effective treatments for this disorder. The current research will use an animal model of a common type of **tinnitus** to explore factors that may be critical to developing the phantom auditory perception. **Tinnitus** will be induced in animals by exposure to noise sufficient induce hearing loss. The **tinnitus** will be detected and characterized in individual subjects using established psychophysical behavioral techniques. The qualitative aspects of **tinnitus** will be measured and correlated with functional and morphological changes in the cochlea induced by the noise exposure. Cochlear function will be measured with auditory brainstem response testing and distortion product otoacoustic emissions, and the pattern of noise-induced hair cell damage evaluate with electron microscopy. This study will determine if noise-induced **tinnitus** is associated with a specific pattern of cochlear damage. The model will also be used to investigate the contribution of the dorsal cochlear nucleus (DCN) to the development of **tinnitus.** The DNA is an auditory structure in the brainstem that has been implicated as a potential **tinnitus** generation site. The current research will directly test this notion by examining the effect of DNA ablation on the auditory perception of **tinnitus.** This research intends to answer fundamental questions concerning mechanisms of **tinnitus** generation. Safe and efficacious therapy for this prevalent and often debilitating problem can only occur with improved understanding of the disorder.

Website: http://crisp.cit.nih.gov/crisp/Crisp_Query.Generate_Screen

- **Project Title: PHARMACOLOGY OF NEUROTRANSMITTERS IN HAIR CELL ORGAN: INNER EAR**

  Principal Investigator & Institution: Sewell, William F.;; Massachusetts Institute of Technology Cambridge, Ma 02139

  Timing: Fiscal Year 2002

  Summary: The primary sensory cell of the inner ear (the hair cell) releases a neurotransmitter to excite auditory nerve fibers. The identification of this transmitter, which may not be one of the known neurotransmitters, is the goal of this project. We have purified, from hair cell tissue and from retina, a substance that can excite afferent nerve fibers innervating hair cells. This substance appears to be a potent, unstable, unknown excitatory amino acid with pharmacological activity similar to glutamate; however, it is clearly not glutamate or any other commonly studied substance. The goals are to identify the chemical structure of the excitatory substance, to analyze its distribution in hair cell organs and in the nervous system and to determine its role in hair cell organ function. In addition to the intrinsic intellectual importance of identifying the neurotransmitter released by hair cells, this work may have significant practical implications for otolaryngology and sh ould have widespread importance for areas of neurobiology beyond the auditory system. If it is possible to develop drugs with some specificity for vestibular fibers, a treatment for motion sickness and intractable vertigo would likely result. Judicious use of a drug with specificity for the auditory system might alleviate some forms of peripheral **tinnitus**. The excitatory amino acid we have isolated from hair cell tissue and from retina is a good candidate to be a neurotransmitter in other parts of the nervous system; we already know that it is concentrated in inner ear and in retina. If it is localized discretely within the nervous system, it will almost assuredly provide a means of selectively studying transmission and function of other regions of the nervous system.

Website: http://crisp.cit.nih.gov/crisp/Crisp_Query.Generate_Screen

- **Project Title: PLASTICITY IN THE DORSAL COCHLEAR NUCLEUS**

Principal Investigator & Institution: Emadi, Gulamali A.; Biomedical Engineering; Johns Hopkins University 3400 N Charles St Baltimore, Md 21218

Timing: Fiscal Year 2002; Project Start 15-SEP-2002; Project End 30-JUN-2004

Summary: (provided by applicant): The proposed research will examine plasticity of responses in the dorsal cochlear nucleus (DCN), one of the first sites of integrative processing within the auditory system. The strengths of inputs from somatosensory brainstem nuclei into the DCN will be manipulated using variations of established protocols for inducing long-term synaptic changes in other brain regions, including but not limited to tetanic electrical stimulation of the input pathways. Input through the somatosensory pathways will be used to investigate whether plastic changes of sound-evoked responses can be induced in the DCN. Finally, the sites of plastic changes will be examined using pharmacological manipulations and stimulation at selected sites within the somatosensory-DCN pathway. This research will provide insight into the association between the somatosensory and auditory systems and into the overall function of the DCN. The work will contribute to the general understanding of the mechanisms and functional significance of plastic changes within the brain, which are relevant to normal development, to pathology (such as somatic tinnitus), and to recovery after damage.

Website: http://crisp.cit.nih.gov/crisp/Crisp_Query.Generate_Screen

- **Project Title: RANDOMIZED TRIAL OF TINNITUS RETRAINING THERAPY**

    Principal Investigator & Institution: Tyler, Richard S.; Professor and Director of Audiology; Otolaryngology; University of Iowa Iowa City, Ia 52242

    Timing: Fiscal Year 2004; Project Start 01-JAN-2003; Project End 30-NOV-2008

    Summary: (provided by applicant): Millions of Americans suffer from **tinnitus.** However, there is no widely accepted treatment that has been shown to be effective in controlled investigations. The purpose of this study is to evaluate the effectiveness of **Tinnitus** Retraining Therapy (TRT) using two controls. TRT, while actively promoted, has not been tested in a controlled investigation. It is based theoretically on a neurophysiological habituation model, where the brain learns to ignore continuous stimuli that are insignificant. TRT involves two main parts: counseling and the use of noise generators set slightly below the perceived loudness of the **tinnitus,** the "mixing point". In order for habituation to occur, the **tinnitus** must be perceived above the noise. This study will investigate the contributions of counseling, the use of devices, and the importance of setting the noise to the mixing point. The proposed study would include six different groups with 30 subjects per group. Subjects with hearing aids will be randomized to Counseling, Masking and Retraining groups. Subjects without hearing aids will be randomized to three different Counseling, Masking and Retraining groups. All groups will receive the same Counseling. In pilot studies we have developed a picture-based counseling protocol. The Retraining group will use binaural noise generators set to the mixing point. The Masking group will use the binaural noise generators set to mask the **tinnitus.** Each patient will be tested on three standardized **tinnitus** handicap scales before the treatment and 18 months after the commencement of treatment. The results of this study will determine if TRT is more effective than masking or counseling. This research will have direct and immediate clinical relevance for professionals and patients. Both are eager to seek out new treatments that promise success. If TRT is more effective than masking or counseling alone, then more professionals will want to use this procedure, and more patients will seek it. If TRT is shown to be no more effective than masking or counseling, professionals should focus on more efficient therapeutic techniques. This experiment will test the neurophysiological model of **tinnitus.**

    Website: http://crisp.cit.nih.gov/crisp/Crisp_Query.Generate_Screen

- **Project Title: RECOVERY OF DAMAGE TO THE VESTIBULAR-AUDITORY SYSTEM**

Principal Investigator & Institution: Barmack, Neal H.; Senior Scientist and Professor; Neurology; Oregon Health & Science University Portland, or 972393098

Timing: Fiscal Year 2002; Project Start 01-JUL-1994; Project End 30-NOV-2003

Summary: Partial recovery of function following a unilateral labyrinthectomy (UL), termed "vestibular compensation," has served as a model for investigations of subcellular investigations of central nervous system plasticity. Previous studies of compensation have "targeted" particular genes for study, using immunohistochemical and hybridization histochemical probes. Rather than target a particular genes, we propose to use the technique of "differential display" (DD-PCR) to screen gene products isolated from vestibular-and auditory-related regions the rabbit brain. Unlike the "targeted gene" approach, DD-PCR screens all differentially transcribed gene products. First, we will screen Scarpa's ganglion, medial vestibular nucleus, nodulus and inferior colliculus following UL. Since the primary vestibular-auditory afferent projects to the nodules and the DCN are unilateral, the structures on the side of the UL will receive a decreased primary afferent input and those on the intact side will receive a normal input. Second, we will use oligonucleotide probes identified by DD-PCR to reveal the tissue distribution and the time course of changes in tissue distribution of different mRNAs in animals that have received a UL. Third, promising molecules will be studied under more physiological conditions. Maintained static tilt will be used to provide asymmetric vestibular stimulation. Unilateral removal of the ossicular chain will be used to create asymmetric acoustic stimulation. Horizontal optokinetic stimulation will be used to provide asymmetric visual climbing fiber inputs to the nodulus. The optokinetic inputs will allow us to screen molecules that are differential expressed in the same structure, the nodulus, under stimulus conditions mediate db two different afferent pathways. Fourth, in analogous screening experiment at the protein level we will use two-dimensional electrophoresis to screen for proteins that are differential expressed following UL. Fifth, some molecules may participate in compensation or plasticity merely by changing their distribution within a cell rather than by changing expression. We will examine such a molecule, PKC-delta, in "activated" Purkinje cells using combined physiological, immunohistochemical and ultrastructural methods. Gene products uncovered by these experiments might play a role in both vestibular and auditory adaptation and provide important clues for the pharmacological treatment of central neural disorders such as motion sickness and **tinnitus.**

Website: http://crisp.cit.nih.gov/crisp/Crisp_Query.Generate_Screen

- **Project Title: TONOTOPIC VARIATIONS IN MECHANO-ELECTRIC TRANSDUCTION**

    Principal Investigator & Institution: Ricci, Anthony J.; Assistant Professor; Neuroscience Ctr of Excellence; Louisiana State Univ Hsc New Orleans New Orleans, La 70112

    Timing: Fiscal Year 2003; Project Start 01-JAN-1999; Project End 31-DEC-2007

    Summary: (provided by applicant): A mechanical tuning mechanism located in the sensory hair cell bundle and intimately associated with the mechano-electric transducer (MET) channels has been described. Termed fast adaptation, this calcium-dependent process has been postulated to underlie in part the cochlea active process, the mechanism responsible for the exquisite sensitivity of the auditory system. Perturbations of this system might result in elevated thresholds, temporary threshold shifts and **tinnitus.** Understanding the mechanisms responsible for the generation and regulation of adaptation of mechano-electric transduction is therefore critical if the long term goal is to design therapeutic treatments for these maladies. To this end, experiments are designed to quantitatively address several critical issues pertaining to the generation and regulation of the ton topic variations in fast adaptation. The first goal is to determine if intrinsic differences in MET channels exist between high and low frequency cells, specifically focusing on channel kinetics and single channel properties. An interaction between MET channels, probably through summation of intraciliary calcium has been postulated as a mechanism underlying the tontopic differences. Experiments are designed to directly test this hypothesis by coupling multiphoton imaging with electrophysiological recordings. A slower component of adaptation has been described that results in an increase in hair bundle compliance. This slow component may serve to prevent saturation and mechanical damage of the sensory hair bundle. Preliminary data suggests this component may be triggered by an intracellular release of stored calcium, and perhaps operate via a myosin motor, experiments are designed to characterize the mechanisms responsible for generating and the biochemical regulation of this slow form of adaptation. Hair cell calcium channels regulate membrane excitability and dictate transmitter release. Differential regulation of calcium channels based on which function the channels serves may be an important tool for signal processing. Characterization of the biophysical, pharmacological and biochemical properties of these channels is the fourth goal of this project and should yield some exciting new information regarding signal processing.

Website: http://crisp.cit.nih.gov/crisp/Crisp_Query.Generate_Screen

E-Journals: PubMed Central[19]

PubMed Central (PMC) is a digital archive of life sciences journal literature developed and managed by the National Center for Biotechnology Information (NCBI) at the U.S. National Library of Medicine (NLM).[20] Access to this growing archive of e-journals is free and unrestricted.[21] To search, go to **http://www.ncbi.nlm.nih.gov/entrez/query.fcgi?db=Pmc**, and type "tinnitus" (or synonyms) into the search box. This search gives you access to full-text articles. The following is a sample of items found for tinnitus in the PubMed Central database:

- **Effectiveness of Ginkgo biloba in treating tinnitus: double blind, placebo controlled trial.** by Drew S, Davies E.; 2001 Jan 13; http://www.pubmedcentral.gov/articlerender.fcgi?tool=pmcentrez&artid=26593

- **Long-term reductions in tinnitus severity.** by Folmer RL.; 2002; http://www.pubmedcentral.gov/articlerender.fcgi?tool=pmcentrez&artid=128822

- **Reorganization of auditory cortex in tinnitus.** by Muhlnickel W, Elbert T, Taub E, Flor H.; 1998 Aug 18; http://www.pubmedcentral.gov/articlerender.fcgi?tool=pmcentrez&artid=21510

The National Library of Medicine: PubMed

One of the quickest and most comprehensive ways to find academic studies in both English and other languages is to use PubMed, maintained by the

---

[19] Adapted from the National Library of Medicine: http://www.pubmedcentral.nih.gov/about/intro.html.

[20] With PubMed Central, NCBI is taking the lead in preservation and maintenance of open access to electronic literature, just as NLM has done for decades with printed biomedical literature. PubMed Central aims to become a world-class library of the digital age.

[21] The value of PubMed Central, in addition to its role as an archive, lies the availability of data from diverse sources stored in a common format in a single repository. Many journals already have online publishing operations, and there is a growing tendency to publish material online only, to the exclusion of print.

National Library of Medicine. The advantage of PubMed over previously mentioned sources is that it covers a greater number of domestic and foreign references. It is also free to the public.[22] If the publisher has a Web site that offers full text of its journals, PubMed will provide links to that site, as well as to sites offering other related data. User registration, a subscription fee, or some other type of fee may be required to access the full text of articles in some journals.

To generate your own bibliography of studies dealing with tinnitus, simply go to the PubMed Web site at **www.ncbi.nlm.nih.gov/pubmed**. Type "tinnitus" (or synonyms) into the search box, and click "Go." The following is the type of output you can expect from PubMed for "tinnitus" (hyperlinks lead to article summaries):

- **A biochemical model of peripheral tinnitus.**
  Author(s): Sahley TL, Nodar RH.
  Source: Hearing Research. 2001 February; 152(1-2): 43-54. Review.
  http://www.ncbi.nlm.nih.gov:80/entrez/query.fcgi?cmd=Retrieve&db=PubMed&list_uids=11223280&dopt=Abstract

- **A protocol of study for tinnitus in childhood.**
  Author(s): Savastano M.
  Source: International Journal of Pediatric Otorhinolaryngology. 2002 May 31; 64(1): 23-7.
  http://www.ncbi.nlm.nih.gov:80/entrez/query.fcgi?cmd=Retrieve&db=PubMed&list_uids=12020910&dopt=Abstract

- **A re-evaluation of tinnitus reliability testing.**
  Author(s): Jacobson GP, Henderson JA, McCaslin DL.
  Source: Journal of the American Academy of Audiology. 2000 March; 11(3): 156-61.
  http://www.ncbi.nlm.nih.gov:80/entrez/query.fcgi?cmd=Retrieve&db=PubMed&list_uids=10755811&dopt=Abstract

---

[22] PubMed was developed by the National Center for Biotechnology Information (NCBI) at the National Library of Medicine (NLM) at the National Institutes of Health (NIH). The PubMed database was developed in conjunction with publishers of biomedical literature as a search tool for accessing literature citations and linking to full-text journal articles at Web sites of participating publishers. Publishers that participate in PubMed supply NLM with their citations electronically prior to or at the time of publication.

- **A retrospective evaluation of the impact of temporomandibular joint arthroscopy on the symptoms of headache, neck pain, shoulder pain, dizziness, and tinnitus.**
  Author(s): Steigerwald DP, Verne SV, Young D.
  Source: Cranio. 1996 January; 14(1): 46-54.
  http://www.ncbi.nlm.nih.gov:80/entrez/query.fcgi?cmd=Retrieve&db=PubMed&list_uids=9086876&dopt=Abstract

- **A review of evidence in support of a role for 5-HT in the perception of tinnitus.**
  Author(s): Simpson JJ, Davies WE.
  Source: Hearing Research. 2000 July; 145(1-2): 1-7. Review.
  http://www.ncbi.nlm.nih.gov:80/entrez/query.fcgi?cmd=Retrieve&db=PubMed&list_uids=10867271&dopt=Abstract

- **A search for evidence of a direct relationship between tinnitus and suicide.**
  Author(s): Jacobson GP, McCaslin DL.
  Source: Journal of the American Academy of Audiology. 2001 November-December; 12(10): 493-6.
  http://www.ncbi.nlm.nih.gov:80/entrez/query.fcgi?cmd=Retrieve&db=PubMed&list_uids=11791935&dopt=Abstract

- **A selective imaging of tinnitus.**
  Author(s): Giraud AL, Chery-Croze S, Fischer G, Fischer C, Vighetto A, Gregoire MC, Lavenne F, Collet L.
  Source: Neuroreport. 1999 January 18; 10(1): 1-5.
  http://www.ncbi.nlm.nih.gov:80/entrez/query.fcgi?cmd=Retrieve&db=PubMed&list_uids=10094123&dopt=Abstract

- **A tinnitus objectivization: how we do it.**
  Author(s): Milicic D, Alcada MN.
  Source: Int Tinnitus J. 1999; 5(1): 5-15.
  http://www.ncbi.nlm.nih.gov:80/entrez/query.fcgi?cmd=Retrieve&db=PubMed&list_uids=10753410&dopt=Abstract

- **A vision for tinnitus research.**
  Author(s): Baguley DM, Davies E, Hazell JW.
  Source: International Journal of Audiology. 2003 January; 42(1): 2-3.
  http://www.ncbi.nlm.nih.gov:80/entrez/query.fcgi?cmd=Retrieve&db=PubMed&list_uids=12564509&dopt=Abstract

- **A warning on venous ligation for pulsatile tinnitus.**
  Author(s): Jackler RK, Brackmann DE, Sismanis A.
  Source: Otology & Neurotology : Official Publication of the American Otological Society, American Neurotology Society [and] European Academy of Otology and Neurotology. 2001 May; 22(3): 427-8.
  http://www.ncbi.nlm.nih.gov:80/entrez/query.fcgi?cmd=Retrieve&db=PubMed&list_uids=11347652&dopt=Abstract

- **A woman with a sudden tinnitus and back pain.**
  Author(s): Berlit P, Loew HH, Kuehne D.
  Source: Journal of the Neurological Sciences. 1999 January 1; 162(1): 89-90.
  http://www.ncbi.nlm.nih.gov:80/entrez/query.fcgi?cmd=Retrieve&db=PubMed&list_uids=10064175&dopt=Abstract

- **Aberrant internal carotid artery as a cause of pulsatile tinnitus and an intratympanic mass.**
  Author(s): Rojas R, Palacios E, D'Antonio M, Correa G.
  Source: Ear, Nose, & Throat Journal. 2003 March; 82(3): 173-4.
  http://www.ncbi.nlm.nih.gov:80/entrez/query.fcgi?cmd=Retrieve&db=PubMed&list_uids=12696233&dopt=Abstract

- **Abrupt onset of sensorineural hearing loss and tinnitus in a patient with capillary telangiectasia of the pons.**
  Author(s): Morinaka S, Hidaka A, Nagata H.
  Source: The Annals of Otology, Rhinology, and Laryngology. 2002 September; 111(9): 855-9.
  http://www.ncbi.nlm.nih.gov:80/entrez/query.fcgi?cmd=Retrieve&db=PubMed&list_uids=12296344&dopt=Abstract

- **Acoustic neuroma surgery and tinnitus.**
  Author(s): Fahy C, Nikolopoulos TP, O'Donoghue GM.
  Source: Eur Arch Otorhinolaryngol. 2002 July;259(6):299-301. Epub 2002 May 01.
  http://www.ncbi.nlm.nih.gov:80/entrez/query.fcgi?cmd=Retrieve&db=PubMed&list_uids=12115076&dopt=Abstract

- **Acupuncture for tinnitus: time to stop?**
  Author(s): Andersson G, Lyttkens L.
  Source: Scandinavian Audiology. 1996; 25(4): 273-5. Review.
  http://www.ncbi.nlm.nih.gov:80/entrez/query.fcgi?cmd=Retrieve&db=PubMed&list_uids=8976001&dopt=Abstract

- **Alternative medications and other treatments for tinnitus: facts from fiction.**
  Author(s): Seidman MD, Babu S.
  Source: Otolaryngologic Clinics of North America. 2003 April; 36(2): 359-81. Review.
  http://www.ncbi.nlm.nih.gov:80/entrez/query.fcgi?cmd=Retrieve&db=PubMed&list_uids=12856304&dopt=Abstract

- **An auditory negative after-image as a human model of tinnitus.**
  Author(s): Norena A, Micheyl C, Chery-Croze S.
  Source: Hearing Research. 2000 November; 149(1-2): 24-32.
  http://www.ncbi.nlm.nih.gov:80/entrez/query.fcgi?cmd=Retrieve&db=PubMed&list_uids=11033244&dopt=Abstract

- **An autosomal dominant disorder with episodic ataxia, vertigo, and tinnitus.**
  Author(s): Steckley JL, Ebers GC, Cader MZ, McLachlan RS.
  Source: Neurology. 2001 October 23; 57(8): 1499-502.
  http://www.ncbi.nlm.nih.gov:80/entrez/query.fcgi?cmd=Retrieve&db=PubMed&list_uids=11673600&dopt=Abstract

- **An unusual cause for tinnitus.**
  Author(s): Khodaei I, Rowley H, Farrell M, Collins CM, Vianni L, Rawluk D.
  Source: Ir Med J. 2001 November-December; 94(10): 312-3.
  http://www.ncbi.nlm.nih.gov:80/entrez/query.fcgi?cmd=Retrieve&db=PubMed&list_uids=11837632&dopt=Abstract

- **Aneurysm of a dural sigmoid sinus: a novel vascular cause of pulsatile tinnitus.**
  Author(s): Houdart E, Chapot R, Merland JJ.
  Source: Annals of Neurology. 2000 October; 48(4): 669-71.
  http://www.ncbi.nlm.nih.gov:80/entrez/query.fcgi?cmd=Retrieve&db=PubMed&list_uids=11026453&dopt=Abstract

- **Anterior communicating artery aneurysm presenting as pulsatile tinnitus.**
  Author(s): Austin JR, Maceri DR.
  Source: Orl; Journal for Oto-Rhino-Laryngology and Its Related Specialties. 1993; 55(1): 54-7. Review.
  http://www.ncbi.nlm.nih.gov:80/entrez/query.fcgi?cmd=Retrieve&db=PubMed&list_uids=8441526&dopt=Abstract

- **A warning on venous ligation for pulsatile tinnitus.**
  Author(s): Jackler RK, Brackmann DE, Sismanis A.
  Source: Otology & Neurotology : Official Publication of the American Otological Society, American Neurotology Society [and] European Academy of Otology and Neurotology. 2001 May; 22(3): 427-8.
  http://www.ncbi.nlm.nih.gov:80/entrez/query.fcgi?cmd=Retrieve&db=PubMed&list_uids=11347652&dopt=Abstract

- **A woman with a sudden tinnitus and back pain.**
  Author(s): Berlit P, Loew HH, Kuehne D.
  Source: Journal of the Neurological Sciences. 1999 January 1; 162(1): 89-90.
  http://www.ncbi.nlm.nih.gov:80/entrez/query.fcgi?cmd=Retrieve&db=PubMed&list_uids=10064175&dopt=Abstract

- **Aberrant internal carotid artery as a cause of pulsatile tinnitus and an intratympanic mass.**
  Author(s): Rojas R, Palacios E, D'Antonio M, Correa G.
  Source: Ear, Nose, & Throat Journal. 2003 March; 82(3): 173-4.
  http://www.ncbi.nlm.nih.gov:80/entrez/query.fcgi?cmd=Retrieve&db=PubMed&list_uids=12696233&dopt=Abstract

- **Abrupt onset of sensorineural hearing loss and tinnitus in a patient with capillary telangiectasia of the pons.**
  Author(s): Morinaka S, Hidaka A, Nagata H.
  Source: The Annals of Otology, Rhinology, and Laryngology. 2002 September; 111(9): 855-9.
  http://www.ncbi.nlm.nih.gov:80/entrez/query.fcgi?cmd=Retrieve&db=PubMed&list_uids=12296344&dopt=Abstract

- Acoustic neuroma surgery and tinnitus.
  Author(s): Fahy C, Nikolopoulos TP, O'Donoghue GM.
  Source: Eur Arch Otorhinolaryngol. 2002 July;259(6):299-301. Epub 2002 May 01.
  http://www.ncbi.nlm.nih.gov:80/entrez/query.fcgi?cmd=Retrieve&db=PubMed&list_uids=12115076&dopt=Abstract

- Acupuncture for tinnitus: time to stop?
  Author(s): Andersson G, Lyttkens L.
  Source: Scandinavian Audiology. 1996; 25(4): 273-5. Review.
  http://www.ncbi.nlm.nih.gov:80/entrez/query.fcgi?cmd=Retrieve&db=PubMed&list_uids=8976001&dopt=Abstract

- **Alternative medications and other treatments for tinnitus: facts from fiction.**
  Author(s): Seidman MD, Babu S.
  Source: Otolaryngologic Clinics of North America. 2003 April; 36(2): 359-81. Review.
  http://www.ncbi.nlm.nih.gov:80/entrez/query.fcgi?cmd=Retrieve&db=PubMed&list_uids=12856304&dopt=Abstract

- **An auditory negative after-image as a human model of tinnitus.**
  Author(s): Norena A, Micheyl C, Chery-Croze S.
  Source: Hearing Research. 2000 November; 149(1-2): 24-32.
  http://www.ncbi.nlm.nih.gov:80/entrez/query.fcgi?cmd=Retrieve&db=PubMed&list_uids=11033244&dopt=Abstract

- **An autosomal dominant disorder with episodic ataxia, vertigo, and tinnitus.**
  Author(s): Steckley JL, Ebers GC, Cader MZ, McLachlan RS.
  Source: Neurology. 2001 October 23; 57(8): 1499-502.
  http://www.ncbi.nlm.nih.gov:80/entrez/query.fcgi?cmd=Retrieve&db=PubMed&list_uids=11673600&dopt=Abstract

- **An unusual cause for tinnitus.**
  Author(s): Khodaei I, Rowley H, Farrell M, Collins CM, Vianni L, Rawluk D.
  Source: Ir Med J. 2001 November-December; 94(10): 312-3.
  http://www.ncbi.nlm.nih.gov:80/entrez/query.fcgi?cmd=Retrieve&db=PubMed&list_uids=11837632&dopt=Abstract

- **Aneurysm of a dural sigmoid sinus: a novel vascular cause of pulsatile tinnitus.**
  Author(s): Houdart E, Chapot R, Merland JJ.
  Source: Annals of Neurology. 2000 October; 48(4): 669-71.
  http://www.ncbi.nlm.nih.gov:80/entrez/query.fcgi?cmd=Retrieve&db=PubMed&list_uids=11026453&dopt=Abstract

- **Anterior communicating artery aneurysm presenting as pulsatile tinnitus.**
  Author(s): Austin JR, Maceri DR.
  Source: Orl; Journal for Oto-Rhino-Laryngology and Its Related Specialties. 1993; 55(1): 54-7. Review.
  http://www.ncbi.nlm.nih.gov:80/entrez/query.fcgi?cmd=Retrieve&db=PubMed&list_uids=8441526&dopt=Abstract

- **Antidepressant treatment of tinnitus patients: report of a randomized clinical trial and clinical prediction of benefit.**
  Author(s): Dobie RA, Sakai CS, Sullivan MD, Katon WJ, Russo J.
  Source: The American Journal of Otology. 1993 January; 14(1): 18-23.
  http://www.ncbi.nlm.nih.gov:80/entrez/query.fcgi?cmd=Retrieve&db=PubMed&list_uids=8424470&dopt=Abstract

- **Arachnoid cyst of the cranial posterior fossa causing sensorineural hearing loss and tinnitus: a case report.**
  Author(s): Ottaviani F, Neglia CB, Scotti A, Capaccio P.
  Source: Eur Arch Otorhinolaryngol. 2002 July;259(6):306-8. Epub 2002 May 09.
  http://www.ncbi.nlm.nih.gov:80/entrez/query.fcgi?cmd=Retrieve&db=PubMed&list_uids=12115078&dopt=Abstract

- **Are there any studies showing whether ginkgo biloba is effective for tinnitus (ringing in the ears)?**
  Author(s): Feinberg AW.
  Source: Health News. 2003 January; 9(1): 12. No Abstract Available.
  http://www.ncbi.nlm.nih.gov:80/entrez/query.fcgi?cmd=Retrieve&db=PubMed&list_uids=12545957&dopt=Abstract

- **Assessment and treatment of tinnitus patients using a "masking approach.".**
  Author(s): Schechter MA, Henry JA.
  Source: Journal of the American Academy of Audiology. 2002 November-December; 13(10): 545-58.
  http://www.ncbi.nlm.nih.gov:80/entrez/query.fcgi?cmd=Retrieve&db=PubMed&list_uids=12503923&dopt=Abstract

- **Assessment of intravenous lidocaine for the treatment of subjective tinnitus.**
  Author(s): Otsuka K, Pulec JL, Suzuki M.
  Source: Ear, Nose, & Throat Journal. 2003 October; 82(10): 781-4.
  http://www.ncbi.nlm.nih.gov:80/entrez/query.fcgi?cmd=Retrieve&db=PubMed&list_uids=14606175&dopt=Abstract

- **Assessment of patients for treatment with tinnitus retraining therapy.**
  Author(s): Henry JA, Jastreboff MM, Jastreboff PJ, Schechter MA, Fausti SA.
  Source: Journal of the American Academy of Audiology. 2002 November-December; 13(10): 523-44.
  http://www.ncbi.nlm.nih.gov:80/entrez/query.fcgi?cmd=Retrieve&db=PubMed&list_uids=12503922&dopt=Abstract

- **Audiologic and psychological profile of Greek patients with tinnitus-- preliminary findings.**
  Author(s): Vallianatou NG, Christodoulou P, Nestoros JN, Helidonis E.
  Source: American Journal of Otolaryngology. 2001 January-February; 22(1): 33-7.
  http://www.ncbi.nlm.nih.gov:80/entrez/query.fcgi?cmd=Retrieve&db=PubMed&list_uids=11172212&dopt=Abstract

- **Audiological problems in patients with tinnitus exposed to noise and vibrations.**
  Author(s): Tzaneva L, Savov A, Damianova V.
  Source: Cent Eur J Public Health. 2000 November; 8(4): 233-5.
  http://www.ncbi.nlm.nih.gov:80/entrez/query.fcgi?cmd=Retrieve&db=PubMed&list_uids=11125978&dopt=Abstract

- **Auditory evoked responses in control subjects and in patients with problem-tinnitus.**
  Author(s): Gerken GM, Hesse PS, Wiorkowski JJ.
  Source: Hearing Research. 2001 July; 157(1-2): 52-64.
  http://www.ncbi.nlm.nih.gov:80/entrez/query.fcgi?cmd=Retrieve&db=PubMed&list_uids=11470185&dopt=Abstract

- **Behavioral treatment of pulsatile tinnitus and headache following traumatic head injury. Objective polygraphic assessment of change.**
  Author(s): Hegel MT, Martin JB.
  Source: Behavior Modification. 1998 October; 22(4): 563-72.
  http://www.ncbi.nlm.nih.gov:80/entrez/query.fcgi?cmd=Retrieve&db=PubMed&list_uids=9755652&dopt=Abstract

- **Bell's palsy and tinnitus during pregnancy: predictors of pre-eclampsia? Three cases and a detailed review of the literature.**
  Author(s): Shapiro JL, Yudin MH, Ray JG.
  Source: Acta Oto-Laryngologica. 1999; 119(6): 647-51. Review.
  http://www.ncbi.nlm.nih.gov:80/entrez/query.fcgi?cmd=Retrieve&db=PubMed&list_uids=10586996&dopt=Abstract

- **Benzodiazepine receptor deficiency and tinnitus.**
  Author(s): Shulman A, Strashun AM, Seibyl JP, Daftary A, Goldstein B.
  Source: Int Tinnitus J. 2000; 6(2): 98-111.
  http://www.ncbi.nlm.nih.gov:80/entrez/query.fcgi?cmd=Retrieve&db=PubMed&list_uids=14689626&dopt=Abstract

- **Benzodiazepines and the ear--tinnitus, hallucinations and schizophrenia.**
  Author(s): Gordon AG.
  Source: Canadian Journal of Psychiatry. Revue Canadienne De Psychiatrie. 1993 March; 38(2): 156-7.
  http://www.ncbi.nlm.nih.gov:80/entrez/query.fcgi?cmd=Retrieve&db=PubMed&list_uids=8467446&dopt=Abstract

- **Bilateral defects of the tegmen tympani associated with brain and dural prolapse in a patient with pulsatile tinnitus.**
  Author(s): Kale SU, Pfleiderer AG, Cradwick JC.
  Source: The Journal of Laryngology and Otology. 2000 November; 114(11): 861-3.
  http://www.ncbi.nlm.nih.gov:80/entrez/query.fcgi?cmd=Retrieve&db=PubMed&list_uids=11144837&dopt=Abstract

- **Biofeedback therapy in the treatment of tinnitus.**
  Author(s): Ogata Y, Sekitani T, Moriya K, Watanabe K.
  Source: Auris, Nasus, Larynx. 1993; 20(2): 95-101.
  http://www.ncbi.nlm.nih.gov:80/entrez/query.fcgi?cmd=Retrieve&db=PubMed&list_uids=8216052&dopt=Abstract

- **Botulinum toxin injection for objective tinnitus from palatal myoclonus: a case report.**
  Author(s): Srirompotong S, Tiamkao S, Jitpimolmard S.
  Source: J Med Assoc Thai. 2002 March; 85(3): 392-5.
  http://www.ncbi.nlm.nih.gov:80/entrez/query.fcgi?cmd=Retrieve&db=PubMed&list_uids=12117033&dopt=Abstract

- **Botulinum toxin treatment of essential palatal myoclonus tinnitus.**
  Author(s): Bryce GE, Morrison MD.
  Source: The Journal of Otolaryngology. 1998 August; 27(4): 213-6.
  http://www.ncbi.nlm.nih.gov:80/entrez/query.fcgi?cmd=Retrieve&db=PubMed&list_uids=9711516&dopt=Abstract

- **Brain imaging of the effects of lidocaine on tinnitus.**
  Author(s): Reyes SA, Salvi RJ, Burkard RF, Coad ML, Wack DS, Galantowicz PJ, Lockwood AH.
  Source: Hearing Research. 2002 September; 171(1-2): 43-50.
  http://www.ncbi.nlm.nih.gov:80/entrez/query.fcgi?cmd=Retrieve&db=PubMed&list_uids=12204348&dopt=Abstract

- **Brainstem auditory evoked responses in patients with tinnitus.**
  Author(s): Lemaire MC, Beutter P.
  Source: Audiology : Official Organ of the International Society of Audiology. 1995 November-December; 34(6): 287-300.
  http://www.ncbi.nlm.nih.gov:80/entrez/query.fcgi?cmd=Retrieve&db=PubMed&list_uids=8833309&dopt=Abstract

- **Caroverine in tinnitus treatment.**
  Author(s): Domeisen H, Hotz MA, Hausler R.
  Source: Acta Oto-Laryngologica. 1998 July; 118(4): 606-8.
  http://www.ncbi.nlm.nih.gov:80/entrez/query.fcgi?cmd=Retrieve&db=PubMed&list_uids=9726691&dopt=Abstract

- **Celebrating a decade of evaluation and treatment: the University of Maryland Tinnitus & Hyperacusis Center.**
  Author(s): Gold SL, Formby C, Gray WC.
  Source: American Journal of Audiology. 2000 December; 9(2): 69-74.
  http://www.ncbi.nlm.nih.gov:80/entrez/query.fcgi?cmd=Retrieve&db=PubMed&list_uids=11200194&dopt=Abstract

- **Central auditory speech test findings in individuals with subjective idiopathic tinnitus.**
  Author(s): Goldstein B, Shulman A.
  Source: Int Tinnitus J. 1999; 5(1): 16-9.
  http://www.ncbi.nlm.nih.gov:80/entrez/query.fcgi?cmd=Retrieve&db=PubMed&list_uids=10753411&dopt=Abstract

- **Central tinnitus.**
  Author(s): Eggermont JJ.
  Source: Auris, Nasus, Larynx. 2003 February; 30 Suppl: S7-12. Review.
  http://www.ncbi.nlm.nih.gov:80/entrez/query.fcgi?cmd=Retrieve&db=PubMed&list_uids=12543153&dopt=Abstract

- **Central tinnitus: a case report.**
  Author(s): Yoneoka Y, Fujii Y, Nakada T.
  Source: Ear, Nose, & Throat Journal. 2001 December; 80(12): 864-6.
  http://www.ncbi.nlm.nih.gov:80/entrez/query.fcgi?cmd=Retrieve&db=PubMed&list_uids=11775517&dopt=Abstract

- **Cerebellar arteriovenous malformation with facial paralysis, hearing loss, and tinnitus: a case report.**
  Author(s): Kikuchi M, Funabiki K, Hasebe S, Takahashi H.
  Source: Otology & Neurotology : Official Publication of the American Otological Society, American Neurotology Society [and] European Academy of Otology and Neurotology. 2002 September; 23(5): 723-6.
  http://www.ncbi.nlm.nih.gov:80/entrez/query.fcgi?cmd=Retrieve&db=PubMed&list_uids=12218626&dopt=Abstract

- **Cerebellopontine angle epidermoid tumor presenting with 'tic convulsif' and tinnitus--case report.**
  Author(s): Desai K, Nadkarni T, Bhayani R, Goel A.
  Source: Neurol Med Chir (Tokyo). 2002 April; 42(4): 162-5.
  http://www.ncbi.nlm.nih.gov:80/entrez/query.fcgi?cmd=Retrieve&db=PubMed&list_uids=12013668&dopt=Abstract

- **Changes in blood serotonin in patients with tinnitus and other vestibular disturbances.**
  Author(s): Sachanska T.
  Source: Int Tinnitus J. 1999; 5(1): 24-6.
  http://www.ncbi.nlm.nih.gov:80/entrez/query.fcgi?cmd=Retrieve&db=PubMed&list_uids=10753413&dopt=Abstract

- **Characteristics and postoperative course of tinnitus in otosclerosis.**
  Author(s): Ayache D, Earally F, Elbaz P.
  Source: Otology & Neurotology : Official Publication of the American Otological Society, American Neurotology Society [and] European Academy of Otology and Neurotology. 2003 January; 24(1): 48-51.
  http://www.ncbi.nlm.nih.gov:80/entrez/query.fcgi?cmd=Retrieve&db=PubMed&list_uids=12544028&dopt=Abstract

- **Characteristics of patients with gaze-evoked tinnitus.**
  Author(s): Coad ML, Lockwood A, Salvi R, Burkard R.
  Source: Otology & Neurotology : Official Publication of the American Otological Society, American Neurotology Society [and] European Academy of Otology and Neurotology. 2001 September; 22(5): 650-4.
  http://www.ncbi.nlm.nih.gov:80/entrez/query.fcgi?cmd=Retrieve&db=PubMed&list_uids=11568674&dopt=Abstract

- **Characteristics of tinnitus induced by acute acoustic trauma: a long-term follow-up.**
  Author(s): Mrena R, Savolainen S, Kuokkanen JT, Ylikoski J.
  Source: Audiology & Neuro-Otology. 2002 March-April; 7(2): 122-30.
  http://www.ncbi.nlm.nih.gov:80/entrez/query.fcgi?cmd=Retrieve&db=PubMed&list_uids=12006740&dopt=Abstract

- **Children's experience of tinnitus: a preliminary survey of children presenting to a psychology department.**
  Author(s): Kentish RC, Crocker SR, McKenna L.
  Source: British Journal of Audiology. 2000 December; 34(6): 335-40.
  http://www.ncbi.nlm.nih.gov:80/entrez/query.fcgi?cmd=Retrieve&db=PubMed&list_uids=11201320&dopt=Abstract

- **Chronic tinnitus as phantom auditory pain.**
  Author(s): Folmer RL, Griest SE, Martin WH.
  Source: Otolaryngology and Head and Neck Surgery. 2001 April; 124(4): 394-400.
  http://www.ncbi.nlm.nih.gov:80/entrez/query.fcgi?cmd=Retrieve&db=PubMed&list_uids=11283496&dopt=Abstract

- **Chronic tinnitus resulting from head or neck injuries.**
  Author(s): Folmer RL, Griest SE.
  Source: The Laryngoscope. 2003 May; 113(5): 821-7.
  http://www.ncbi.nlm.nih.gov:80/entrez/query.fcgi?cmd=Retrieve&db=PubMed&list_uids=12792317&dopt=Abstract

- **Classification and epidemiology of tinnitus.**
  Author(s): Heller AJ.
  Source: Otolaryngologic Clinics of North America. 2003 April; 36(2): 239-48. Review.
  http://www.ncbi.nlm.nih.gov:80/entrez/query.fcgi?cmd=Retrieve&db=PubMed&list_uids=12856294&dopt=Abstract

- **Client centred hypnotherapy in the management of tinnitus--is it better than counselling?**
  Author(s): Mason JD, Rogerson DR, Butler JD.
  Source: The Journal of Laryngology and Otology. 1996 February; 110(2): 117-20.
  http://www.ncbi.nlm.nih.gov:80/entrez/query.fcgi?cmd=Retrieve&db=PubMed&list_uids=8729491&dopt=Abstract

- **Clinical associations between tinnitus and chronic pain.**
  Author(s): Isaacson JE, Moyer MT, Schuler HG, Blackall GF.
  Source: Otolaryngology and Head and Neck Surgery. 2003 May; 128(5): 706-10.
  http://www.ncbi.nlm.nih.gov:80/entrez/query.fcgi?cmd=Retrieve&db=PubMed&list_uids=12748565&dopt=Abstract

- **Cochlear implantation for tinnitus suppression.**
  Author(s): Miyamoto RT, Bichey BG.
  Source: Otolaryngologic Clinics of North America. 2003 April; 36(2): 345-52. Review.
  http://www.ncbi.nlm.nih.gov:80/entrez/query.fcgi?cmd=Retrieve&db=PubMed&list_uids=12856302&dopt=Abstract

- **Cochlear-motor, transduction and signal-transfer tinnitus: models for three types of cochlear tinnitus.**
  Author(s): Zenner HP, Ernst A.
  Source: European Archives of Oto-Rhino-Laryngology : Official Journal of the European Federation of Oto-Rhino-Laryngological Societies (Eufos) : Affiliated with the German Society for Oto-Rhino-Laryngology - Head and Neck Surgery. 1993; 249(8): 447-54. Review.
  http://www.ncbi.nlm.nih.gov:80/entrez/query.fcgi?cmd=Retrieve&db=PubMed&list_uids=7680210&dopt=Abstract

- **Combined laser-EGb 761 tinnitus therapy.**
  Author(s): Hahn A, Sejna I, Stolbova K, Cocek A.
  Source: Acta Otolaryngol Suppl. 2001; 545: 92-3.
  http://www.ncbi.nlm.nih.gov:80/entrez/query.fcgi?cmd=Retrieve&db=PubMed&list_uids=11677752&dopt=Abstract

- **Comparison of tinnitus masking and tinnitus retraining therapy.**
  Author(s): Henry JA, Schechter MA, Nagler SM, Fausti SA.
  Source: Journal of the American Academy of Audiology. 2002 November-December; 13(10): 559-81.
  http://www.ncbi.nlm.nih.gov:80/entrez/query.fcgi?cmd=Retrieve&db=PubMed&list_uids=12503924&dopt=Abstract

- **Comparison of two computer-automated procedures for tinnitus pitch matching.**
  Author(s): Henry JA, Flick CL, Gilbert A, Ellingson RM, Fausti SA.
  Source: Journal of Rehabilitation Research and Development. 2001 September-October; 38(5): 557-66.
  http://www.ncbi.nlm.nih.gov:80/entrez/query.fcgi?cmd=Retrieve&db=PubMed&list_uids=11732833&dopt=Abstract

- **Computer-automated clinical technique for tinnitus quantification.**
  Author(s): Henry JA, Fausti SA, Flick CL, Helt WJ, Ellingson RM.
  Source: American Journal of Audiology. 2000 June; 9(1): 36-49.
  http://www.ncbi.nlm.nih.gov:80/entrez/query.fcgi?cmd=Retrieve&db=PubMed&list_uids=10943023&dopt=Abstract

- **Continuous, high-frequency objective tinnitus caused by middle ear myoclonus.**
  Author(s): Bento RF, Sanchez TG, Miniti A, Tedesco-Marchesi AJ.
  Source: Ear, Nose, & Throat Journal. 1998 October; 77(10): 814-8.
  http://www.ncbi.nlm.nih.gov:80/entrez/query.fcgi?cmd=Retrieve&db=PubMed&list_uids=9818532&dopt=Abstract

- **Convergent validity of the tinnitus handicap inventory and the tinnitus questionnaire.**
  Author(s): Baguley DM, Humphriss RL, Hodgson CA.
  Source: The Journal of Laryngology and Otology. 2000 November; 114(11): 840-3.
  http://www.ncbi.nlm.nih.gov:80/entrez/query.fcgi?cmd=Retrieve&db=PubMed&list_uids=11144832&dopt=Abstract

- **Correlates of sleep disturbance in chronic distressing tinnitus.**
  Author(s): Hallam RS.
  Source: Scandinavian Audiology. 1996; 25(4): 263-6.
  http://www.ncbi.nlm.nih.gov:80/entrez/query.fcgi?cmd=Retrieve&db=PubMed&list_uids=8975999&dopt=Abstract

- **Cortical networks subserving the perception of tinnitus--a PET study.**
  Author(s): Mirz F, Gjedde A, Ishizu K, Pedersen CB.
  Source: Acta Otolaryngol Suppl. 2000; 543: 241-3.
  http://www.ncbi.nlm.nih.gov:80/entrez/query.fcgi?cmd=Retrieve&db=PubMed&list_uids=10909031&dopt=Abstract

- **Current perspectives on tinnitus.**
  Author(s): Baguley DM, McFerran DJ.
  Source: Archives of Disease in Childhood. 2002 March; 86(3): 141-3.
  http://www.ncbi.nlm.nih.gov:80/entrez/query.fcgi?cmd=Retrieve&db=PubMed&list_uids=11861225&dopt=Abstract

- **Cutaneous-evoked tinnitus. I. Phenomenology, psychophysics and functional imaging.**
  Author(s): Cacace AT, Cousins JP, Parnes SM, Semenoff D, Holmes T, McFarland DJ, Davenport C, Stegbauer K, Lovely TJ.
  Source: Audiology & Neuro-Otology. 1999 September-October; 4(5): 247-57.
  http://www.ncbi.nlm.nih.gov:80/entrez/query.fcgi?cmd=Retrieve&db=PubMed&list_uids=10436317&dopt=Abstract

- **Cutaneous-evoked tinnitus. II. Review Of neuroanatomical, physiological and functional imaging studies.**
  Author(s): Cacace AT, Cousins JP, Parnes SM, McFarland DJ, Semenoff D, Holmes T, Davenport C, Stegbauer K, Lovely TJ.
  Source: Audiology & Neuro-Otology. 1999 September-October; 4(5): 258-68. Review.
  http://www.ncbi.nlm.nih.gov:80/entrez/query.fcgi?cmd=Retrieve&db=PubMed&list_uids=10436318&dopt=Abstract

- **Dental pulpalgia contributing to bilateral preauricular pain and tinnitus.**
  Author(s): Wright EF, Gullickson DC.
  Source: J Orofac Pain. 1996 Spring; 10(2): 166-8.
  http://www.ncbi.nlm.nih.gov:80/entrez/query.fcgi?cmd=Retrieve&db=PubMed&list_uids=9133861&dopt=Abstract

- **Depression and tinnitus.**
  Author(s): Dobie RA.
  Source: Otolaryngologic Clinics of North America. 2003 April; 36(2): 383-8. Review.
  http://www.ncbi.nlm.nih.gov:80/entrez/query.fcgi?cmd=Retrieve&db=PubMed&list_uids=12856305&dopt=Abstract

- **Depression, palpitations, and unilateral pulsatile tinnitus due to a dopamine-secreting glomus jugulare tumor.**
  Author(s): Troughton RW, Fry D, Allison RS, Nicholls MG.
  Source: The American Journal of Medicine. 1998 March; 104(3): 310-1.
  http://www.ncbi.nlm.nih.gov:80/entrez/query.fcgi?cmd=Retrieve&db=PubMed&list_uids=9552094&dopt=Abstract

- **Descending auditory system/cerebellum/tinnitus.**
  Author(s): Shulman A, Strashun A.
  Source: Int Tinnitus J. 1999; 5(2): 92-106. Review.
  http://www.ncbi.nlm.nih.gov:80/entrez/query.fcgi?cmd=Retrieve&db=PubMed&list_uids=10753427&dopt=Abstract

- **Detailed analysis of auditory brainstem responses in patients with noise-induced tinnitus.**
  Author(s): Attias J, Pratt H, Reshef I, Bresloff I, Horowitz G, Polyakov A, Shemesh Z.
  Source: Audiology : Official Organ of the International Society of Audiology. 1996 September-October; 35(5): 259-70.
  http://www.ncbi.nlm.nih.gov:80/entrez/query.fcgi?cmd=Retrieve&db=PubMed&list_uids=8937658&dopt=Abstract

- **Detrimental effects of alcohol on tinnitus.**
  Author(s): Stephens D.
  Source: Clinical Otolaryngology and Allied Sciences. 1999 April; 24(2): 114-6.
  http://www.ncbi.nlm.nih.gov:80/entrez/query.fcgi?cmd=Retrieve&db=PubMed&list_uids=10225155&dopt=Abstract

- **Development of the Tinnitus Handicap Inventory.**
  Author(s): Newman CW, Jacobson GP, Spitzer JB.
  Source: Archives of Otolaryngology--Head & Neck Surgery. 1996 February; 122(2): 143-8.
  http://www.ncbi.nlm.nih.gov:80/entrez/query.fcgi?cmd=Retrieve&db=PubMed&list_uids=8630207&dopt=Abstract

- **Diagnostic approach to tinnitus.**
  Author(s): Crummer RW, Hassan GA.
  Source: American Family Physician. 2004 January 1; 69(1): 120-6. Review.
  http://www.ncbi.nlm.nih.gov:80/entrez/query.fcgi?cmd=Retrieve&db=PubMed&list_uids=14727828&dopt=Abstract

- **Diaries of tinnitus sufferers.**
  Author(s): Kemp S, George RN.
  Source: British Journal of Audiology. 1992 December; 26(6): 381-6.
  http://www.ncbi.nlm.nih.gov:80/entrez/query.fcgi?cmd=Retrieve&db=PubMed&list_uids=1292822&dopt=Abstract

- **Differences in resting state regional cerebral blood flow assessed with 99mTc-HMPAO SPECT and brain atlas matching between depressed patients with and without tinnitus.**
  Author(s): Gardner A, Pagani M, Jacobsson H, Lindberg G, Larsson SA, Wagner A, Hallstrom T.
  Source: Nuclear Medicine Communications. 2002 May; 23(5): 429-39.
  http://www.ncbi.nlm.nih.gov:80/entrez/query.fcgi?cmd=Retrieve&db=PubMed&list_uids=11973483&dopt=Abstract

- **Different treatment modalities of tinnitus at the EuromedClinic.**
  Author(s): Gul H, Nowak R, Buchner FA, Nagel D, Haid CT.
  Source: Int Tinnitus J. 2000; 6(1): 50-3.
  http://www.ncbi.nlm.nih.gov:80/entrez/query.fcgi?cmd=Retrieve&db=PubMed&list_uids=14689618&dopt=Abstract

- **Distinguishing levels of tinnitus distress.**
  Author(s): Andersson G, Lyttkens L, Larsen HC.
  Source: Clinical Otolaryngology and Allied Sciences. 1999 September; 24(5): 404-10.
  http://www.ncbi.nlm.nih.gov:80/entrez/query.fcgi?cmd=Retrieve&db=PubMed&list_uids=10542919&dopt=Abstract

- **Distortion products in normal hearing patients with tinnitus.**
  Author(s): Castello E.
  Source: Boll Soc Ital Biol Sper. 1997 May-June; 73(5-6): 93-100.
  http://www.ncbi.nlm.nih.gov:80/entrez/query.fcgi?cmd=Retrieve&db=PubMed&list_uids=9796127&dopt=Abstract

- **Doppler sonography of vertebral arteries in patients with tinnitus.**
  Author(s): Koyuncu M, Celik O, Luleci C, Inan E, Ozturk A.
  Source: Auris, Nasus, Larynx. 1995; 22(1): 24-8.
  http://www.ncbi.nlm.nih.gov:80/entrez/query.fcgi?cmd=Retrieve&db=PubMed&list_uids=7677632&dopt=Abstract

- **Drug treatments for tinnitus: the Tulane experience.**
  Author(s): Amedee RG, Risey J.
  Source: Int Tinnitus J. 2000; 6(1): 63-6. Review.
  http://www.ncbi.nlm.nih.gov:80/entrez/query.fcgi?cmd=Retrieve&db=PubMed&list_uids=14689621&dopt=Abstract

- **Drug-induced tinnitus and other hearing disorders.**
  Author(s): Seligmann H, Podoshin L, Ben-David J, Fradis M, Goldsher M.
  Source: Drug Safety : an International Journal of Medical Toxicology and Drug Experience. 1996 March; 14(3): 198-212. Review.
  http://www.ncbi.nlm.nih.gov:80/entrez/query.fcgi?cmd=Retrieve&db=PubMed&list_uids=8934581&dopt=Abstract

- **Effect of hyperbaric oxygen therapy in comparison to conventional or placebo therapy or no treatment in idiopathic sudden hearing loss, acoustic trauma, noise-induced hearing loss and tinnitus. A literature survey.**
  Author(s): Lamm K, Lamm H, Arnold W.
  Source: Advances in Oto-Rhino-Laryngology. 1998; 54: 86-99. Review.
  http://www.ncbi.nlm.nih.gov:80/entrez/query.fcgi?cmd=Retrieve&db=PubMed&list_uids=9547879&dopt=Abstract

- **Effect of intratympanic gentamicin on hearing and tinnitus in Meniere's disease.**
  Author(s): Eklund S, Pyykko I, Aalto H, Ishizaki H, Vasama JP.
  Source: The American Journal of Otology. 1999 May; 20(3): 350-6.
  http://www.ncbi.nlm.nih.gov:80/entrez/query.fcgi?cmd=Retrieve&db=PubMed&list_uids=10337977&dopt=Abstract

- **Effect of melatonin on tinnitus.**
  Author(s): Rosenberg SI, Silverstein H, Rowan PT, Olds MJ.
  Source: The Laryngoscope. 1998 March; 108(3): 305-10.
  http://www.ncbi.nlm.nih.gov:80/entrez/query.fcgi?cmd=Retrieve&db=PubMed&list_uids=9504599&dopt=Abstract

- **Effect of stapedectomy on subjective tinnitus.**
  Author(s): Szymanski M, Golabek W, Mills R.
  Source: The Journal of Laryngology and Otology. 2003 April; 117(4): 261-4.
  http://www.ncbi.nlm.nih.gov:80/entrez/query.fcgi?cmd=Retrieve&db=PubMed&list_uids=12816213&dopt=Abstract

- **Effect of traditional Chinese acupuncture on severe tinnitus: a double-blind, placebo-controlled, clinical investigation with open therapeutic control.**
  Author(s): Vilholm OJ, Moller K, Jorgensen K.
  Source: British Journal of Audiology. 1998 June; 32(3): 197-204.
  http://www.ncbi.nlm.nih.gov:80/entrez/query.fcgi?cmd=Retrieve&db=PubMed&list_uids=9710337&dopt=Abstract

- **Effectiveness of Ginkgo biloba in treating tinnitus: double blind, placebo controlled trial.**
  Author(s): Drew S, Davies E.
  Source: Bmj (Clinical Research Ed.). 2001 January 13; 322(7278): 73.
  http://www.ncbi.nlm.nih.gov:80/entrez/query.fcgi?cmd=Retrieve&db=PubMed&list_uids=11154618&dopt=Abstract

- **Effects of greater occipital nerve block on tinnitus and dizziness.**
  Author(s): Matsushima JI, Sakai N, Uemi N, Ifukube T.
  Source: Int Tinnitus J. 1999; 5(1): 40-6.
  http://www.ncbi.nlm.nih.gov:80/entrez/query.fcgi?cmd=Retrieve&db=PubMed&list_uids=10753418&dopt=Abstract

- **Effects of tinnitus on posture: a study of electrical tinnitus suppression.**
  Author(s): Matsushima JI, Sakai N, Ifukube T.
  Source: Int Tinnitus J. 1999; 5(1): 35-9.
  http://www.ncbi.nlm.nih.gov:80/entrez/query.fcgi?cmd=Retrieve&db=PubMed&list_uids=10753417&dopt=Abstract

- **Effects of tinnitus retraining therapy (TRT) for patients with tinnitus and subjective hearing loss versus tinnitus only.**
  Author(s): Bartnik G, Fabijanska A, Rogowski M.
  Source: Scand Audiol Suppl. 2001; (52): 206-8.
  http://www.ncbi.nlm.nih.gov:80/entrez/query.fcgi?cmd=Retrieve&db=PubMed&list_uids=11318470&dopt=Abstract

- **Efficacy of acupuncture as a treatment for tinnitus: a systematic review.**
  Author(s): Park J, White AR, Ernst E.
  Source: Archives of Otolaryngology--Head & Neck Surgery. 2000 April; 126(4): 489-92. Review.
  http://www.ncbi.nlm.nih.gov:80/entrez/query.fcgi?cmd=Retrieve&db=PubMed&list_uids=10772302&dopt=Abstract

- **Efficacy of amitriptyline in the treatment of subjective tinnitus.**
  Author(s): Bayar N, Boke B, Turan E, Belgin E.
  Source: The Journal of Otolaryngology. 2001 October; 30(5): 300-3.
  http://www.ncbi.nlm.nih.gov:80/entrez/query.fcgi?cmd=Retrieve&db=PubMed&list_uids=11771024&dopt=Abstract

- **Efficacy of transmeatal low power laser irradiation on tinnitus: a preliminary report.**
  Author(s): Shiomi Y, Takahashi H, Honjo I, Kojima H, Naito Y, Fujiki N.
  Source: Auris, Nasus, Larynx. 1997; 24(1): 39-42.
  http://www.ncbi.nlm.nih.gov:80/entrez/query.fcgi?cmd=Retrieve&db=PubMed&list_uids=9148726&dopt=Abstract

- **Electrical suppression of tinnitus with high-rate pulse trains.**
  Author(s): Rubinstein JT, Tyler RS, Johnson A, Brown CJ.
  Source: Otology & Neurotology : Official Publication of the American Otological Society, American Neurotology Society [and] European Academy of Otology and Neurotology. 2003 May; 24(3): 478-85.
  http://www.ncbi.nlm.nih.gov:80/entrez/query.fcgi?cmd=Retrieve&db=PubMed&list_uids=12806303&dopt=Abstract

- **Electrocochleographic analysis of the suppression of tinnitus by electrical promontory stimulation.**
  Author(s): Watanabe K, Okawara D, Baba S, Yagi T.
  Source: Audiology : Official Organ of the International Society of Audiology. 1997 May-June; 36(3): 147-54.
  http://www.ncbi.nlm.nih.gov:80/entrez/query.fcgi?cmd=Retrieve&db=PubMed&list_uids=9193732&dopt=Abstract

- **Electroencephalography correlates in tinnitus.**
  Author(s): Weiler EW, Brill K, Tachiki KH, Wiegand R.
  Source: Int Tinnitus J. 2000; 6(1): 21-4.
  http://www.ncbi.nlm.nih.gov:80/entrez/query.fcgi?cmd=Retrieve&db=PubMed&list_uids=14689613&dopt=Abstract

- **Electronic access to tinnitus data: the Oregon Tinnitus Data Archive.**
  Author(s): Meikle MB.
  Source: Otolaryngology and Head and Neck Surgery. 1997 December; 117(6): 698-700.
  http://www.ncbi.nlm.nih.gov:80/entrez/query.fcgi?cmd=Retrieve&db=PubMed&list_uids=9419101&dopt=Abstract

- **Electronystagmography: vestibular findings in a patient with tinnitus.**
  Author(s): Brookler KH.
  Source: Ear, Nose, & Throat Journal. 2003 September; 82(9): 673.
  http://www.ncbi.nlm.nih.gov:80/entrez/query.fcgi?cmd=Retrieve&db=PubMed&list_uids=14569699&dopt=Abstract

- **Electrophysiological indices of selective auditory attention in subjects with and without tinnitus.**
  Author(s): Jacobson GP, Calder JA, Newman CW, Peterson EL, Wharton JA, Ahmad BK.
  Source: Hearing Research. 1996 August; 97(1-2): 66-74.
  http://www.ncbi.nlm.nih.gov:80/entrez/query.fcgi?cmd=Retrieve&db=PubMed&list_uids=8844187&dopt=Abstract

- **Endogenous dynorphins: possible role in peripheral tinnitus.**
  Author(s): Sahley TL, Nodar RH, Musiek FE.
  Source: Int Tinnitus J. 1999; 5(2): 76-91. Review.
  http://www.ncbi.nlm.nih.gov:80/entrez/query.fcgi?cmd=Retrieve&db=PubMed&list_uids=10753426&dopt=Abstract

- **Epidermoid cyst of the skull with nonpulsatile tinnitus.**
  Author(s): Piotin M, Gailloud P, Reverdin A, Schneider PA, Pizzolato G, Rufenacht DA.
  Source: Neuroradiology. 1998 July; 40(7): 452-4.
  http://www.ncbi.nlm.nih.gov:80/entrez/query.fcgi?cmd=Retrieve&db=PubMed&list_uids=9730346&dopt=Abstract

- **Estimation of the loudness of tinnitus from matching tests.**
  Author(s): Matsuhira T, Yamashita K, Yasuda M.
  Source: British Journal of Audiology. 1992 December; 26(6): 387-95.
  http://www.ncbi.nlm.nih.gov:80/entrez/query.fcgi?cmd=Retrieve&db=PubMed&list_uids=1292823&dopt=Abstract

- **Evaluating tinnitus.**
  Author(s): Jerger J.
  Source: Journal of the American Academy of Audiology. 1999 October; 10(9): 466.
  http://www.ncbi.nlm.nih.gov:80/entrez/query.fcgi?cmd=Retrieve&db=PubMed&list_uids=10522619&dopt=Abstract

- **Evaluation of cochlear function in patients with normal hearing and tinnitus: a distortion product otoacoustic emission study.**
  Author(s): Satar B, Kapkin O, Ozkaptan Y.
  Source: Kulak Burun Bogaz Ihtis Derg. 2003 May; 10(5): 177-82.
  http://www.ncbi.nlm.nih.gov:80/entrez/query.fcgi?cmd=Retrieve&db=PubMed&list_uids=12970589&dopt=Abstract

- **Evaluation of tinnitus patients by peroral multi-drug treatment.**
  Author(s): Ohsaki K, Ueno M, Zheng HX, Wang QC, Nishizaki K, Nobuto Y, Fujimura T.
  Source: Auris, Nasus, Larynx. 1998 May; 25(2): 149-54.
  http://www.ncbi.nlm.nih.gov:80/entrez/query.fcgi?cmd=Retrieve&db=PubMed&list_uids=9673727&dopt=Abstract

- **Expanding the biological basis of tinnitus: crossmodal origins and the role of neuroplasticity.**
  Author(s): Cacace AT.
  Source: Hearing Research. 2003 January; 175(1-2): 112-32. Review.
  http://www.ncbi.nlm.nih.gov:80/entrez/query.fcgi?cmd=Retrieve&db=PubMed&list_uids=12527130&dopt=Abstract

- **Experiences in the treatment of patients with tinnitus and/or hyperacusis using the habituation method.**
  Author(s): Bartnik G, Fabijanska A, Rogowski M.
  Source: Scand Audiol Suppl. 2001; (52): 187-90.
  http://www.ncbi.nlm.nih.gov:80/entrez/query.fcgi?cmd=Retrieve&db=PubMed&list_uids=11318464&dopt=Abstract

- **Explosive tinnitus: an underrecognized disorder.**
  Author(s): Teixido MT, Connolly K.
  Source: Otolaryngology and Head and Neck Surgery. 1998 January; 118(1): 108-9. Review.
  http://www.ncbi.nlm.nih.gov:80/entrez/query.fcgi?cmd=Retrieve&db=PubMed&list_uids=9450839&dopt=Abstract

- **Facial spasm and paroxysmal tinnitus associated with an arachnoid cyst of the cerebellopontine angle--case report.**
  Author(s): Takano S, Maruno T, Shirai S, Nose T.
  Source: Neurol Med Chir (Tokyo). 1998 February; 38(2): 100-3.
  http://www.ncbi.nlm.nih.gov:80/entrez/query.fcgi?cmd=Retrieve&db=PubMed&list_uids=9557537&dopt=Abstract

- **Factor analysis of the Tinnitus Handicap Inventory.**
  Author(s): Baguley DM, Andersson G.
  Source: American Journal of Audiology. 2003 June; 12(1): 31-4.
  http://www.ncbi.nlm.nih.gov:80/entrez/query.fcgi?cmd=Retrieve&db=PubMed&list_uids=12894865&dopt=Abstract

- **Fluoxetine for treatment of tinnitus.**
  Author(s): Shemen L.
  Source: Otolaryngology and Head and Neck Surgery. 1998 March; 118(3 Pt 1): 421.
  http://www.ncbi.nlm.nih.gov:80/entrez/query.fcgi?cmd=Retrieve&db=PubMed&list_uids=9527133&dopt=Abstract

- **Forensic aspects of tinnitus in Belgium and France.**
  Author(s): Boniver R.
  Source: Int Tinnitus J. 1999; 5(1): 67-70.
  http://www.ncbi.nlm.nih.gov:80/entrez/query.fcgi?cmd=Retrieve&db=PubMed&list_uids=10753425&dopt=Abstract

- **Functional brain imaging of tinnitus-like perception induced by aversive auditory stimuli.**
  Author(s): Mirz F, Gjedde A, Sodkilde-Jrgensen H, Pedersen CB.
  Source: Neuroreport. 2000 February 28; 11(3): 633-7.
  http://www.ncbi.nlm.nih.gov:80/entrez/query.fcgi?cmd=Retrieve&db=PubMed&list_uids=10718327&dopt=Abstract

- **Further validation of the Iowa tinnitus handicap questionnaire.**
  Author(s): Bouscau-Faure F, Keller P, Dauman R.
  Source: Acta Oto-Laryngologica. 2003 January; 123(2): 227-31.
  http://www.ncbi.nlm.nih.gov:80/entrez/query.fcgi?cmd=Retrieve&db=PubMed&list_uids=12701746&dopt=Abstract

- **Gabapentin for the treatment of tinnitus: a case report.**
  Author(s): Zapp JJ.
  Source: Ear, Nose, & Throat Journal. 2001 February; 80(2): 114-6.
  http://www.ncbi.nlm.nih.gov:80/entrez/query.fcgi?cmd=Retrieve&db=PubMed&list_uids=11233342&dopt=Abstract

- **Gaze-evoked tinnitus following acoustic neuroma resection: a de-afferentation plasticity phenomenon?**
  Author(s): Biggs ND, Ramsden RT.
  Source: Clinical Otolaryngology and Allied Sciences. 2002 October; 27(5): 338-43.
  http://www.ncbi.nlm.nih.gov:80/entrez/query.fcgi?cmd=Retrieve&db=PubMed&list_uids=12383293&dopt=Abstract

- **Gingko biloba (Rokan) therapy in tinnitus patients and measurable interactions between tinnitus and vestibular disturbances.**
  Author(s): Schneider D, Schneider L, Shulman A, Claussen CF, Just E, Koltchev C, Kersebaum M, Dehler R, Goldstein B, Claussen E.
  Source: Int Tinnitus J. 2000; 6(1): 56-62.
  http://www.ncbi.nlm.nih.gov:80/entrez/query.fcgi?cmd=Retrieve&db=PubMed&list_uids=14689620&dopt=Abstract

- **Ginkgo biloba extract for the treatment of tinnitus.**
  Author(s): Holgers KM, Axelsson A, Pringle I.
  Source: Audiology : Official Organ of the International Society of Audiology. 1994 March-April; 33(2): 85-92.
  http://www.ncbi.nlm.nih.gov:80/entrez/query.fcgi?cmd=Retrieve&db=PubMed&list_uids=8179518&dopt=Abstract

- **Ginkgo biloba for tinnitus: a review.**
  Author(s): Ernst E, Stevinson C.
  Source: Clinical Otolaryngology and Allied Sciences. 1999 June; 24(3): 164-7. Review.
  http://www.ncbi.nlm.nih.gov:80/entrez/query.fcgi?cmd=Retrieve&db=PubMed&list_uids=10384838&dopt=Abstract

- **Ginkgo ineffective for tinnitus.**
  Author(s): DeBisschop M.
  Source: The Journal of Family Practice. 2003 October; 52(10): 766, 769.
  http://www.ncbi.nlm.nih.gov:80/entrez/query.fcgi?cmd=Retrieve&db=PubMed&list_uids=14529599&dopt=Abstract

- **Growth behavior of the 2 f1-f2 distortion product otoacoustic emission in tinnitus.**
  Author(s): Janssen T, Kummer P, Arnold W.
  Source: The Journal of the Acoustical Society of America. 1998 June; 103(6): 3418-30.
  http://www.ncbi.nlm.nih.gov:80/entrez/query.fcgi?cmd=Retrieve&db=PubMed&list_uids=9637029&dopt=Abstract

- **Guidelines for the grading of tinnitus severity: the results of a working group commissioned by the British Association of Otolaryngologists, Head and Neck Surgeons, 1999.**
  Author(s): McCombe A, Baguley D, Coles R, McKenna L, McKinney C, Windle-Taylor P; British Association of Otolaryngologists, Head and Neck Surgeons.
  Source: Clinical Otolaryngology and Allied Sciences. 2001 October; 26(5): 388-93.
  http://www.ncbi.nlm.nih.gov:80/entrez/query.fcgi?cmd=Retrieve&db=PubMed&list_uids=11678946&dopt=Abstract

- **Health and Nutrition Examination Survey of 1971-75: Part II. Tinnitus, subjective hearing loss, and well-being.**
  Author(s): Cooper JC Jr.
  Source: Journal of the American Academy of Audiology. 1994 January; 5(1): 37-43.
  http://www.ncbi.nlm.nih.gov:80/entrez/query.fcgi?cmd=Retrieve&db=PubMed&list_uids=8155893&dopt=Abstract

- **Hearing impairment and tinnitus pitch in patients with unilateral tinnitus: comparison of sudden hearing loss and chronic tinnitus.**
  Author(s): Ochi K, Ohashi T, Kenmochi M.
  Source: The Laryngoscope. 2003 March; 113(3): 427-31.
  http://www.ncbi.nlm.nih.gov:80/entrez/query.fcgi?cmd=Retrieve&db=PubMed&list_uids=12616191&dopt=Abstract

- **Hearing loss and tinnitus in acute acoustic trauma.**
  Author(s): Temmel AF, Kierner AC, Steurer M, Riedl S, Innitzer J.
  Source: Wiener Klinische Wochenschrift. 1999 November 12; 111(21): 891-3.
  http://www.ncbi.nlm.nih.gov:80/entrez/query.fcgi?cmd=Retrieve&db=PubMed&list_uids=10599152&dopt=Abstract

- **Hearing loss and tinnitus in Meniere's disease.**
  Author(s): Havia M, Kentala E, Pyykko I.
  Source: Auris, Nasus, Larynx. 2002 April; 29(2): 115-9.
  http://www.ncbi.nlm.nih.gov:80/entrez/query.fcgi?cmd=Retrieve&db=PubMed&list_uids=11893444&dopt=Abstract

- **Hearing loss and tinnitus with carbimazole.**
  Author(s): Hill D, Whittet H, Simpson H.
  Source: Bmj (Clinical Research Ed.). 1994 October 8; 309(6959): 929.
  http://www.ncbi.nlm.nih.gov:80/entrez/query.fcgi?cmd=Retrieve&db=PubMed&list_uids=7950664&dopt=Abstract

- **Hypnosis as an aid for tinnitus patients.**
  Author(s): Kaye JM, Marlowe FI, Ramchandani D, Berman S, Schindler B, Loscalzo G.
  Source: Ear, Nose, & Throat Journal. 1994 May; 73(5): 309-12, 315.
  http://www.ncbi.nlm.nih.gov:80/entrez/query.fcgi?cmd=Retrieve&db=PubMed&list_uids=8045234&dopt=Abstract

- **Iatrogenic pulsatile tinnitus.**
  Author(s): Agrawal R, Flood LM, Bradey N.
  Source: The Journal of Laryngology and Otology. 1993 May; 107(5): 445-7.
  http://www.ncbi.nlm.nih.gov:80/entrez/query.fcgi?cmd=Retrieve&db=PubMed&list_uids=8326228&dopt=Abstract

- **Imaging of neurovascular compression in tinnitus.**
  Author(s): Meaney JF, Miles JB, Mackenzie IJ.
  Source: Lancet. 1994 July 16; 344(8916): 200-1.
  http://www.ncbi.nlm.nih.gov:80/entrez/query.fcgi?cmd=Retrieve&db=PubMed&list_uids=7912800&dopt=Abstract

- **Imaging of pulsatile tinnitus: basic examination versus comprehensive examination package.**
  Author(s): Hasso AN.
  Source: Ajnr. American Journal of Neuroradiology. 1994 May; 15(5): 890-2.
  http://www.ncbi.nlm.nih.gov:80/entrez/query.fcgi?cmd=Retrieve&db=PubMed&list_uids=8059656&dopt=Abstract

- **Imaging of tinnitus: a review.**
  Author(s): Weissman JL, Hirsch BE.
  Source: Radiology. 2000 August; 216(2): 342-9. Review.
  http://www.ncbi.nlm.nih.gov:80/entrez/query.fcgi?cmd=Retrieve&db=PubMed&list_uids=10924551&dopt=Abstract

- **Impact of a relaxation training on psychometric and immunologic parameters in tinnitus sufferers.**
  Author(s): Weber C, Arck P, Mazurek B, Klapp BF.
  Source: Journal of Psychosomatic Research. 2002 January; 52(1): 29-33.
  http://www.ncbi.nlm.nih.gov:80/entrez/query.fcgi?cmd=Retrieve&db=PubMed&list_uids=11801262&dopt=Abstract

- **Impaired brain processing in noise-induced tinnitus patients as measured by auditory and visual event-related potentials.**
  Author(s): Attias J, Furman V, Shemesh Z, Bresloff I.
  Source: Ear and Hearing. 1996 August; 17(4): 327-33.
  http://www.ncbi.nlm.nih.gov:80/entrez/query.fcgi?cmd=Retrieve&db=PubMed&list_uids=8862970&dopt=Abstract

- **Importance of behavior in response to tinnitus symptoms.**
  Author(s): Savastano M, Maron MB.
  Source: Int Tinnitus J. 1999; 5(2): 121-4.
  http://www.ncbi.nlm.nih.gov:80/entrez/query.fcgi?cmd=Retrieve&db=PubMed&list_uids=10753430&dopt=Abstract

- **Improved word perception following electrical stimulation of the ear in hearing-impaired patients without tinnitus.**
  Author(s): Matsushima J, Kumagai M, Takeichi N, Uemi N, Miyoshi S, Sakajiri M, Ifukube T, Sakai N.
  Source: Acta Otolaryngol Suppl. 1997; 532: 119-22.
  http://www.ncbi.nlm.nih.gov:80/entrez/query.fcgi?cmd=Retrieve&db=PubMed&list_uids=9442858&dopt=Abstract

- **Improved word perception in tinnitus patients following electrical stimulation of the ear: a preliminary report.**
  Author(s): Matsushima J, Kumagai M, Takeichi N, Miyoshi S, Sakajiri M, Uemi N, Ifukube T, Sakai N.
  Source: Acta Otolaryngol Suppl. 1997; 532: 115-8.
  http://www.ncbi.nlm.nih.gov:80/entrez/query.fcgi?cmd=Retrieve&db=PubMed&list_uids=9442857&dopt=Abstract

- **Increases in spontaneous neural activity in the hamster dorsal cochlear nucleus following cisplatin treatment: a possible basis for cisplatin-induced tinnitus.**
  Author(s): Rachel JD, Kaltenbach JA, Janisse J.
  Source: Hearing Research. 2002 February; 164(1-2): 206-14.
  http://www.ncbi.nlm.nih.gov:80/entrez/query.fcgi?cmd=Retrieve&db=PubMed&list_uids=11950539&dopt=Abstract

- **Indirect carotid cavernous fistula presenting as pulsatile tinnitus.**
  Author(s): Mohyuddin A.
  Source: The Journal of Laryngology and Otology. 2000 October; 114(10): 788-9.
  http://www.ncbi.nlm.nih.gov:80/entrez/query.fcgi?cmd=Retrieve&db=PubMed&list_uids=11127153&dopt=Abstract

- **Internet administration of the Hospital Anxiety and Depression Scale in a sample of tinnitus patients.**
  Author(s): Andersson G, Kaldo-Sandstrom V, Strom L, Stromgren T.
  Source: Journal of Psychosomatic Research. 2003 September; 55(3): 259-62.
  http://www.ncbi.nlm.nih.gov:80/entrez/query.fcgi?cmd=Retrieve&db=PubMed&list_uids=12932800&dopt=Abstract

- **Intracochlear electrical tinnitus reduction.**
  Author(s): Dauman R, Tyler RS, Aran JM.
  Source: Acta Oto-Laryngologica. 1993 May; 113(3): 291-5.
  http://www.ncbi.nlm.nih.gov:80/entrez/query.fcgi?cmd=Retrieve&db=PubMed&list_uids=8517130&dopt=Abstract

- **Intradermal injection vs. oral treatment of tinnitus.**
  Author(s): Savastano M, Tomaselli F, Maggiori S.
  Source: Therapie. 2001 July-August; 56(4): 403-7.
  http://www.ncbi.nlm.nih.gov:80/entrez/query.fcgi?cmd=Retrieve&db=PubMed&list_uids=11677863&dopt=Abstract

- **Intratympanic drug therapy with steroids for tinnitus control: a preliminary report.**
  Author(s): Shulman A, Goldstein B.
  Source: Int Tinnitus J. 2000; 6(1): 10-20.
  http://www.ncbi.nlm.nih.gov:80/entrez/query.fcgi?cmd=Retrieve&db=PubMed&list_uids=14689612&dopt=Abstract

- **Intratympanic gentamicin in Meniere's disease: the impact on tinnitus.**
  Author(s): Yetiser S, Kertmen M.
  Source: International Journal of Audiology. 2002 September; 41(6): 363-70.
  http://www.ncbi.nlm.nih.gov:80/entrez/query.fcgi?cmd=Retrieve&db=PubMed&list_uids=12353609&dopt=Abstract

- **Intratympanic steroid treatment of inner ear disease and tinnitus (preliminary report).**
  Author(s): Silverstein H, Choo D, Rosenberg SI, Kuhn J, Seidman M, Stein I.
  Source: Ear, Nose, & Throat Journal. 1996 August; 75(8): 468-71, 474, 476 Passim.
  http://www.ncbi.nlm.nih.gov:80/entrez/query.fcgi?cmd=Retrieve&db=PubMed&list_uids=8828271&dopt=Abstract

- **Is biofeedback effective for chronic tinnitus? An intensive study with seven subjects.**
  Author(s): Landis B, Landis E.
  Source: American Journal of Otolaryngology. 1992 November-December; 13(6): 349-56.
  http://www.ncbi.nlm.nih.gov:80/entrez/query.fcgi?cmd=Retrieve&db=PubMed&list_uids=1443390&dopt=Abstract

- **Is perilymphatic pressure altered in tinnitus?**
  Author(s): Wable J, Museux F, Collet L, Morgon A, Chery-Croze S.
  Source: Acta Oto-Laryngologica. 1996 March; 116(2): 205-8.
  http://www.ncbi.nlm.nih.gov:80/entrez/query.fcgi?cmd=Retrieve&db=PubMed&list_uids=8725515&dopt=Abstract

- **Is the test of medial efferent system function a relevant investigation in tinnitus?**
  Author(s): Chery-Croze S, Moulin A, Collet L, Morgon A.
  Source: British Journal of Audiology. 1994 February; 28(1): 13-25.
  http://www.ncbi.nlm.nih.gov:80/entrez/query.fcgi?cmd=Retrieve&db=PubMed&list_uids=7987268&dopt=Abstract

- **Late course of preserved hearing and tinnitus after acoustic neurilemoma surgery.**
  Author(s): Goel A, Sekhar LN, Langheinrich W, Kamerer D, Hirsch B.
  Source: Journal of Neurosurgery. 1992 November; 77(5): 685-9.
  http://www.ncbi.nlm.nih.gov:80/entrez/query.fcgi?cmd=Retrieve&db=PubMed&list_uids=1403107&dopt=Abstract

- **Lateral inhibition in the auditory cortex: an EEG index of tinnitus?**
  Author(s): Kadner A, Viirre E, Wester DC, Walsh SF, Hestenes J, Vankov A, Pineda JA.
  Source: Neuroreport. 2002 March 25; 13(4): 443-6.
  http://www.ncbi.nlm.nih.gov:80/entrez/query.fcgi?cmd=Retrieve&db=PubMed&list_uids=11930157&dopt=Abstract

- **Lateralized carotid artery: an unusual cause of pulsatile tinnitus.**
  Author(s): Pak MW, Kew J, Andrew van Hasselt C.
  Source: Ear, Nose, & Throat Journal. 2001 March; 80(3): 148-9.
  http://www.ncbi.nlm.nih.gov:80/entrez/query.fcgi?cmd=Retrieve&db=PubMed&list_uids=11269217&dopt=Abstract

- **Lateralized tinnitus studied with functional magnetic resonance imaging: abnormal inferior colliculus activation.**
  Author(s): Melcher JR, Sigalovsky IS, Guinan JJ Jr, Levine RA.
  Source: Journal of Neurophysiology. 2000 February; 83(2): 1058-72.
  http://www.ncbi.nlm.nih.gov:80/entrez/query.fcgi?cmd=Retrieve&db=PubMed&list_uids=10669517&dopt=Abstract

- **Lemonade out of lemons--tinnitus retraining therapy.**
  Author(s): Nagler S.
  Source: J Med Assoc Ga. 1998 September; 87(3): 220-3. No Abstract Available.
  http://www.ncbi.nlm.nih.gov:80/entrez/query.fcgi?cmd=Retrieve&db=PubMed&list_uids=9747080&dopt=Abstract

- **Lidocaine test in patients with tinnitus: rationale of accomplishment and relation to the treatment with carbamazepine.**
  Author(s): Sanchez TG, Balbani AP, Bittar RS, Bento RF, Camara J.
  Source: Auris, Nasus, Larynx. 1999 October; 26(4): 411-7.
  http://www.ncbi.nlm.nih.gov:80/entrez/query.fcgi?cmd=Retrieve&db=PubMed&list_uids=10530736&dopt=Abstract

- **Life-threatening tinnitus.**
  Author(s): Javaheri S, Cohen V, Libman I, Sandor V.
  Source: Lancet. 2000 July 22; 356(9226): 308.
  http://www.ncbi.nlm.nih.gov:80/entrez/query.fcgi?cmd=Retrieve&db=PubMed&list_uids=11071187&dopt=Abstract

- **Ligation of the internal jugular vein in venous hum tinnitus.**
  Author(s): Nehru VI, al-Khaboori MJ, Kishore K.
  Source: The Journal of Laryngology and Otology. 1993 November; 107(11): 1037-8.
  http://www.ncbi.nlm.nih.gov:80/entrez/query.fcgi?cmd=Retrieve&db=PubMed&list_uids=8288976&dopt=Abstract

- **Longitudinal follow-up of occupational status in tinnitus patients.**
  Author(s): Andersson G.
  Source: Int Tinnitus J. 2000; 6(2): 127-9.
  http://www.ncbi.nlm.nih.gov:80/entrez/query.fcgi?cmd=Retrieve&db=PubMed&list_uids=14689630&dopt=Abstract

- **Longitudinal follow-up of tinnitus complaints.**
  Author(s): Andersson G, Vretblad P, Larsen HC, Lyttkens L.
  Source: Archives of Otolaryngology--Head & Neck Surgery. 2001 February; 127(2): 175-9.
  http://www.ncbi.nlm.nih.gov:80/entrez/query.fcgi?cmd=Retrieve&db=PubMed&list_uids=11177034&dopt=Abstract

- **Long-term effect of hyperbaric oxygenation treatment on chronic distressing tinnitus.**
  Author(s): Tan J, Tange RA, Dreschler WA, vd Kleij A, Tromp EC.
  Source: Scandinavian Audiology. 1999; 28(2): 91-6.
  http://www.ncbi.nlm.nih.gov:80/entrez/query.fcgi?cmd=Retrieve&db=PubMed&list_uids=10384896&dopt=Abstract

- **Magnetic resonance imaging and tinnitus.**
  Author(s): Vernon J, Press L, McLaughlin T.
  Source: Otolaryngology and Head and Neck Surgery. 1996 December; 115(6): 587-8.
  http://www.ncbi.nlm.nih.gov:80/entrez/query.fcgi?cmd=Retrieve&db=PubMed&list_uids=8969772&dopt=Abstract

- **Magnetic resonance imaging in patients with sudden hearing loss, tinnitus and vertigo.**
  Author(s): Schick B, Brors D, Koch O, Schafers M, Kahle G.
  Source: Otology & Neurotology : Official Publication of the American Otological Society, American Neurotology Society [and] European Academy of Otology and Neurotology. 2001 November; 22(6): 808-12.
  http://www.ncbi.nlm.nih.gov:80/entrez/query.fcgi?cmd=Retrieve&db=PubMed&list_uids=11698800&dopt=Abstract

- **Managing tinnitus: a comparison of different approaches to tinnitus management training.**
  Author(s): Dineen R, Doyle J, Bench J.
  Source: British Journal of Audiology. 1997 October; 31(5): 331-44.
  http://www.ncbi.nlm.nih.gov:80/entrez/query.fcgi?cmd=Retrieve&db=PubMed&list_uids=9373742&dopt=Abstract

- **Masking devices and alprazolam treatment for tinnitus.**
  Author(s): Vernon JA, Meikle MB.
  Source: Otolaryngologic Clinics of North America. 2003 April; 36(2): 307-20, Vii. Review.
  http://www.ncbi.nlm.nih.gov:80/entrez/query.fcgi?cmd=Retrieve&db=PubMed&list_uids=12856299&dopt=Abstract

- **Masking effects and tinnitus as explanatory variables in hearing disability.**
  Author(s): Corthals P, Vinck B, De Vel E, Van Cauwenberge P.
  Source: Scandinavian Audiology. 1998; 27(1): 31-6.
  http://www.ncbi.nlm.nih.gov:80/entrez/query.fcgi?cmd=Retrieve&db=PubMed&list_uids=9505289&dopt=Abstract

- **Masking of tinnitus and mental activity.**
  Author(s): Andersson G, Khakpoor A, Lyttkens L.
  Source: Clinical Otolaryngology and Allied Sciences. 2002 August; 27(4): 270-4.
  http://www.ncbi.nlm.nih.gov:80/entrez/query.fcgi?cmd=Retrieve&db=PubMed&list_uids=12169130&dopt=Abstract

- **Masking of tinnitus through a cochlear implant.**
  Author(s): Vernon JA.
  Source: Journal of the American Academy of Audiology. 2000 June; 11(6): 293-4.
  http://www.ncbi.nlm.nih.gov:80/entrez/query.fcgi?cmd=Retrieve&db=PubMed&list_uids=10857999&dopt=Abstract

- **Measures of tinnitus: step size, matches to imagined tones, and masking patterns.**
  Author(s): Penner MJ, Klafter EJ.
  Source: Ear and Hearing. 1992 December; 13(6): 410-6.
  http://www.ncbi.nlm.nih.gov:80/entrez/query.fcgi?cmd=Retrieve&db=PubMed&list_uids=1487103&dopt=Abstract

- **Mechanisms of tinnitus.**
  Author(s): Baguley DM.
  Source: British Medical Bulletin. 2002; 63: 195-212. Review.
  http://www.ncbi.nlm.nih.gov:80/entrez/query.fcgi?cmd=Retrieve&db=PubMed&list_uids=12324394&dopt=Abstract

- **Medical evaluation of tinnitus.**
  Author(s): Schwaber MK.
  Source: Otolaryngologic Clinics of North America. 2003 April; 36(2): 287-92, Vi. Review.
  http://www.ncbi.nlm.nih.gov:80/entrez/query.fcgi?cmd=Retrieve&db=PubMed&list_uids=12856297&dopt=Abstract

- **Medicolegal aspects of tinnitus.**
  Author(s): Hart CW.
  Source: Int Tinnitus J. 1999; 5(1): 63-6. Review. No Abstract Available.
  http://www.ncbi.nlm.nih.gov:80/entrez/query.fcgi?cmd=Retrieve&db=PubMed&list_uids=10753424&dopt=Abstract

- **Meeting the expectations of chronic tinnitus patients: comparison of a structured group therapy program for tinnitus management with a problem-solving group.**
  Author(s): Wise K, Rief W, Goebel G.
  Source: Journal of Psychosomatic Research. 1998 June; 44(6): 681-5.
  http://www.ncbi.nlm.nih.gov:80/entrez/query.fcgi?cmd=Retrieve&db=PubMed&list_uids=9678749&dopt=Abstract

- **Meningeal metastases from malignant melanoma presenting with gaze-evoked tinnitus.**
  Author(s): Caraceni A, Scolari S, Gallino G, Simonetti F.
  Source: Neurology. 1999 December 10; 53(9): 2207-8.
  http://www.ncbi.nlm.nih.gov:80/entrez/query.fcgi?cmd=Retrieve&db=PubMed&list_uids=10599812&dopt=Abstract

- **Microvascular decompression for tinnitus.**
  Author(s): Ko Y, Park CW.
  Source: Stereotactic and Functional Neurosurgery. 1997; 68(1-4 Pt 1): 266-9.
  http://www.ncbi.nlm.nih.gov:80/entrez/query.fcgi?cmd=Retrieve&db=PubMed&list_uids=9711727&dopt=Abstract

- **Microvascular decompression of the cochlear nerve in patients with severe tinnitus. Preoperative findings and operative outcome in 22 patients.**
    Author(s): Vasama JP, Moller MB, Moller AR.
    Source: Neurological Research. 1998 April; 20(3): 242-8.
    http://www.ncbi.nlm.nih.gov:80/entrez/query.fcgi?cmd=Retrieve&db=PubMed&list_uids=9583586&dopt=Abstract

- **Minnesota Multiphasic Personality Inventory profile of patients with subjective tinnitus.**
    Author(s): Bayar N, Oguzturk O, Koc C.
    Source: The Journal of Otolaryngology. 2002 October; 31(5): 317-22.
    http://www.ncbi.nlm.nih.gov:80/entrez/query.fcgi?cmd=Retrieve&db=PubMed&list_uids=12512898&dopt=Abstract

- **Modulation of tinnitus by voluntary jaw movements.**
    Author(s): Pinchoff RJ, Burkard RF, Salvi RJ, Coad ML, Lockwood AH.
    Source: The American Journal of Otology. 1998 November; 19(6): 785-9.
    http://www.ncbi.nlm.nih.gov:80/entrez/query.fcgi?cmd=Retrieve&db=PubMed&list_uids=9831155&dopt=Abstract

- **Movement-induced transient tinnitus.**
    Author(s): Kunkle EC.
    Source: The Annals of Otology, Rhinology, and Laryngology. 2001 May; 110(5 Pt 1): 494.
    http://www.ncbi.nlm.nih.gov:80/entrez/query.fcgi?cmd=Retrieve&db=PubMed&list_uids=11372937&dopt=Abstract

- **Myths in neurotology, revisited: smoke and mirrors in tinnitus therapy.**
    Author(s): Nagler SM.
    Source: Otology & Neurotology : Official Publication of the American Otological Society, American Neurotology Society [and] European Academy of Otology and Neurotology. 2002 March; 23(2): 239-40.
    http://www.ncbi.nlm.nih.gov:80/entrez/query.fcgi?cmd=Retrieve&db=PubMed&list_uids=11875359&dopt=Abstract

- **Myths in neurotology, revisited: smoke and mirrors in tinnitus therapy.**
  Author(s): Howard ML.
  Source: Otology & Neurotology : Official Publication of the American Otological Society, American Neurotology Society [and] European Academy of Otology and Neurotology. 2001 November; 22(6): 711-4.
  http://www.ncbi.nlm.nih.gov:80/entrez/query.fcgi?cmd=Retrieve&db=PubMed&list_uids=11698785&dopt=Abstract

- **Neural mechanisms of tinnitus.**
  Author(s): Lenarz T, Schreiner C, Snyder RL, Ernst A.
  Source: European Archives of Oto-Rhino-Laryngology : Official Journal of the European Federation of Oto-Rhino-Laryngological Societies (Eufos) : Affiliated with the German Society for Oto-Rhino-Laryngology - Head and Neck Surgery. 1993; 249(8): 441-6. Review.
  http://www.ncbi.nlm.nih.gov:80/entrez/query.fcgi?cmd=Retrieve&db=PubMed&list_uids=8442938&dopt=Abstract

- **Neuroanatomy of tinnitus.**
  Author(s): Lockwood AH, Salvi RJ, Burkard RF, Galantowicz PJ, Coad ML, Wack DS.
  Source: Scand Audiol Suppl. 1999; 51: 47-52.
  http://www.ncbi.nlm.nih.gov:80/entrez/query.fcgi?cmd=Retrieve&db=PubMed&list_uids=10803913&dopt=Abstract

- **Neuronavigated repetitive transcranial magnetic stimulation in patients with tinnitus: a short case series.**
  Author(s): Eichhammer P, Langguth B, Marienhagen J, Kleinjung T, Hajak G.
  Source: Biological Psychiatry. 2003 October 15; 54(8): 862-5.
  http://www.ncbi.nlm.nih.gov:80/entrez/query.fcgi?cmd=Retrieve&db=PubMed&list_uids=14550687&dopt=Abstract

- **Neuronavigated rTMS in a patient with chronic tinnitus. Effects of 4 weeks treatment.**
  Author(s): Langguth B, Eichhammer P, Wiegand R, Marienhegen J, Maenner P, Jacob P, Hajak G.
  Source: Neuroreport. 2003 May 23; 14(7): 977-80.
  http://www.ncbi.nlm.nih.gov:80/entrez/query.fcgi?cmd=Retrieve&db=PubMed&list_uids=12802186&dopt=Abstract

- **Neurophysiologic mechanisms of tinnitus.**
  Author(s): Kaltenbach JA.
  Source: Journal of the American Academy of Audiology. 2000 March; 11(3): 125-37. Review.
  http://www.ncbi.nlm.nih.gov:80/entrez/query.fcgi?cmd=Retrieve&db=PubMed&list_uids=10755809&dopt=Abstract

- **Neurophysiological approach to tinnitus patients.**
  Author(s): Baguley D.
  Source: The American Journal of Otology. 1997 March; 18(2): 265-6.
  http://www.ncbi.nlm.nih.gov:80/entrez/query.fcgi?cmd=Retrieve&db=PubMed&list_uids=9093687&dopt=Abstract

- **Neurophysiological approach to tinnitus patients.**
  Author(s): Jastreboff PJ, Gray WC, Gold SL.
  Source: The American Journal of Otology. 1996 March; 17(2): 236-40. Review.
  http://www.ncbi.nlm.nih.gov:80/entrez/query.fcgi?cmd=Retrieve&db=PubMed&list_uids=8723954&dopt=Abstract

- **Neurophysiological model of tinnitus: dependence of the minimal masking level on treatment outcome.**
  Author(s): Jastreboff PJ, Hazell JW, Graham RL.
  Source: Hearing Research. 1994 November; 80(2): 216-32.
  http://www.ncbi.nlm.nih.gov:80/entrez/query.fcgi?cmd=Retrieve&db=PubMed&list_uids=7896580&dopt=Abstract

- **Neurovascular decompression for tinnitus.**
  Author(s): Bayazit Y.
  Source: Journal of Neurosurgery. 1998 December; 89(6): 1072-3.
  http://www.ncbi.nlm.nih.gov:80/entrez/query.fcgi?cmd=Retrieve&db=PubMed&list_uids=9833843&dopt=Abstract

- **Neurovascular decompression of the eighth cranial nerve in patients with hemifacial spasm and incidental tinnitus: an alternative way to study tinnitus.**
  Author(s): Ryu H, Yamamoto S, Sugiyama K, Uemura K, Nozue M.
  Source: Journal of Neurosurgery. 1998 February; 88(2): 232-6.
  http://www.ncbi.nlm.nih.gov:80/entrez/query.fcgi?cmd=Retrieve&db=PubMed&list_uids=9452229&dopt=Abstract

- **Nutrition, biochemistry, and tinnitus.**
  Author(s): Rubin W.
  Source: Int Tinnitus J. 1999; 5(2): 144-5. Review.
  http://www.ncbi.nlm.nih.gov:80/entrez/query.fcgi?cmd=Retrieve&db=PubMed&list_uids=10753435&dopt=Abstract

- **Objective pulsatile tinnitus caused by intrapetrous dissecting aneurysm.**
  Author(s): Depauw P, Caekebeke J, Vanhoenacker P.
  Source: Clinical Neurology and Neurosurgery. 2001 October; 103(3): 197-9.
  http://www.ncbi.nlm.nih.gov:80/entrez/query.fcgi?cmd=Retrieve&db=PubMed&list_uids=11532564&dopt=Abstract

- **Objective tinnitus associated with essential laryngeal myoclonus: report of two cases.**
  Author(s): Bertholon P, Convers P, Antoine JC, Mayaud R, Prades JM, Michel D, Martin C.
  Source: Movement Disorders : Official Journal of the Movement Disorder Society. 2002 January; 17(1): 218-20.
  http://www.ncbi.nlm.nih.gov:80/entrez/query.fcgi?cmd=Retrieve&db=PubMed&list_uids=11835471&dopt=Abstract

- **Objective tinnitus caused by an aberrant internal carotid artery.**
  Author(s): Koizuka I, Hattori K, Tsutsumi K, Sakuma A, Katsumi N, Kikuchi H, Kato I.
  Source: Auris, Nasus, Larynx. 1998 September; 25(3): 323-7.
  http://www.ncbi.nlm.nih.gov:80/entrez/query.fcgi?cmd=Retrieve&db=PubMed&list_uids=9800001&dopt=Abstract

- **Objective tinnitus in children.**
  Author(s): Fritsch MH, Wynne MK, Matt BH, Smith WL, Smith CM.
  Source: Otology & Neurotology : Official Publication of the American Otological Society, American Neurotology Society [and] European Academy of Otology and Neurotology. 2001 September; 22(5): 644-9.
  http://www.ncbi.nlm.nih.gov:80/entrez/query.fcgi?cmd=Retrieve&db=PubMed&list_uids=11568673&dopt=Abstract

- **Objective tinnitus in patients with atherosclerotic carotid artery disease.**
  Author(s): Sismanis A, Stamm MA, Sobel M.
  Source: The American Journal of Otology. 1994 May; 15(3): 404-7.
  http://www.ncbi.nlm.nih.gov:80/entrez/query.fcgi?cmd=Retrieve&db=PubMed&list_uids=8579149&dopt=Abstract

- **Objective tinnitus resulting from internal carotid artery stenosis.**
  Author(s): Carlin RE, McGraw DJ, Anderson CB.
  Source: Journal of Vascular Surgery : Official Publication, the Society for Vascular Surgery [and] International Society for Cardiovascular Surgery, North American Chapter. 1997 March; 25(3): 581-3.
  http://www.ncbi.nlm.nih.gov:80/entrez/query.fcgi?cmd=Retrieve&db=PubMed&list_uids=9081143&dopt=Abstract

- **On the evidence of auditory evoked magnetic fields as an objective measure of tinnitus.**
  Author(s): Colding-Jorgensen E, Lauritzen M, Johnsen NJ, Mikkelsen KB, Saermark K.
  Source: Electroencephalography and Clinical Neurophysiology. 1992 November; 83(5): 322-7.
  http://www.ncbi.nlm.nih.gov:80/entrez/query.fcgi?cmd=Retrieve&db=PubMed&list_uids=1385088&dopt=Abstract

- **Organization of tinnitus management in Poland.**
  Author(s): Skarzynski H, Rogowski M, Bartnik G, Fabijanska A.
  Source: Acta Oto-Laryngologica. 2000 March; 120(2): 225-6.
  http://www.ncbi.nlm.nih.gov:80/entrez/query.fcgi?cmd=Retrieve&db=PubMed&list_uids=11603778&dopt=Abstract

- **Orthostatic tinnitus: an otological presentation of spontaneous intracranial hypotension.**
  Author(s): Arai M, Takada T, Nozue M.
  Source: Auris, Nasus, Larynx. 2003 February; 30(1): 85-7.
  http://www.ncbi.nlm.nih.gov:80/entrez/query.fcgi?cmd=Retrieve&db=PubMed&list_uids=12589857&dopt=Abstract

- **Otosclerosis and chronic tinnitus.**
  Author(s): Gristwood RE, Venables WN.
  Source: The Annals of Otology, Rhinology, and Laryngology. 2003 May; 112(5): 398-403.
  http://www.ncbi.nlm.nih.gov:80/entrez/query.fcgi?cmd=Retrieve&db=PubMed&list_uids=12784976&dopt=Abstract

- **Outcome after microvascular decompression for typical trigeminal neuralgia, hemifacial spasm, tinnitus, disabling positional vertigo, and glossopharyngeal neuralgia (honored guest lecture).**
  Author(s): Jannetta PJ.
  Source: Clin Neurosurg. 1997; 44: 331-83. Review. No Abstract Available.
  http://www.ncbi.nlm.nih.gov:80/entrez/query.fcgi?cmd=Retrieve&db=PubMed&list_uids=10080016&dopt=Abstract

- **Outcome of using magnetic resonance imaging as an initial screen to exclude vestibular schwannoma in patients presenting with unilateral tinnitus.**
  Author(s): Dawes PJ, Basiouny HE.
  Source: The Journal of Laryngology and Otology. 1999 September; 113(9): 818-22.
  http://www.ncbi.nlm.nih.gov:80/entrez/query.fcgi?cmd=Retrieve&db=PubMed&list_uids=10664684&dopt=Abstract

- **Paroxetine in the treatment of tinnitus.**
  Author(s): Christensen RC.
  Source: Otolaryngology and Head and Neck Surgery. 2001 October; 125(4): 436-8.
  http://www.ncbi.nlm.nih.gov:80/entrez/query.fcgi?cmd=Retrieve&db=PubMed&list_uids=11593197&dopt=Abstract

- **Pathophysiology of tinnitus.**
  Author(s): Moller AR.
  Source: Otolaryngologic Clinics of North America. 2003 April; 36(2): 249-66, V-Vi. Review.
  http://www.ncbi.nlm.nih.gov:80/entrez/query.fcgi?cmd=Retrieve&db=PubMed&list_uids=12856295&dopt=Abstract

- **Patient-based outcomes in patients with primary tinnitus undergoing tinnitus retraining therapy.**
  Author(s): Berry JA, Gold SL, Frederick EA, Gray WC, Staecker H.
  Source: Archives of Otolaryngology--Head & Neck Surgery. 2002 October; 128(10): 1153-7.
  http://www.ncbi.nlm.nih.gov:80/entrez/query.fcgi?cmd=Retrieve&db=PubMed&list_uids=12365886&dopt=Abstract

- **Pharmacological approach of tinnitus.**
  Author(s): Oestreicher E.
  Source: Acta Otorhinolaryngol Belg. 2002; 56(4): 353-4. Review. No Abstract Available.
  http://www.ncbi.nlm.nih.gov:80/entrez/query.fcgi?cmd=Retrieve&db=PubMed&list_uids=12674088&dopt=Abstract

- **Postdural puncture tinnitus.**
  Author(s): Wong AY, Irwin MG.
  Source: British Journal of Anaesthesia. 2003 November; 91(5): 762-3.
  http://www.ncbi.nlm.nih.gov:80/entrez/query.fcgi?cmd=Retrieve&db=PubMed&list_uids=14570815&dopt=Abstract

- **Predictive factors for the severity of tinnitus.**
  Author(s): Holgers KM, Erlandsson SI, Barrenas ML.
  Source: Audiology : Official Organ of the International Society of Audiology. 2000 September-October; 39(5): 284-91. Review.
  http://www.ncbi.nlm.nih.gov:80/entrez/query.fcgi?cmd=Retrieve&db=PubMed&list_uids=11093613&dopt=Abstract

- **Prevalence and 5-year incidence of tinnitus among older adults: the epidemiology of hearing loss study.**
  Author(s): Nondahl DM, Cruickshanks KJ, Wiley TL, Klein R, Klein BE, Tweed TS.
  Source: Journal of the American Academy of Audiology. 2002 June; 13(6): 323-31.
  http://www.ncbi.nlm.nih.gov:80/entrez/query.fcgi?cmd=Retrieve&db=PubMed&list_uids=12141389&dopt=Abstract

- **Prevalence and characteristics of tinnitus in older adults: the Blue Mountains Hearing Study.**
  Author(s): Sindhusake D, Mitchell P, Newall P, Golding M, Rochtchina E, Rubin G.
  Source: International Journal of Audiology. 2003 July; 42(5): 289-94.
  http://www.ncbi.nlm.nih.gov:80/entrez/query.fcgi?cmd=Retrieve&db=PubMed&list_uids=12916702&dopt=Abstract

- **Psychiatric comorbidity in a population of outpatients affected by tinnitus.**
  Author(s): Marciano E, Carrabba L, Giannini P, Sementina C, Verde P, Bruno C, Di Pietro G, Ponsillo NG.
  Source: International Journal of Audiology. 2003 January; 42(1): 4-9.
  http://www.ncbi.nlm.nih.gov:80/entrez/query.fcgi?cmd=Retrieve&db=PubMed&list_uids=12564510&dopt=Abstract

- **Psychiatric disorders in tinnitus patients without severe hearing impairment: 24 month follow-up of patients at an audiological clinic.**
  Author(s): Zoger S, Svedlund J, Holgers KM.
  Source: Audiology : Official Organ of the International Society of Audiology. 2001 May-June; 40(3): 133-40.
  http://www.ncbi.nlm.nih.gov:80/entrez/query.fcgi?cmd=Retrieve&db=PubMed&list_uids=11465295&dopt=Abstract

- **Psychoacoustic characterization of the tinnitus spectrum: implications for the underlying mechanisms of tinnitus.**
  Author(s): Norena A, Micheyl C, Chery-Croze S, Collet L.
  Source: Audiology & Neuro-Otology. 2002 November-December; 7(6): 358-69.
  http://www.ncbi.nlm.nih.gov:80/entrez/query.fcgi?cmd=Retrieve&db=PubMed&list_uids=12401967&dopt=Abstract

- **Psychoacoustic measures of tinnitus.**
  Author(s): Henry JA, Meikle MB.
  Source: Journal of the American Academy of Audiology. 2000 March; 11(3): 138-55. Review.
  http://www.ncbi.nlm.nih.gov:80/entrez/query.fcgi?cmd=Retrieve&db=PubMed&list_uids=10755810&dopt=Abstract

- **Psychologic profile of tinnitus patients using the SCL-90-R and Tinnitus Handicap Inventory.**
  Author(s): Lynn SG, Bauch CD, Williams DE, Beatty CW, Mellon MW, Weaver AL.
  Source: Otology & Neurotology : Official Publication of the American Otological Society, American Neurotology Society [and] European Academy of Otology and Neurotology. 2003 November; 24(6): 878-81.
  http://www.ncbi.nlm.nih.gov:80/entrez/query.fcgi?cmd=Retrieve&db=PubMed&list_uids=14600467&dopt=Abstract

- **Psychological aspects of tinnitus and the application of cognitive-behavioral therapy.**
  Author(s): Andersson G.
  Source: Clinical Psychology Review. 2002 September; 22(7): 977-90. Review.
  http://www.ncbi.nlm.nih.gov:80/entrez/query.fcgi?cmd=Retrieve&db=PubMed&list_uids=12238249&dopt=Abstract

- **Pulsatile and nonpulsatile tinnitus: a systemic approach.**
  Author(s): Marsot-Dupuch K.
  Source: Semin Ultrasound Ct Mr. 2001 June; 22(3): 250-70. Review.
  http://www.ncbi.nlm.nih.gov:80/entrez/query.fcgi?cmd=Retrieve&db=PubMed&list_uids=11451099&dopt=Abstract

- **Pulsatile audible tinnitus and metastatic breast carcinoma of the temporal bone.**
  Author(s): Vasama JP, Pitkaranta A, Piilonen A.
  Source: Orl; Journal for Oto-Rhino-Laryngology and Its Related Specialties. 2001 January-February; 63(1): 56-7.
  http://www.ncbi.nlm.nih.gov:80/entrez/query.fcgi?cmd=Retrieve&db=PubMed&list_uids=11174064&dopt=Abstract

- **Pulsatile tinnitus alleviated by contralateral neck compression: a case report.**
  Author(s): Jun BH, Choi IS, Lee GJ.
  Source: Auris, Nasus, Larynx. 2003 February; 30(1): 89-91.
  http://www.ncbi.nlm.nih.gov:80/entrez/query.fcgi?cmd=Retrieve&db=PubMed&list_uids=12589858&dopt=Abstract

- **Pulsatile tinnitus in patients with morbid obesity: the effectiveness of weight reduction surgery.**
  Author(s): Michaelides EM, Sismanis A, Sugerman HJ, Felton WL 3rd.
  Source: The American Journal of Otology. 2000 September; 21(5): 682-5.
  http://www.ncbi.nlm.nih.gov:80/entrez/query.fcgi?cmd=Retrieve&db=PubMed&list_uids=10993458&dopt=Abstract

- **Pulsatile tinnitus.**
  Author(s): Sismanis A.
  Source: Otolaryngologic Clinics of North America. 2003 April; 36(2): 389-402, Viii. Review.
  http://www.ncbi.nlm.nih.gov:80/entrez/query.fcgi?cmd=Retrieve&db=PubMed&list_uids=12856306&dopt=Abstract

- **Pulsatile tinnitus.**
  Author(s): Corr P, Tsheole-Marishane L.
  Source: The British Journal of Radiology. 2001 July; 74(883): 669-70. Review.
  http://www.ncbi.nlm.nih.gov:80/entrez/query.fcgi?cmd=Retrieve&db=PubMed&list_uids=11509407&dopt=Abstract

- **Quantitative electroencephalography and tinnitus: a case study.**
  Author(s): Weiler EW, Brill K, Tachiki KH.
  Source: Int Tinnitus J. 2000; 6(2): 124-6.
  http://www.ncbi.nlm.nih.gov:80/entrez/query.fcgi?cmd=Retrieve&db=PubMed&list_uids=14689629&dopt=Abstract

- **Randomized controlled trial of internet-based cognitive behavior therapy for distress associated with tinnitus.**
  Author(s): Andersson G, Stromgren T, Strom L, Lyttkens L.
  Source: Psychosomatic Medicine. 2002 September-October; 64(5): 810-6.
  http://www.ncbi.nlm.nih.gov:80/entrez/query.fcgi?cmd=Retrieve&db=PubMed&list_uids=12271112&dopt=Abstract

- **Re: myths in neurotology, revisited: smoke and mirrors in tinnitus therapy.**
  Author(s): Seidman MD, Keate B.
  Source: Otology & Neurotology : Official Publication of the American Otological Society, American Neurotology Society [and] European Academy of Otology and Neurotology. 2002 November; 23(6): 1013-5; Author Reply 1015-6.
  http://www.ncbi.nlm.nih.gov:80/entrez/query.fcgi?cmd=Retrieve&db=PubMed&list_uids=12438873&dopt=Abstract

- **Recent advances in the pharmacological treatment of tinnitus.**
  Author(s): Simpson JJ, Davies WE.
  Source: Trends in Pharmacological Sciences. 1999 January; 20(1): 12-8. Review.
  http://www.ncbi.nlm.nih.gov:80/entrez/query.fcgi?cmd=Retrieve&db=PubMed&list_uids=10101957&dopt=Abstract

- **Regional cerebral blood flow during tinnitus: a PET case study with lidocaine and auditory stimulation.**
  Author(s): Andersson G, Lyttkens L, Hirvela C, Furmark T, Tillfors M, Fredrikson M.
  Source: Acta Oto-Laryngologica. 2000 October; 120(8): 967-72.
  http://www.ncbi.nlm.nih.gov:80/entrez/query.fcgi?cmd=Retrieve&db=PubMed&list_uids=11200593&dopt=Abstract

- **Regional glucose metabolic increases in left auditory cortex in tinnitus patients: a preliminary study with positron emission tomography.**
  Author(s): Wang H, Tian J, Yin D, Jiang S, Yang W, Han D, Yao S, Shao M.
  Source: Chinese Medical Journal. 2001 August; 114(8): 848-51.
  http://www.ncbi.nlm.nih.gov:80/entrez/query.fcgi?cmd=Retrieve&db=PubMed&list_uids=11780365&dopt=Abstract

- **Relationships among psychoacoustic judgments, speech understanding ability and self-perceived handicap in tinnitus subjects.**
  Author(s): Newman CW, Wharton JA, Shivapuja BG, Jacobson GP.
  Source: Audiology : Official Organ of the International Society of Audiology. 1994 January-February; 33(1): 47-60.
  http://www.ncbi.nlm.nih.gov:80/entrez/query.fcgi?cmd=Retrieve&db=PubMed&list_uids=8129680&dopt=Abstract

- **Reliability and validity of a Danish adaptation of the Tinnitus Handicap Inventory.**
  Author(s): Zachariae R, Mirz F, Johansen LV, Andersen SE, Bjerring P, Pedersen CB.
  Source: Scandinavian Audiology. 2000; 29(1): 37-43.
  http://www.ncbi.nlm.nih.gov:80/entrez/query.fcgi?cmd=Retrieve&db=PubMed&list_uids=10718675&dopt=Abstract

- **Reliability of self-rated tinnitus distress and association with psychological symptom patterns.**
  Author(s): Hiller W, Goebel G, Rief W.
  Source: The British Journal of Clinical Psychology / the British Psychological Society. 1994 May; 33 (Pt 2): 231-9.
  http://www.ncbi.nlm.nih.gov:80/entrez/query.fcgi?cmd=Retrieve&db=PubMed&list_uids=8038742&dopt=Abstract

- **Reliability of tinnitus loudness matches under procedural variation.**
  Author(s): Henry JA, Flick CL, Gilbert A, Ellingson RM, Fausti SA.
  Source: Journal of the American Academy of Audiology. 1999 October; 10(9): 502-20.
  http://www.ncbi.nlm.nih.gov:80/entrez/query.fcgi?cmd=Retrieve&db=PubMed&list_uids=10522624&dopt=Abstract

- **Reorganization of auditory cortex in tinnitus.**
  Author(s): Muhlnickel W, Elbert T, Taub E, Flor H.
  Source: Proceedings of the National Academy of Sciences of the United States of America. 1998 August 18; 95(17): 10340-3.
  http://www.ncbi.nlm.nih.gov:80/entrez/query.fcgi?cmd=Retrieve&db=PubMed&list_uids=9707649&dopt=Abstract

- **Results of combined low-power laser therapy and extracts of Ginkgo biloba in cases of sensorineural hearing loss and tinnitus.**
  Author(s): Plath P, Olivier J.
  Source: Advances in Oto-Rhino-Laryngology. 1995; 49: 101-4.
  http://www.ncbi.nlm.nih.gov:80/entrez/query.fcgi?cmd=Retrieve&db=PubMed&list_uids=7653339&dopt=Abstract

- **Retest stability of the tinnitus handicap questionnaire.**
  Author(s): Newman CW, Wharton JA, Jacobson GP.
  Source: The Annals of Otology, Rhinology, and Laryngology. 1995 September; 104(9 Pt 1): 718-23.
  http://www.ncbi.nlm.nih.gov:80/entrez/query.fcgi?cmd=Retrieve&db=PubMed&list_uids=7661523&dopt=Abstract

- **Retraining therapy for chronic tinnitus. A critical analysis of its status.**
  Author(s): Kroener-Herwig B, Biesinger E, Gerhards F, Goebel G, Verena Greimel K, Hiller W.
  Source: Scandinavian Audiology. 2000; 29(2): 67-78. Review.
  http://www.ncbi.nlm.nih.gov:80/entrez/query.fcgi?cmd=Retrieve&db=PubMed&list_uids=10888343&dopt=Abstract

- **Role of angiography in the evaluation of patients with pulsatile tinnitus.**
  Author(s): Shin EJ, Lalwani AK, Dowd CF.
  Source: The Laryngoscope. 2000 November; 110(11): 1916-20.
  http://www.ncbi.nlm.nih.gov:80/entrez/query.fcgi?cmd=Retrieve&db=PubMed&list_uids=11081610&dopt=Abstract

- **Secondary tinnitus as a symptom of instability of the upper cervical spine: operative management.**
  Author(s): Montazem A.
  Source: Int Tinnitus J. 2000; 6(2): 130-3.
  http://www.ncbi.nlm.nih.gov:80/entrez/query.fcgi?cmd=Retrieve&db=PubMed&list_uids=14689631&dopt=Abstract

- **Selective cochlear neurectomy for debilitating tinnitus.**
  Author(s): Wazen JJ, Foyt D, Sisti M.
  Source: The Annals of Otology, Rhinology, and Laryngology. 1997 July; 106(7 Pt 1): 568-70.
  http://www.ncbi.nlm.nih.gov:80/entrez/query.fcgi?cmd=Retrieve&db=PubMed&list_uids=9228857&dopt=Abstract

- **Self-reports about tinnitus and about cochlear implants.**
  Author(s): Noble W.
  Source: Ear and Hearing. 2000 August; 21(4 Suppl): 50S-59S. Review.
  http://www.ncbi.nlm.nih.gov:80/entrez/query.fcgi?cmd=Retrieve&db=PubMed&list_uids=10981594&dopt=Abstract

- **Similarities between chronic pain and tinnitus.**
  Author(s): Moller AR.
  Source: The American Journal of Otology. 1997 September; 18(5): 577-85. Review.
  http://www.ncbi.nlm.nih.gov:80/entrez/query.fcgi?cmd=Retrieve&db=PubMed&list_uids=9303153&dopt=Abstract

- **Similarities between severe tinnitus and chronic pain.**
  Author(s): Moller AR.
  Source: Journal of the American Academy of Audiology. 2000 March; 11(3): 115-24. Review.
  http://www.ncbi.nlm.nih.gov:80/entrez/query.fcgi?cmd=Retrieve&db=PubMed&list_uids=10755808&dopt=Abstract

- **Sleepiness and sleep in elderly persons with tinnitus.**
  Author(s): Asplund R.
  Source: Archives of Gerontology and Geriatrics. 2003 September-October; 37(2): 139-45.
  http://www.ncbi.nlm.nih.gov:80/entrez/query.fcgi?cmd=Retrieve&db=PubMed&list_uids=12888227&dopt=Abstract

- **Sodium valproate for tinnitus.**
  Author(s): Menkes DB, Larson PM.
  Source: Journal of Neurology, Neurosurgery, and Psychiatry. 1998 November; 65(5): 803.
  http://www.ncbi.nlm.nih.gov:80/entrez/query.fcgi?cmd=Retrieve&db=PubMed&list_uids=9810969&dopt=Abstract

- **Somatic (craniocervical) tinnitus and the dorsal cochlear nucleus hypothesis.**
  Author(s): Levine RA.
  Source: American Journal of Otolaryngology. 1999 November-December; 20(6): 351-62.
  http://www.ncbi.nlm.nih.gov:80/entrez/query.fcgi?cmd=Retrieve&db=PubMed&list_uids=10609479&dopt=Abstract

- **Some psychological aspects of tinnitus.**
  Author(s): Reiss M, Reiss G.
  Source: Percept Mot Skills. 1999 June; 88(3 Pt 1): 790-2. Review.
  http://www.ncbi.nlm.nih.gov:80/entrez/query.fcgi?cmd=Retrieve&db=PubMed&list_uids=10407886&dopt=Abstract

- **Sound stimulation via bone conduction for tinnitus relief: a pilot study.**
  Author(s): Holgers KM, Hakansson BE.
  Source: International Journal of Audiology. 2002 July; 41(5): 293-300.
  http://www.ncbi.nlm.nih.gov:80/entrez/query.fcgi?cmd=Retrieve&db=PubMed&list_uids=12166689&dopt=Abstract

- **Spontaneous carotico-cavernous fistula presenting as pulsatile tinnitus.**
  Author(s): Robertson A, Nicolaides AR, Taylor RH.
  Source: The Journal of Laryngology and Otology. 1999 August; 113(8): 744-6.
  http://www.ncbi.nlm.nih.gov:80/entrez/query.fcgi?cmd=Retrieve&db=PubMed&list_uids=10748852&dopt=Abstract

- **Spontaneous dissection of the internal carotid artery presenting with pulsatile tinnitus.**
  Author(s): Vories A, Liening D.
  Source: American Journal of Otolaryngology. 1998 May-June; 19(3): 213-5.
  http://www.ncbi.nlm.nih.gov:80/entrez/query.fcgi?cmd=Retrieve&db=PubMed&list_uids=9617936&dopt=Abstract

- **Standard variant venous dysplasia of the cerebellum in a patient suffering from Muenke's syndrome and tinnitus.**
  Author(s): Dunne AA, Bien S, Folz BJ, Werner JA.
  Source: Auris, Nasus, Larynx. 2001 August; 28(3): 249-52.
  http://www.ncbi.nlm.nih.gov:80/entrez/query.fcgi?cmd=Retrieve&db=PubMed&list_uids=11489370&dopt=Abstract

- **Stress and the onset of sudden hearing loss and tinnitus.**
  Author(s): Schmitt C, Patak M, Kroner-Herwig B.
  Source: Int Tinnitus J. 2000; 6(1): 41-9.
  http://www.ncbi.nlm.nih.gov:80/entrez/query.fcgi?cmd=Retrieve&db=PubMed&list_uids=14689617&dopt=Abstract

- **Subjective idiopathic tinnitus.**
  Author(s): Billue JS.
  Source: Clin Excell Nurse Pract. 1998 March; 2(2): 73-82. Review.
  http://www.ncbi.nlm.nih.gov:80/entrez/query.fcgi?cmd=Retrieve&db=PubMed&list_uids=10451267&dopt=Abstract

- **Subjective pulsatile tinnitus associated with extensive pneumatization of temporal bone.**
  Author(s): Tuz M, Dogru H, Yesildag A.
  Source: Auris, Nasus, Larynx. 2003 May; 30(2): 183-5.
  http://www.ncbi.nlm.nih.gov:80/entrez/query.fcgi?cmd=Retrieve&db=PubMed&list_uids=12753991&dopt=Abstract

- **Sudden-onset tinnitus associated with arterial dissection of the vertebrobasilar system.**
  Author(s): Yokota M, Ito T, Hosoya T, Suzuki Y, Aoyagi M.
  Source: Acta Otolaryngol Suppl. 2000; 542: 29-33.
  http://www.ncbi.nlm.nih.gov:80/entrez/query.fcgi?cmd=Retrieve&db=PubMed&list_uids=10897396&dopt=Abstract

- **Support for the central theory of tinnitus generation: a military epidemiological study.**
  Author(s): Attias J, Reshef I, Shemesh Z, Salomon G.
  Source: International Journal of Audiology. 2002 July; 41(5): 301-7. Erratum In: Int J Audiol. 2003 January; 42(1): 57.
  http://www.ncbi.nlm.nih.gov:80/entrez/query.fcgi?cmd=Retrieve&db=PubMed&list_uids=12166690&dopt=Abstract

- **Surgical treatment of the high jugular bulb in patients with Meniere's disease and pulsatile tinnitus.**
  Author(s): Couloigner V, Grayeli AB, Bouccara D, Julien N, Sterkers O.
  Source: European Archives of Oto-Rhino-Laryngology : Official Journal of the European Federation of Oto-Rhino-Laryngological Societies (Eufos) : Affiliated with the German Society for Oto-Rhino-Laryngology - Head and Neck Surgery. 1999; 256(5): 224-9.
  http://www.ncbi.nlm.nih.gov:80/entrez/query.fcgi?cmd=Retrieve&db=PubMed&list_uids=10392295&dopt=Abstract

- **Survey of the perceived benefits and shortcomings of a specialist tinnitus clinic.**
  Author(s): Sanchez L, Stephens D.
  Source: Audiology : Official Organ of the International Society of Audiology. 2000 November-December; 39(6): 333-9.
  http://www.ncbi.nlm.nih.gov:80/entrez/query.fcgi?cmd=Retrieve&db=PubMed&list_uids=11766693&dopt=Abstract

- **The influence of voluntary muscle contractions upon the onset and modulation of tinnitus.**
  Author(s): Sanchez TG, Guerra GC, Lorenzi MC, Brandao AL, Bento RF.
  Source: Audiology & Neuro-Otology. 2002 November-December; 7(6): 370-5.
  http://www.ncbi.nlm.nih.gov:80/entrez/query.fcgi?cmd=Retrieve&db=PubMed&list_uids=12401968&dopt=Abstract

- **The management of chronic tinnitus: comparison of an outpatient cognitive-behavioral group training to minimal-contact interventions.**
  Author(s): Kroner-Herwig B, Frenzel A, Fritsche G, Schilkowsky G, Esser G.
  Source: Journal of Psychosomatic Research. 2003 April; 54(4): 381-9.
  http://www.ncbi.nlm.nih.gov:80/entrez/query.fcgi?cmd=Retrieve&db=PubMed&list_uids=12670617&dopt=Abstract

- **The role of zinc in management of tinnitus.**
  Author(s): Yetiser S, Tosun F, Satar B, Arslanhan M, Akcam T, Ozkaptan Y.
  Source: Auris, Nasus, Larynx. 2002 October; 29(4): 329-33.
  http://www.ncbi.nlm.nih.gov:80/entrez/query.fcgi?cmd=Retrieve&db=PubMed&list_uids=12393036&dopt=Abstract

- **The role of zinc in the treatment of tinnitus.**
  Author(s): Arda HN, Tuncel U, Akdogan O, Ozluoglu LN.
  Source: Otology & Neurotology : Official Publication of the American Otological Society, American Neurotology Society [and] European Academy of Otology and Neurotology. 2003 January; 24(1): 86-9.
  http://www.ncbi.nlm.nih.gov:80/entrez/query.fcgi?cmd=Retrieve&db=PubMed&list_uids=12544035&dopt=Abstract

- **Tinnitus after cycling.**
  Author(s): Lanczik O, Szabo K, Gass A, Hennerici MG.
  Source: Lancet. 2003 July 26; 362(9380): 292.
  http://www.ncbi.nlm.nih.gov:80/entrez/query.fcgi?cmd=Retrieve&db=PubMed&list_uids=12892960&dopt=Abstract

- **Tinnitus and bruxing.**
  Author(s): Miyano K.
  Source: The Journal of the American Dental Association. 2003 August; 134(8): 1036, 1038.
  http://www.ncbi.nlm.nih.gov:80/entrez/query.fcgi?cmd=Retrieve&db=PubMed&list_uids=12956337&dopt=Abstract

- **Tinnitus evaluation and treatment: assessment of quality of life indicators.**
  Author(s): H S.
  Source: Acta Otorhinolaryngol Belg. 2002; 56(4): 355-6. Review. No Abstract Available.
  http://www.ncbi.nlm.nih.gov:80/entrez/query.fcgi?cmd=Retrieve&db=PubMed&list_uids=12674089&dopt=Abstract

- **Tinnitus impact: three different measurement tools.**
  Author(s): Bauch CD, Lynn SG, Williams DE, Mellon MW, Weaver AL.
  Source: Journal of the American Academy of Audiology. 2003 May-June; 14(4): 181-7.
  http://www.ncbi.nlm.nih.gov:80/entrez/query.fcgi?cmd=Retrieve&db=PubMed&list_uids=12940702&dopt=Abstract

- **Tinnitus in 7-year-old children.**
  Author(s): Holgers KM.
  Source: European Journal of Pediatrics. 2003 April; 162(4): 276-8. Epub 2003 February 26.
  http://www.ncbi.nlm.nih.gov:80/entrez/query.fcgi?cmd=Retrieve&db=PubMed&list_uids=12647204&dopt=Abstract

- **Tinnitus in cochlear implant patients--a comparison with other hearing-impaired patients.**
  Author(s): Mo B, Harris S, Lindbaek M.
  Source: International Journal of Audiology. 2002 December; 41(8): 527-34.
  http://www.ncbi.nlm.nih.gov:80/entrez/query.fcgi?cmd=Retrieve&db=PubMed&list_uids=12477173&dopt=Abstract

- **Tinnitus loudness matchings in relation to annoyance and grading of severity.**
  Author(s): Andersson G.
  Source: Auris, Nasus, Larynx. 2003 May; 30(2): 129-33.
  http://www.ncbi.nlm.nih.gov:80/entrez/query.fcgi?cmd=Retrieve&db=PubMed&list_uids=12753982&dopt=Abstract

- **Tinnitus reduction using transcutaneous electrical stimulation.**
  Author(s): Steenerson RL, Cronin GW.
  Source: Otolaryngologic Clinics of North America. 2003 April; 36(2): 337-44.
  http://www.ncbi.nlm.nih.gov:80/entrez/query.fcgi?cmd=Retrieve&db=PubMed&list_uids=12856301&dopt=Abstract

- **Tinnitus retraining therapy for patients with tinnitus and decreased sound tolerance.**
  Author(s): Jastreboff PJ, Jastreboff MM.
  Source: Otolaryngologic Clinics of North America. 2003 April; 36(2): 321-36. Review.
  http://www.ncbi.nlm.nih.gov:80/entrez/query.fcgi?cmd=Retrieve&db=PubMed&list_uids=12856300&dopt=Abstract

- **Tinnitus. A patient's perspective.**
  Author(s): Nagler SM.
  Source: Otolaryngologic Clinics of North America. 2003 April; 36(2): 235-8, V.
  http://www.ncbi.nlm.nih.gov:80/entrez/query.fcgi?cmd=Retrieve&db=PubMed&list_uids=12856293&dopt=Abstract

- **Tinnitus. Advances in evaluation and management.**
  Author(s): Sismanis A.
  Source: Otolaryngologic Clinics of North America. 2003 April; 36(2): Xi-Xii.
  http://www.ncbi.nlm.nih.gov:80/entrez/query.fcgi?cmd=Retrieve&db=PubMed&list_uids=12856292&dopt=Abstract

- **Tinnitus. Diagnosis and treatment of this elusive symptom.**
  Author(s): Noell CA, Meyerhoff WL.
  Source: Geriatrics. 2003 February; 58(2): 28-34. Review.
  http://www.ncbi.nlm.nih.gov:80/entrez/query.fcgi?cmd=Retrieve&db=PubMed&list_uids=12596495&dopt=Abstract

- **Tinnitus: clinical measurement.**
  Author(s): Vernon JA, Meikle MB.
  Source: Otolaryngologic Clinics of North America. 2003 April; 36(2): 293-305, Vi. Review.
  http://www.ncbi.nlm.nih.gov:80/entrez/query.fcgi?cmd=Retrieve&db=PubMed&list_uids=12856298&dopt=Abstract

- **Transient suppression of tinnitus by transcranial magnetic stimulation.**
  Author(s): Plewnia C, Bartels M, Gerloff C.
  Source: Annals of Neurology. 2003 February; 53(2): 263-6.
  http://www.ncbi.nlm.nih.gov:80/entrez/query.fcgi?cmd=Retrieve&db=PubMed&list_uids=12557296&dopt=Abstract

- **Transtympanic management of tinnitus.**
  Author(s): Hoffer ME, Wester D, Kopke RD, Weisskopf P, Gottshall K.
  Source: Otolaryngologic Clinics of North America. 2003 April; 36(2): 353-8.
  http://www.ncbi.nlm.nih.gov:80/entrez/query.fcgi?cmd=Retrieve&db=PubMed&list_uids=12856303&dopt=Abstract

- **Transtympanic pilocarpine in tinnitus.**
  Author(s): DeLucchi E.
  Source: Int Tinnitus J. 2000; 6(1): 37-40.
  http://www.ncbi.nlm.nih.gov:80/entrez/query.fcgi?cmd=Retrieve&db=PubMed&list_uids=14689616&dopt=Abstract

- **Unilateral pulsatile tinnitus relieved by contralateral carotid endarterectomy.**
  Author(s): Norman LK, West PD, Perry PM.
  Source: Journal of the Royal Society of Medicine. 1999 August; 92(8): 406-7.
  http://www.ncbi.nlm.nih.gov:80/entrez/query.fcgi?cmd=Retrieve&db=PubMed&list_uids=10656006&dopt=Abstract

- **Unilateral tinnitus occurring with a peripheral vestibular disorder in the contralateral ear.**
  Author(s): Brookler KH.
  Source: Ear, Nose, & Throat Journal. 2001 December; 80(12): 860-1.
  http://www.ncbi.nlm.nih.gov:80/entrez/query.fcgi?cmd=Retrieve&db=PubMed&list_uids=11775515&dopt=Abstract

- **Unique case of pulsatile tinnitus.**
  Author(s): Harris JP, Horlbeck DM, Brew KH.
  Source: The Annals of Otology, Rhinology, and Laryngology. 2000 December; 109(12 Pt 1): 1103-6.
  http://www.ncbi.nlm.nih.gov:80/entrez/query.fcgi?cmd=Retrieve&db=PubMed&list_uids=11130819&dopt=Abstract

- **Update on tinnitus.**
  Author(s): Seidman MD, Jacobson GP.
  Source: Otolaryngologic Clinics of North America. 1996 June; 29(3): 455-65. Review.
  http://www.ncbi.nlm.nih.gov:80/entrez/query.fcgi?cmd=Retrieve&db=PubMed&list_uids=8743344&dopt=Abstract

- **Use of alprazolam for relief of tinnitus. A double-blind study.**
  Author(s): Johnson RM, Brummett R, Schleuning A.
  Source: Archives of Otolaryngology--Head & Neck Surgery. 1993 August; 119(8): 842-5.
  http://www.ncbi.nlm.nih.gov:80/entrez/query.fcgi?cmd=Retrieve&db=PubMed&list_uids=8343245&dopt=Abstract

- Use of homeopathy in the treatment of tinnitus.
  Author(s): Simpson JJ, Donaldson I, Davies WE.
  Source: British Journal of Audiology. 1998 August; 32(4): 227-33.
  http://www.ncbi.nlm.nih.gov:80/entrez/query.fcgi?cmd=Retrieve&db=PubMed&list_uids=9923984&dopt=Abstract

- Vagal schwannoma of the cerebello-medullary cistern presenting with hoarseness and intractable tinnitus: a rare case of intra-operative bradycardia and cardiac asystole.
  Author(s): Sharma RR, Pawar SJ, Dev E, Chackochan EK, Suri N.
  Source: Journal of Clinical Neuroscience : Official Journal of the Neurosurgical Society of Australasia. 2001 November; 8(6): 577-80.
  http://www.ncbi.nlm.nih.gov:80/entrez/query.fcgi?cmd=Retrieve&db=PubMed&list_uids=11683613&dopt=Abstract

- Validation assessment of a French version of the tinnitus reaction questionnaire: a comparison between data from English and French versions.
  Author(s): Meric C, Pham E, Chery-Croze S.
  Source: Journal of Speech, Language, and Hearing Research : Jslhr. 2000 February; 43(1): 184-90.
  http://www.ncbi.nlm.nih.gov:80/entrez/query.fcgi?cmd=Retrieve&db=PubMed&list_uids=10668661&dopt=Abstract

- **Valproate-induced tinnitus misinterpreted as psychotic symptoms.**
  Author(s): Reeves RR, Mustain DW, Pendarvis JE.
  Source: Southern Medical Journal. 2000 October; 93(10): 1030-1.
  http://www.ncbi.nlm.nih.gov:80/entrez/query.fcgi?cmd=Retrieve&db=PubMed&list_uids=11147471&dopt=Abstract

- **Vascular decompression surgery for severe tinnitus: selection criteria and results.**
  Author(s): Moller MB, Moller AR, Jannetta PJ, Jho HD.
  Source: The Laryngoscope. 1993 April; 103(4 Pt 1): 421-7.
  http://www.ncbi.nlm.nih.gov:80/entrez/query.fcgi?cmd=Retrieve&db=PubMed&list_uids=8459751&dopt=Abstract

- **Vascular-decompression surgery for severe tinnitus.**
  Author(s): Brookes GB.
  Source: The American Journal of Otology. 1996 July; 17(4): 569-76.
  http://www.ncbi.nlm.nih.gov:80/entrez/query.fcgi?cmd=Retrieve&db=PubMed&list_uids=8841702&dopt=Abstract

- **Venlafaxine and severe tinnitus.**
  Author(s): Ahmad S.
  Source: American Family Physician. 1995 June; 51(8): 1830.
  http://www.ncbi.nlm.nih.gov:80/entrez/query.fcgi?cmd=Retrieve&db=PubMed&list_uids=7762476&dopt=Abstract

- **Vertigo, hearing loss, and tinnitus.**
  Author(s): Raza SA, Phillipps JJ.
  Source: Postgraduate Medical Journal. 1998 June; 74(872): 375-7.
  http://www.ncbi.nlm.nih.gov:80/entrez/query.fcgi?cmd=Retrieve&db=PubMed&list_uids=9799900&dopt=Abstract

- **Vertigo, tinnitus, and hearing loss in the geriatric patient.**
  Author(s): Kessinger RC, Boneva DV.
  Source: Journal of Manipulative and Physiological Therapeutics. 2000 June; 23(5): 352-62.
  http://www.ncbi.nlm.nih.gov:80/entrez/query.fcgi?cmd=Retrieve&db=PubMed&list_uids=10863256&dopt=Abstract

- **Vestibular findings in a patient with a history of tinnitus before developing Meniere's disease.**
  Author(s): Brookler KH.
  Source: Ear, Nose, & Throat Journal. 2003 August; 82(8): 552.
  http://www.ncbi.nlm.nih.gov:80/entrez/query.fcgi?cmd=Retrieve&db=PubMed&list_uids=14503087&dopt=Abstract

- **Vestibular schwannoma, tinnitus and cellular telephones.**
  Author(s): Hardell L, Hansson Mild K, Sandstrom M, Carlberg M, Hallquist A, Pahlson A.
  Source: Neuroepidemiology. 2003 March-April; 22(2): 124-9. Review.
  http://www.ncbi.nlm.nih.gov:80/entrez/query.fcgi?cmd=Retrieve&db=PubMed&list_uids=12629278&dopt=Abstract

- **Vitamin B12 deficiency in patients with chronic-tinnitus and noise-induced hearing loss.**
  Author(s): Shemesh Z, Attias J, Ornan M, Shapira N, Shahar A.
  Source: American Journal of Otolaryngology. 1993 March-April; 14(2): 94-9.
  http://www.ncbi.nlm.nih.gov:80/entrez/query.fcgi?cmd=Retrieve&db=PubMed&list_uids=8484483&dopt=Abstract

- **What MR sequences should be used in the evaluation of pulsatile tinnitus?**
  Author(s): Brunberg JA.
  Source: Ajr. American Journal of Roentgenology. 1995 July; 165(1): 226.
  http://www.ncbi.nlm.nih.gov:80/entrez/query.fcgi?cmd=Retrieve&db=PubMed&list_uids=7785612&dopt=Abstract

Vocabulary Builder

Ablation: The removal of an organ by surgery. [NIH]

Adjustment: The dynamic process wherein the thoughts, feelings, behavior, and biophysiological mechanisms of the individual continually change to adjust to the environment. [NIH]

Afferent: Concerned with the transmission of neural impulse toward the central part of the nervous system. [NIH]

Amplification: The production of additional copies of a chromosomal DNA sequence, found as either intrachromosomal or extrachromosomal DNA. [NIH]

Autoradiography: A process in which radioactive material within an object produces an image when it is in close proximity to a radiation sensitive emulsion. [NIH]

Axonal: Condition associated with metabolic derangement of the entire neuron and is manifest by degeneration of the distal portion of the nerve fiber. [NIH]

Basalis: Chiasmatic cistern. [NIH]

Binaural: Used of the two ears functioning together. [NIH]

Bioluminescence: The emission of light by living organisms such as the firefly, certain mollusks, beetles, fish, bacteria, fungi and protozoa. [NIH]

Broadband: A wide frequency range. Sound whose energy is distributed over a broad range of frequency (generally, more than one octave). [NIH]

CDNA: Synthetic DNA reverse transcribed from a specific RNA through the action of the enzyme reverse transcriptase. DNA synthesized by reverse transcriptase using RNA as a template. [NIH]

Clamp: A u-shaped steel rod used with a pin or wire for skeletal traction in the treatment of certain fractures. [NIH]

Clavicle: A long bone of the shoulder girdle. [NIH]

Deletion: A genetic rearrangement through loss of segments of DNA (chromosomes), bringing sequences, which are normally separated, into close proximity. [NIH]

Density: The logarithm to the base 10 of the opacity of an exposed and processed film. [NIH]

Dissection: Cutting up of an organism for study. [NIH]

Dyslexia: Partial alexia in which letters but not words may be read, or in which words may be read but not understood. [NIH]

EEG: A graphic recording of the changes in electrical potential associated with the activity of the cerebral cortex made with the electroencephalogram. [NIH]

Efferent: Nerve fibers which conduct impulses from the central nervous system to muscles and glands. [NIH]

Enzymatic: Phase where enzyme cuts the precursor protein. [NIH]

Equalization: The reduction of frequency and/or phase distortion, or modification of gain and or phase versus frequency characteristics of a transducer, by the use of attenuation circuits whose loss or delay is a function of frequency. [NIH]

Excitatory: When cortical neurons are excited, their output increases and each new input they receive while they are still excited raises their output markedly. [NIH]

Fossa: A cavity, depression, or pit. [NIH]

Generator: Any system incorporating a fixed parent radionuclide from which is produced a daughter radionuclide which is to be removed by elution or by any other method and used in a radiopharmaceutical. [NIH]

Genetics: The biological science that deals with the phenomena and mechanisms of heredity. [NIH]

Glutamate: Excitatory neurotransmitter of the brain. [NIH]

Gravis: Eruption of watery blisters on the skin among those handling animals and animal products. [NIH]

Growth: The progressive development of a living being or part of an organism from its earliest stage to maturity. [NIH]

Handicap: A handicap occurs as a result of disability, but disability does not always constitute a handicap. A handicap may be said to exist when a disability causes a substantial and continuing reduction in a person's capacity to function socially and vocationally. [NIH]

Hereditary: Of, relating to, or denoting factors that can be transmitted genetically from one generation to another. [NIH]

Homozygotes: An individual having a homozygous gene pair. [NIH]

Hybrid: Cross fertilization between two varieties or, more usually, two species of vines, see also crossing. [NIH]

Hypnotherapy: Sleeping-cure. [NIH]

Immunologic: The ability of the antibody-forming system to recall a previous experience with an antigen and to respond to a second exposure with the prompt production of large amounts of antibody. [NIH]

Initiation: Mutation induced by a chemical reactive substance causing cell changes; being a step in a carcinogenic process. [NIH]

Joint: The point of contact between elements of an animal skeleton with the parts that surround and support it. [NIH]

Kb: A measure of the length of DNA fragments, 1 Kb = 1000 base pairs. The largest DNA fragments are up to 50 kilobases long. [NIH]

Koch: It was an early form of tuberculin of low specificity, devised by Robert Koch and made by heat concentration of a broth culture of Mycobacterium tuberculosis. [NIH]

Loop: A wire usually of platinum bent at one end into a small loop (usually 4 mm inside diameter) and used in transferring microorganisms. [NIH]

Medial: Lying near the midsaggital plane of the body; opposed to lateral. [NIH]

Metabotropic: A glutamate receptor which triggers an increase in production of 2 intracellular messengers: diacylglycerol and inositol 1, 4, 5-triphosphate. [NIH]

Modeling: A treatment procedure whereby the therapist presents the target behavior which the learner is to imitate and make part of his repertoire. [NIH]

Modification: A change in an organism, or in a process in an organism, that is acquired from its own activity or environment. [NIH]

Monoamine: Enzyme that breaks down dopamine in the astrocytes and microglia. [NIH]

Morphological: Relating to the configuration or the structure of live organs. [NIH]

MRNA: The RNA molecule that conveys from the DNA the information that is to be translated into the structure of a particular polypeptide molecule. [NIH]

Naive: Used to describe an individual who has never taken a certain drug or class of drugs (e. g., AZT-naive, antiretroviral-naive), or to refer to an undifferentiated immune system cell. [NIH]

Networks: Pertaining to a nerve or to the nerves, a meshlike structure of interlocking fibers or strands. [NIH]

Nuclei: A body of specialized protoplasm found in nearly all cells and containing the chromosomes. [NIH]

Nucleus: A body of specialized protoplasm found in nearly all cells and containing the chromosomes. [NIH]

Orderly: A male hospital attendant. [NIH]

Otology: The branch of medicine which deals with the diagnosis and treatment of the disorders and diseases of the ear. [NIH]

Outpatient: A patient who is not an inmate of a hospital but receives diagnosis or treatment in a clinic or dispensary connected with the hospital. [NIH]

Palsy: Disease of the peripheral nervous system occurring usually after many years of increased lead absorption. [NIH]

Paralysis: Loss or impairment of muscle function or sensation. [NIH]

Pathologies: The study of abnormality, especially the study of diseases. [NIH]

Pediatrics: The branch of medical science concerned with children and their diseases. [NIH]

Perilymph: The fluid contained within the space separating the membranous from the osseous labyrinth of the ear. [NIH]

Phantom: Used to absorb and/or scatter radiation equivalently to a patient, and hence to estimate radiation doses and test imaging systems without actually exposing a patient. It may be an anthropomorphic or a physical test object. [NIH]

Plasticity: In an individual or a population, the capacity for adaptation: a) through gene changes (genetic plasticity) or b) through internal physiological modifications in response to changes of environment (physiological plasticity). [NIH]

Polymerase: An enzyme which catalyses the synthesis of DNA using a single DNA strand as a template. The polymerase copies the template in the 5'-3'direction provided that sufficient quantities of free nucleotides, dATP and dTTP are present. [NIH]

Postsynaptic: Nerve potential generated by an inhibitory hyperpolarizing stimulation. [NIH]

Potassium: It is essential to the ability of muscle cells to contract. [NIH]

Presumptive: A treatment based on an assumed diagnosis, prior to receiving confirmatory laboratory test results. [NIH]

Probe: An instrument used in exploring cavities, or in the detection and dilatation of strictures, or in demonstrating the potency of channels; an elongated instrument for exploring or sounding body cavities. [NIH]

Promoter: A chemical substance that increases the activity of a carcinogenic process. [NIH]

Reassurance: A procedure in psychotherapy that seeks to give the client confidence in a favorable outcome. It makes use of suggestion, of the prestige of the therapist. [NIH]

Recombination: The formation of new combinations of genes as a result of segregation in crosses between genetically different parents; also the rearrangement of linked genes due to crossing-over. [NIH]

Rehabilitative: Instruction of incapacitated individuals or of those affected with some mental disorder, so that some or all of their lost ability may be regained. [NIH]

Reliability: Used technically, in a statistical sense, of consistency of a test with itself, i. e. the extent to which we can assume that it will yield the same result if repeated a second time. [NIH]

Schizophrenia: A mental disorder characterized by a special type of disintegration of the personality. [NIH]

Specificity: Degree of selectivity shown by an antibody with respect to the number and types of antigens with which the antibody combines, as well as with respect to the rates and the extents of these reactions. [NIH]

Stereotactic: Radiotherapy that treats brain tumors by using a special frame affixed directly to the patient's cranium. By aiming the X-ray source with respect to the rigid frame, technicians can position the beam extremely precisely during each treatment. [NIH]

Stimulus: That which can elicit or evoke action (response) in a muscle, nerve, gland or other excitable issue, or cause an augmenting action upon any function or metabolic process. [NIH]

Suppression: A conscious exclusion of disapproved desire contrary with repression, in which the process of exclusion is not conscious. [NIH]

Synapse: The region where the processes of two neurons come into close contiguity, and the nervous impulse passes from one to the other; the fibers of the two are intermeshed, but, according to the general view, there is no direct contiguity. [NIH]

Temporal: One of the two irregular bones forming part of the lateral surfaces and base of the skull, and containing the organs of hearing. [NIH]

Tetanic: Having the characteristics of, or relating to tetanus. [NIH]

Therapeutics: The branch of medicine which is concerned with the treatment of diseases, palliative or curative. [NIH]

Threshold: For a specified sensory modality (e. g. light, sound, vibration), the lowest level (absolute threshold) or smallest difference (difference threshold, difference limen) or intensity of the stimulus discernible in prescribed conditions of stimulation. [NIH]

Tonal: Based on special tests used for a topographic diagnosis of perceptive deafness (damage of the Corti organ, peripheral or central damage, i. e. the auditive cortex). [NIH]

Transduction: The transfer of genes from one cell to another by means of a viral (in the case of bacteria, a bacteriophage) vector or a vector which is similar to a virus particle (pseudovirion). [NIH]

Translational: The cleavage of signal sequence that directs the passage of the protein through a cell or organelle membrane. [NIH]

Transmitter: A chemical substance which effects the passage of nerve impulses from one cell to the other at the synapse. [NIH]

Trigeminal: Cranial nerve V. It is sensory for the eyeball, the conjunctiva, the eyebrow, the skin of face and scalp, the teeth, the mucous membranes in the mouth and nose, and is motor to the muscles of mastication. [NIH]

Vasodilators: Any nerve or agent which induces dilatation of the blood vessels. [NIH]

Vitro: Descriptive of an event or enzyme reaction under experimental investigation occurring outside a living organism. Parts of an organism or microorganism are used together with artificial substrates and/or conditions. [NIH]

Zoster: A virus infection of the Gasserian ganglion and its nerve branches, characterized by discrete areas of vesiculation of the epithelium of the forehead, the nose, the eyelids, and the cornea together with subepithelial infiltration. [NIH]

CHAPTER 5. PATENTS ON TINNITUS

Overview

You can learn about innovations relating to tinnitus by reading recent patents and patent applications. Patents can be physical innovations (e.g. chemicals, pharmaceuticals, medical equipment) or processes (e.g. treatments or diagnostic procedures). The United States Patent and Trademark Office defines a patent as a grant of a property right to the inventor, issued by the Patent and Trademark Office.[23] Patents, therefore, are intellectual property. For the United States, the term of a new patent is 20 years from the date when the patent application was filed. If the inventor wishes to receive economic benefits, it is likely that the invention will become commercially available to patients with tinnitus within 20 years of the initial filing. It is important to understand, therefore, that an inventor's patent does not indicate that a product or service is or will be commercially available to patients with tinnitus. The patent implies only that the inventor has "the right to exclude others from making, using, offering for sale, or selling" the invention in the United States. While this relates to U.S. patents, similar rules govern foreign patents.

In this chapter, we show you how to locate information on patents and their inventors. If you find a patent that is particularly interesting to you, contact the inventor or the assignee for further information.

---

[23] Adapted from The U. S. Patent and Trademark Office: http://www.uspto.gov/web/offices/pac/doc/general/whatis.htm.

Patents on Tinnitus

By performing a patent search focusing on tinnitus, you can obtain information such as the title of the invention, the names of the inventor(s), the assignee(s) or the company that owns or controls the patent, a short abstract that summarizes the patent, and a few excerpts from the description of the patent. The abstract of a patent tends to be more technical in nature, while the description is often written for the public. Full patent descriptions contain much more information than is presented here (e.g. claims, references, figures, diagrams, etc.). We will tell you how to obtain this information later in the chapter. The following is an example of the type of information that you can expect to obtain from a patent search on tinnitus:

- **Apparatus and method for an open ear auditory pathway stimulator to manage tinnitus and hyperacusis**

    Inventor(s): Bauman; Natan (New Haven, CT), Juneau; Roger P. (Destrehan, LA)

    Assignee(s): Natan Bauman (new Haven, Ct)

    Patent Number: 6,048,305

    Date filed: August 7, 1998

    Abstract: An open-in-the-ear auditory pathway stimulator device includes a noise generator in the device for generating noise and controls in the device for adjusting the volume of the noise. The device is preferably open ear. The device is preferably programmable. The device can also include a hearing aid for amplifying ambient sounds.

    Excerpt(s): The present invention relates to an Auditory Pathway Stimulator for management through central habituation of patients suffering from **Tinnitus** or Hyperacusis, or both. More particularly, the present invention relates to a system and method for reducing the debilitating effects of **tinnitus** by means of an all-in-the-canal, open-ear, noise stimulus of the auditory pathway.... Over 300 research projects funded by public and private agencies have been conducted to address **tinnitus** and its harmful effects during the last two decades. A cure is still unforeseen in the near future. This invention is an important step to a systematic solution with long-term significant results.... The concept of **tinnitus** is difficult to convey since it is a "Phantom Auditory Perception" representing lack of certain neuro activity in the auditory system rather than an increased activity. It is also a symptom associated with many auditory and non auditory pathologies.

    Web site: http://www.delphion.com/details?pn=US06048305__

- **Apparatus and method for the treatment of disorders of tissue and/or the joints**

    Inventor(s): Markoll; Richard (Boca Raton, FL)

    Assignee(s): Bio-magnetic Therapy Systems, Inc. (west Palm Beach, Fl)

    Patent Number: 6,447,440

    Date filed: February 8, 2000

    Abstract: In this apparatus and method a U-shaped hollow housing containing a plurality of electromagnets with their cores directed inward is placed with its arms on the opposite sides of the patient's head. The magnets are energized to treat paradentosis, TMJ arthrosis, **tinnitus**, etc. A power supply connected to the magnets provides pulsed D.C. current pulsing at 1-30 cps to generate a pulsing field of less than 20 Gauss.

    Excerpt(s): This invention relates to an apparatus for the treatment of tissue disorders and/or disorders of tissue and joints in the area of a patient's head, particularly the jaw, neck or ears, using one or more electromagnetic fields.... The application of an electromagnetic field for the treatment of chronic disorders of the locomotor system, such as the joints, ligaments and back, is known in principle. Such disorders include, for example, arthroses, i.e. degenerative joint trouble, as well as tendinoses, degenerative ligamentary and tendinous trouble, rheumatic disorders, such as inflammatory disorders of the joints, and acute injuries caused by sports-related or industrial accidents.... In this way, the Applicant's patents U.S. Pat. No. 5,131,94 or U.S. Pat. No. 5,453,07, for example, show an apparatus for the application of an electromagnetic field in order to treat inflammatory or degenerative disorders of the joints, especially arthrosis.

    Web site: http://www.delphion.com/details?pn=US06447440

- **Apparatus for producing alternating magnetic fields for inducing eddy currents in an organism**

    Inventor(s): Neuwirth; Gerald (Ponauer Str. 35/VI/3, Spittal/Drau 9800, AT)

    Assignee(s): None Reported

    Patent Number: 6,162,166

    Date filed: March 17, 1999

Abstract: In an apparatus for producing alternating magnetic fields for inducing eddy currents in an organism, wherein the apparatus (1) is designed to produce and deliver alternating magnetic fields of an adjustable, low frequency at pulses having steep pulse edges with harmonic wave portions, it is provided that the magnetic field strength of the alternating magnetic fields delivered by the apparatus (1) is chosen to be smaller than 300 A/m and, in particular, between 100 and 250 A/m, preferably in an adjustable manner, in order to induce eddy currents in an organisms by such alternating magnetic fields by way of a simple system, for instance, for treating ear noises, **tinnitus** or the like.

Excerpt(s): The present invention relates to an apparatus for producing alternating magnetic fields for inducing eddy currents in an organism as well as the use of such an apparatus, wherein the apparatus is designed to produce and deliver alternating magnetic fields of an adjustable, low frequency at pulses having steep pulse edges with harmonic wave portions.... Various apparatus for producing and delivering alternating electromagnetic waves for treating and examining organisms are known, wherein it is to be generally anticipated that the depth of penetration of such alternating electromagnetic fields is a function of the frequency. An apparatus of the initially defined kind has become known, for instance, from EP-A 0 084 019. In general, the electric field may be neglected as long as the frequency is within a very low range, i.e., in the range of what is called an extremely low frequency. By contrast, an alternating magnetic field induces eddy currents in the whole organism, which result in charge transfers in the cell membranes, thereby provoking stimulations of the vegetative nervous system capable of, for instance, reducing blockages present in the organism.... The present invention aims at providing an apparatus for producing alternating magnetic fields for inducing eddy currents in an organisms, which enables the concerted and dangerless production of eddy currents in an organism in a structurally simple manner so as to cause the purposeful influence of potential charge transfers in the cell membranes and eliminate or relax existing blockages by aid of the thus induced stimulation of the vegetative nervous system. To solve these objects, the apparatus according to the invention essentially is characterized in that the magnetic field strength of the alternating magnetic fields delivered by the apparatus is chosen to be smaller than 300 A/m and, in particular, between 100 and 250 A/m, preferably in an adjustable manner. Since alternating magnetic fields of an adjustable, low frequency are delivered by the apparatus according to the invention, simple adaptation to the varying sensitivities of different organisms is feasible, it having been found that the sensitivity is maximal at the frequency that corresponds with the EEG.alpha. rhythm of the person to be treated. The low field strengths selected according to the invention, moreover, ensure that the desired effects with a view to inducing eddy currents in an organism are achieved by problem-free and absolutely dangerless handling. Pulses are produced and delivered in the form of waves having pulsating steep edges with harmonic wave portions, wherein the pulses inherent in an organism are incited and assisted to the optimum degree by such induced pulses delivered to the organism, if the frequency of the alternating magnetic field externally applied is synchronous with the pulses inherent in the organism, thereby assisting in the vegetative nervous system stimulations sought.

Web site: http://www.delphion.com/details?pn=US06162166__

- **Apparatus for treating people afflicted with tinnitus**

   Inventor(s): Upham; George W. (2 Williams Rd., Lynnfield, MA 01940)

   Assignee(s): None Reported

   Patent Number: 5,628,330

   Date filed: March 15, 1995

   Abstract: Methods and means of treating a person afflicted with **Tinnitus** in order to relieve the discomfort and aggravation of the affliction uses apparatus that includes: a metal shell of generally hemispherical shape and diameter about the same as a person's head, nested in a similarly shaped larger shell, the space between the nested shells being filled with a natural, soft, flexible, thermally insulating material that may be animal or plant, the two shells being figures of revolution about a common axis and attached together along the common axis with the material in between, compressed somewhat by the attachment, and a handle, whereby the afflicted person can hold the apparatus against his afflicted ear for repeated intervals to relief is noted by the user after several days of these treatments in order to relieve the discomfort and aggravation of the affliction.

   Excerpt(s): This invention relates to apparatus for treating a person afflicted with **Tinnitus** in order to relieve the discomfort and aggravation of the affliction.... Tinnitus is the sound one hears when there is no external cause for that sound. The most common description of **tinnitus** is "ringing", but sounds such as roaring, hissing, whistling, music, steam, and numerous others have been reported by those afflicted with **tinnitus**.... There are many causes of **tinnitus.** The most frequent cause recognized by all authorities is exposure to loud sounds. Tinnitus-like symptoms are associated with just about every thing which can go wrong in the human auditory system. If arteriosclerosis produces obstructions to blood flow in vessels near the ear, a special form of tinnitus-like otoacoustic emissions, called pulsatile emissions (also improperly called pulsatile tinnitus), may result. Pulsatile emissions are a noise in the ear that is synchronous with the heart beat. People with pulsatile should probably see a cardiovascular specialist. Pulsatile **tinnitus** has been treated with some success with Masking techniques (described hereinbelow).

Web site: http://www.delphion.com/details?pn=US05628330__

- **Composition to treat ear disorders**

    Inventor(s): Petrus; Edward J. (Austin, TX)

    Assignee(s): Advanced Medical Instruments (austin, Tx)

    Patent Number: 6,093,417

    Date filed: January 11, 1999

    Abstract: A topical ear composition that uses penetration enhancers to diffuse the therapeutic agents through the tympanic membrane into the middle and inner ear for the purpose of reducing the inflammation of ear tissues, providing pain relief, and introducing agents with antimicrobial activity to combat infection. The composition reduces swelling of the lining membranes of the middle and inner ear, prevent the destructive effects of inflamation, inhibit the production of prostaglandins, reduce symptoms of **tinnitus** and vertigo, improve and prevent paralysis of the facial nerve, relieve labyrinthitis, and prevent hearing loss.

    Excerpt(s): A therapeutic composition for the relief and prevention of symptoms associated with ear disorders in humans and animals.... Most ear disorders are the result of an inflammatory response to infections, allergic reactions, or trauma. The infection may be of bacterial, fungal or viral origin and determination of the precise etiology is not practical since the causative organism is often difficult to isolate and culture. The determination of a viral cause is even more difficult to establish. Trauma, as a cause of ear disorders is made on the basis of a medical history and radiological confirmation.... It is important to treat the inflammation as soon as possible to reduce the sequella of hearing loss, **tinnitus,** facial nerve palsy, mastoiditis, labyrinthitis, vertigo, and possible encephalitis. Otitis is a non-specific term that describes a symptom and indicates an inflammation of the ear. The ear is anatomically divided into the external, middle and inner ear.

    Web site: http://www.delphion.com/details?pn=US06093417__

- **Computer implemented methods for reducing the effects of tinnitus**

    Inventor(s): Calhoun; Barbara (Berkeley, CA), Merzenich; Michael M. (San Francisco, CA), Peterson; Bret E. (Lafayette, CA)

    Assignee(s): Scientific Learning Corporation (berkeley, Ca)

    Patent Number: 6,155,971

    Date filed: January 29, 1999

    Abstract: A computer-implemented method for diagnosing and/or treating **tinnitus** in a human subject is disclosed. The method includes generating tonal stimuli for characterizing the intensity and frequency range of the **tinnitus**. The method further includes generating a set of tonal stimuli used in tests comprised of tasks designed to treat the **tinnitus** of the human subject. The tests may be readministered at varying levels of difficulty based on the performance of the human subject. The computer-implemented method further includes providing the set of tests to the human being and receiving a response from the human being. The response from the human subject is compared to a performance threshold before potential modification of the tests. The computer-implemented method includes administration using at least two computers where at least one is local and the other is remote.

    Excerpt(s): The present invention relates generally to techniques for treating hearing disorders in people. More particularly, the present invention relates to computer implemented methods for characterizing and treating **tinnitus**.... Tinnitus is commonly referred to as "ringing of the ear." It is a perceived sound that cannot be attributed to an external source. One cause of **tinnitus**, common in hearing loss, is believed to be damage to the hair cells of the cochlea responsible for reception of sound. As an example, damage can be to the hair cells responsible for reception in the 4 kHz to 8 kHz range. As a result, sound in this frequency range may not be transformed adequately into voltage potentials that can be conducted by neurons and processed by the central auditory system. In general, **tinnitus** will commonly occur at the lower frequency end of the malfunctioning range, or 4 kHz in the above example. **Tinnitus** can vary in intensity and, as an example, may be perceived as an intensity from 5 to 10 dB, although some **tinnitus** sufferers have reported a higher intensity level.... Most people have experienced **tinnitus,** for example, after hearing a traumatically loud noise or series of loud noises over time. The effects of **tinnitus** have been associated with hearing loss; approximately one third of elderly people experience the problem on a regular basis. Of greater concern is the one-half to one percent of people who are considered disabled by **tinnitus.** For these people, **tinnitus** impairs their ability to lead a normal and healthy lifestyle. As a result, numerous techniques have been used to reduce the effects of **tinnitus.**

Web site: http://www.delphion.com/details?pn=US06155971__

- **Computerized method and device for remediating exaggerated sensory response in an individual with an impaired sensory modality**

Inventor(s): Merzenich; Michael M. (San Francisco, CA)

Assignee(s): Scientific Learning Corporation (berkeley, Ca)

Patent Number: 6,234,979

Date filed: March 31, 1998

Abstract: The present invention provides a method and apparatus for implementing a training regimen which alleviates exaggerated sensory, perceptual, cognitive and/or emotional response problems. For example, in the aural domain, some autistic individuals are hypersensitive to one of the senses, e.g., sound. As discussed above, sounds at the specific frequency can cause discomfort to these autistic individuals even when presented at an intensity level which normally is not perceived as being too loud by most individuals. Similarly, **tinnitus** afflicted individuals also suffer from disconcerting perceived ringing sensations in their ears. The present invention hypothesizes that a catastrophic cascade of responses within a "supergroup" of auditory neurons is triggered by a hypersensitive response to a particular frequency or range of frequencies. The self sustaining cascade is very much like an epileptic seizure in which the sudden involuntary response of a relatively small group of neurons trigger responses in a supergroup of neurons located in the motor control region of the brain. In accordance with the present invention, the abnormally sensitive response problem associated with supergroups can be substantially alleviated via a remedial training regimen which emphasizes the redevelopment of the afflicted individual's ability to make fine sensory distinctions and/or the improvement of the individual's differential sensory acuteness. Providing the regimen to the individual consistently over a period of time increases the likelihood of normal or near normal sensory ability returning.

Excerpt(s): The present invention relates to alleviation of abnormal response problems. More particularly, the present invention relates to a computerized method for the remediation of exaggerated responses, such as in sensory, perceptual, cognitive and/or emotional domains of an individual.... Some integrated such as sensory, perceptual, cognitive and/or emotional response problems in individuals are associated with neural dysfunction. Examples include autism, epilepsy, dyslexia, PDD, attention deficit disorder (ADD) including ADD with hyperactivity disorder (ADD/HD), focal dystonias and obsessive/compulsive disorders (OCD).... For example, in some autistic individuals, an exaggerated integrated sensory response problem manifests itself as a hypersensitivity to a specific audible frequency (or frequencies). Sounds at the specific frequency can cause discomfort to these autistic individuals even when presented at a sound level not perceived as being too loud by most individuals. Unfortunately these frequencies belong within the frequency spectrum of normal speech. As a result, these autistic individuals consciously avoid exposure to the "painful" sounds. In the case of a young autistic child, the conscious avoidance of "painful" sounds greatly impedes the child's development of spoken language skills, and hence delays the child's acquisition of social skills.

Web site: http://www.delphion.com/details?pn=US06234979

- **Dextromethorphan and an oxidase inhibitor for treating intractable conditions**

Inventor(s): Licht; Jonathan M. (San Diego, CA), Smith; Richard Alan (La Jolla, CA)

Assignee(s): Center for Neurologic Study (la Jolla, Ca)

Patent Number: 5,863,927

Date filed: September 19, 1996

Abstract: Methods are disclosed for increasing the effectiveness of dextromethorphan in treating chronic or intractable pain, for treating **tinnitus** and for treating sexual dysfunction comprising administering dextromethorphan in combination with a therapeutically effective dosage of a debrisoquin hydroxylase inhibitor. A preferred combination is dextromethorphan and the oxidative inhibitor quinidine.

Excerpt(s): This application is a 371 of PCT/US94/10771, filed Sep. 22, 1994.... This invention relates to pharmacology. More specifically, the invention relates to compositions of matter useful for preparing medicaments for the treatment of various disorders.... A number of chronic disorders have symptoms which are known to be very difficult to treat, and often fail to respond to safe, non-addictive, and non-steroid medications. Such disorders, such as intractable coughing, fail to respond to conventional medicines and must be treated by such drugs as codeine, morphine, or the anti-inflammatory steroid prednisone. These drugs are unacceptable for long-term treatment due to dangerous side-effects, long-term risks to the patient's health, or the danger of addiction. Other disorders, such as dermatitis, have no satisfactory treatment for the severe itching and rash at this time. Drugs such as prednisone and even tricyclic antidepressants, as well as topical applications, have been tried, but do not appear to offer substantial and consistent relief.

Web site: http://www.delphion.com/details?pn=US05863927__

- **Electronic stimulation system for treating tinnitus disorders**

Inventor(s): Mino; Alfonso Di (15 Arcadia Rd., Woodcliff Lake, NJ 07675)

Assignee(s): None Reported

Patent Number: 5,788,656

Date filed: February 28, 1997

Abstract: An electronic stimulation system for treating a patient suffering from a **tinnitus** disorder in which the patient hears ringing or other sounds originating in the ear. The system includes an electronically actuated probe to which is applied a complex signal in the auditory range to cause the probe to vibrate in accordance with the signal. The probe is placed at a site on the patient in proximity to the cochlea of the inner ear whereby the probe vibrations are transmitted to the cochlea to stimulate this organ and thereby alleviate the **tinnitus** disorder. In this system, use is made of two adjustable audio-frequency oscillators, one operating in a low frequency range whose upper limit is about 400 Hz, the other operating in a high-frequency whose upper limit is about 1000 Hz. The outputs of these oscillators are combined and amplified to produce the complex signal applied to the probe. The mechanical vibrations transmitted by the probe in accordance with the complex signal must be properly related to the sonic frequencies of the **tinnitus** sounds being heard by the patient.

Excerpt(s): This invention relates generally to the treatment of **tinnitus** disorders, and more particularly to an electronic stimulation system in which a complex signal in the audio range is applied to an electromagnetically actuated probe to cause the probe to vibrate in accordance with the signal, the vibrations of the probe being transmitted to the cochlea of the inner ear of a patient to stimulate this organ and thereby alleviate the **tinnitus** disorder suffered by the patient.... The human ear functions as an auditory system for converting incoming sound vibrations into electrical energy which triggers nerve impulses in the auditory nerve connected to the brain. In this auditory system, sounds picked up by the outer ear (auriole) are conducted through an auditory canal to a tympanic membrane or eardrum. The middle ear which is separated from the outer ear by the eardrum, contains three small bones which as sounds strike the eardrum are then caused to vibrate. These bone vibrations set up corresponding vibrations in an oval window from which the vibrations are conveyed to the three fluid-filled canals contained in the cochlea of the inner ear.... At the base of the central canal of the cochlea is a basilar membrane, and supported on this membrane is the organ of Corti and its hair cells. These cells are the true receptors of hearing, for proliferations from the fibers of the auditory nerve extend up the center of the cochlea and connect with these hair cells.

Web site: http://www.delphion.com/details?pn=US05788656__

- **Herbal composition for treatment of tinnitus**

Inventor(s): Neville, II; Delmar S. (1300 Bernita Rd., El Cajon, CA 92020), Ozog, III; Stanley T. (4651 Pico St., #111, San Diego, CA 92109)

Assignee(s): None Reported

Patent Number: 6,358,540

Date filed: November 7, 2000

Abstract: A method for treating **tinnitus** comprising the step of administering to a subject requiring such treatment a therapeutically effective amount of an herbal composition comprising Radix Puerariae, Radix Platycodi Grandiflori, Radix Angelicae Dahuricae, Semen Coicis Lachryma-jobi, Rhizoma Zigiberis Officinalis Recens, Radix Ligustici Chuanxiong, Radix Paeoniae Lactiflorae, Folium Perillae Frutescentis, Flos Magnoliae, Herba cum Radice Asari, Ramulus Cinnamomi Cassiae, Radix Scutellariae Baicalensis, and Radix Glycyrrhizae Uralensis.

Excerpt(s): This invention relates to new medicinal compositions and methods for treating ear disorders, in particular the treatment of **tinnitus**.... Tinnitus, or ringing in the ears, is the sensation of hearing ringing, buzzing, hissing, chirping, whistling or other sounds. The noise can be intermittent or continuous, and can vary in loudness. It is often worse when background noise is low, so you may be most aware of it at night when you're trying to fall asleep in a quiet room. In rare cases, the sound beats in sync with your heart. **Tinnitus** is very common, affecting an estimated 50 million adults in the United States. For most people the condition is merely an annoyance. In severe cases, however, **tinnitus** can cause people to have difficulty concentrating and sleeping. It may eventually interfere with work and personal relationships, resulting in psychological distress. About 12 million people seek medical help for severe **tinnitus** every year.... A wide variety of conditions and illnesses can lead to **tinnitus**. Blockages of the ear due to a buildup of wax, an infection, or rarely, a tumor of the auditory nerve can cause the unwanted sounds, as can a perforated eardrum. But perhaps the most common source of chronic **tinnitus** is prolonged exposure to loud sounds. The noise causes permanent damage to the sound-sensitive cells of the cochlea, a spiral-shaped organ in the inner ear. Carpenters, pilots, rock musicians and street-repair workers are among those whose jobs put them at risk, as are people who work with chain saws, guns or other loud devices or who repeatedly listen to loud music. A single exposure to a sudden extremely loud noise can also cause **tinnitus.**

Web site: http://www.delphion.com/details?pn=US06358540__

- **Human drug delivery device for tinnitus**

Inventor(s): Bauer; Carol A. (Houston, TX), Howard, III; Matthew A. (Iowa City, IA), McCulloch; Timothy M. (Iowa City, IA)

Assignee(s): The University of Iowa Research Foundation (iowa City, Ia)

Patent Number: 5,713,847

Date filed: February 6, 1996

Abstract: A neural prosthetic drug delivery apparatus for reducing or eliminating the effects of **tinnitus**. The apparatus includes a catheter which is inserted into the patient's auditory cortex or thalamus. The catheter microinfuses drugs which suppress or eliminate abnormal neural activity into geometrically separate locations of the patient's brain, thereby reducing or eliminating the effects of **tinnitus.** In one embodiment the apparatus includes a stimulation device for outputting processed electrical signals and an electrode having a plurality of electrical contacts which is arranged in a target zone of the patient's brain. Each of the plurality of electrical contacts independently outputs electrical discharges in accordance with the electrical signals.

Excerpt(s): This invention relates generally to an apparatus for treating **tinnitus,** and in particular, to a prosthetic drug delivery device for microinfusing portions of drugs at geometrically separate locations of the patient's primary auditory cortex or the patient's thalamus.... Tinnitus is a disorder where a patient experiences a sound sensation within the head ("a ringing in the ears") in the absence of an external stimulus. This uncontrollable ringing can be extremely uncomfortable and often results in severe disability. **Tinnitus** is a very common disorder affecting an estimated. 15% of the U.S. population according to the National Institutes for Health, 1989 National Strategic Research Plan. Hence, approximately 9 million Americans have clinically significant **tinnitus** with 2 million of those being severely disabled by the disorder.... There are no treatments currently available that consistently eliminate **tinnitus** although many different types of treatments have been attempted. This wide variety of attempted treatments attests to the unsatisfactory state of current **tinnitus** therapy. Several more common attempts will be discussed below.

Web site: http://www.delphion.com/details?pn=US05713847__

- **Implantable device for treatment of tinnitus**

    Inventor(s): Leysieffer; Hans (Taufkirchen, DE)

    Assignee(s): Implex Aktiengesellschaft Hearing Technology (ismaning, De)

    Patent Number: 6,251,062

    Date filed: August 11, 1999

    Abstract: An implantable device for treatment of **tinnitus** is provided comprising an electronic signal generation unit and a power source for supplying power. A hermetically gas-tight, biocompatible and implantable electroacoustic transducer is also provided as the sound-delivering output transducer which, after an at least partial mastoidectomy, can be positioned in the mastoid cavity such that the sound emitted from the electroacoustic transducer travels from the mastoid to the tympanic cavity via the natural passage of the aditus ad antrum.

    Excerpt(s): The invention relates to an implantable device for treatment of **tinnitus** which includes an electronic signal generation unit and a power source for power supply of the device.... Many individuals suffer from intermittent or permanent **tinnitus** which cannot be cured by surgery. Also, to date, there have been no approved drug forms of treatment for **tinnitus**. However, so-called **tinnitus** maskers are known, such as disclosed in published PCT application 90/07251. These maskers are small, battery-operated devices which are worn like a hearing aid behind or in the ear and cover (mask) the **tinnitus** psychoacoustically by artificial sounds which are emitted, for example, via a hearing aid speaker into the auditory canal and which reduce the disturbing **tinnitus** as far as possible below the threshold of perception. The artificial sounds are often narrowband noise (for example, third octave noise) which in its spectral position and its loudness level can be adjusted via a programming device to enable the maximum possible adaptation to the individual **tinnitus** situation.... Moreover, recently the so-called "retraining method" has been provided according to which, by combination of a metal training program and presentation of broadband sound (noise) near the hearing threshold, the perceptibility of the **tinnitus** is supposed to be largely suppressed (see the journal "Hoerakustik" 2/97, pages 26 and 27).

Web site: http://www.delphion.com/details?pn=US06251062__

- **Implantable hearing aid with tinnitus masker or noiser**

    Inventor(s): Leysieffer; Hans (Taufkirchen, DE)

    Assignee(s): Cochlear Limited (lane Cove Nsw, Au)

    Patent Number: 6,394,947

    Date filed: December 21, 1999

    Abstract: Partially or fully implantable hearing aid for rehabilitation of an inner ear hearing disorder, with a microphone (10) which delivers an audio signal, an electronic signal processing and amplification unit (40, 50, 80, 140, 141) which is located in an audio signal-processing electronic hearing aid path, an implantable electromechanical output converter (20) and a unit (60) for power supply of the implant. The hearing aid is provided with an electronic module (90, 140, 141) for rehabilitation of **tinnitus** and it generates the signals necessary for a **tinnitus** masking or noiser function and feeds them into the audio signal processing path of the hearing implant.

    Excerpt(s): The present invention relates to partially or fully implantable hearing aids for rehabilitation of an inner ear hearing disorder, which have a microphone which delivers an audio signal, an electronic signal processing and amplification unit which is located in an audio signal processing electronic hearing aid path, an implantable electromechanical output converter and a unit for supplying power to the hearing aid.... Partially and fully implantable hearing aids for rehabilitation of inner ear damage with mechanical stimulation of the damaged inner ear have recently been available or will soon be available on the market journal HNO 46:844-852, 10-1998, H. P. Zenner et al., "Initial implantations of a completely implantable electronic hearing system in patients with an inner ear hearing disorder"; journal HNO 46:853-863, 10-1998,. Leysieffer et al., "A completely implantable hearing system for inner ear hearing handicapped: TICA LZ 3001"); U.S. Pat. Nos. 5,277,694; 5,788,711; 5,814,095; 5,554,096; and 5,624,376.... Especially in filly implantable systems is the visibility of the system not an issue, so that in addition to the advantages of high sound quality, the open auditory canal and full suitability for everyday use, high future patient acceptance can be assumed.

    Web site: http://www.delphion.com/details?pn=US06394947__

- **Method and apparatus for treatment of monofrequency tinnitus utilizing sound wave cancellation techniques**

Inventor(s): Choy; Daniel S. J. (170 E. 77th St., New York, NY 10021)

Assignee(s): Choy; Daniel S. J. (new York, Ny)

Patent Number: 6,610,019

Date filed: March 1, 2002

Abstract: Tinnitus is defined as sound(s) heard by an individual when no external sound is present and often takes the form of a hissing, ringing, chirping or clicking sound which may be either intermittent or constant. According to the American **Tinnitus** Association, **tinnitus** affects tens of millions of Americans and many suffer so severely from **tinnitus** they are not able to function normally on a daily basis. Unfortunately the exact cause or causes of **tinnitus** are not understood by the medical community and thus many **tinnitus** sufferers are told by their doctors to "learn to live with it".In accordance with novel aspects of Applicant's monofrequency **tinnitus** patient treatment apparatus and process, phase cancellation effects are achieved by utilizing an externally generated sound which is subjectively selected by the monofrequency **tinnitus** patient to match in both tone and loudness his or her **tinnitus** sound. This subjectively selected externally generated sound wave which matches in tone and loudness the patient's **tinnitus** sound, is either (i) sequentially phase shifted through a plurality of phase shift sequence steps totaling at least 180 degrees or (ii) alternatively is directly phase shifted in essentially a single step motion into a 180 degree, out-of-phase reciprocal, canceling relationship with the patient determined **tinnitus** tone. The sequential steps of the phase shifted tone or the directly phase shifted tone are applied to the **tinnitus** patient to effect cancellation or diminishment of the patient's **tinnitus**.

Excerpt(s): Applicant's inventions are related to the treatment of **tinnitus** patients and more particularly to improved methods and apparatus for treatment of monofrequency **tinnitus** patients utilizing phase shift cancellation principles.... Tinnitus is defined as the perception of sound by an individual when no external sound is present, and often takes the form of a hissing, ringing, roaring, chirping or clicking sound which may be intermittent or constant. According to the American **Tinnitus** Association, **tinnitus** afflicts more than 50 million Americans and more than 12 million of those suffer so severely from **tinnitus** that they seek medical attention and many cannot function normally on a day-to-day basis.... Tinnitus, often referred to as ringing in the ears, is estimated to be present in approximately 50% of the US population over 65 years of age. In general, **tinnitus** takes many and varied forms which may be related to its underlying cause. **Tinnitus** may be caused by or related to such diverse factors as trauma, drugs, hearing loss, the normal aging process or other unknown causes.

Web site: http://www.delphion.com/details?pn=US06610019__

- **Method and composition of a topical treatment of inner ear and labyrinth symptoms**

Inventor(s): Liedtke; Rainer K. (Postfach 306 D-82027 Gruenwald b., Munich, DE)

Assignee(s): None Reported

Patent Number: 5,863,941

Date filed: July 8, 1996

Abstract: Periauricularly administered topical therapy with a carrier system containing local anesthetics is a new and effective treatment of disorders of the inner ear and labyrinth, which has a low incidence of side effects. The use of this type of therapy applies especially to a non-invasive topical treatment of **tinnitus,** vertigo, lack of balance, and nausea.

Excerpt(s): The subject of this invention relates to a method and composition of a non-invasive, topical treatment and prevention of pathological symptoms of the inner ear and labyrinth, in particular of **tinnitus,** vertigo, lack of balance, and nausea.... It is known that in the majority of cases, persistent **tinnitus** and vertigo, accompanied by a lack of balance and nausea, are due to a disorder or disease of the organs of the inner ear or of the auditory nerves. **Tinnitus** may occur both in the low-frequency and in the high-frequency range; in the low-frequency range, it occurs especially in the presence of disorders of the auditory canal and the middle ear, in the high-frequency, mainly in the presence of disorders of the labyrinth. These persistent symptoms have an extremely negative effect on those affected. One characteristic complex of symptoms, which includes **tinnitus,** vertigo and lack of balance, possibly in association with nystagmus, hearing impairment and vomiting, is seen, for example, in Meniere's disease. The sudden attacks of the symptoms may be attributable to vasomotor disorders of labyrinth vessels or temporary disorders of the secretion and composition of the labyrinthine liquor. Under the influence of permanent **tinnitus** and impaired hearing, the persons affected often become irritable, they suffer from anxiety, and, in some cases, develop considerable psychosomatic problems as this illness proceeds.... The therapeutic methods used so far to treat these problems are not sufficiently effective. If it is not possible to identify an underlying disease, only symptomatic measures, such as stimulus deprivation, rest and pharmacological sedation, can be taken. The pharmacological principle frequently used for this purpose is the orally administered dimenhydrinate which has a sedative effect. Scopolamine, a parasympatholytic agent, may also be used; however, this agent is primarily used to treat the pathophysiologically associated phenomenon of motion-induced nausea, i.e., kinetosis, which develops on exposure to externally moving objects. This sickness is also known as motion or sea sickness and is associated with vegetative phenomena, mainly with nausea. In systemic therapy, scopolamine is also administered by transdermal route (Y. W. Chien, Novel Drug Delivery Systems, Drugs and the Pharmaceutical Sciences, Vol. 14, 1982, Marcel Decker, New York), which, when compared to the intramuscular administration of scopolamine, results in a lower and more uniform blood concentration in the body. In spite of this, however, the typical undesirable side effects of scopolamine, in particular, impaired vision, very dry mouth, changes in the ability to concentrate, and somnolence, are observed. The undesirable side effect mentioned last is, among other things, also present after an oral administration of dimenhydrinate which is also used to treat kinetoses but which is less effective. Thus, overall, the administration of scopolamine as a therapeutic principle is very restricted indeed.

Web site: http://www.delphion.com/details?pn=US05863941__

- **Method for coupling an electromechanical transducer of an implantable hearing aid or tinnitus masker to a middle ear ossicle**

Inventor(s): Leysieffer; Hans (Taufkirchen, DE)

Assignee(s): Implex Gmbh Spezialhorgerate (ismaning, De)

Patent Number: 6,077,215

Date filed: October 8, 1998

Abstract: A method for coupling an electromechanical transducer of a partially or totally implantable hearing aid and/or **tinnitus** masker to a middle ear ossicle of a hearing impaired person which is to be stimulated. The hearing aid and/or **tinnitus** masker includes the electromechanical transducer, a transducer positioning and fixing device, and an elongated coupling rod driven by the transducer, the elongated coupling rod having a tip. The method of the present invention includes performing a mastoidectomy to provide a mastoid cavity adapted for receiving the hearing aid and/or **tinnitus** masker transducer, passing the coupling rod through the natural passage of the aditus ad antrum, positioning and fixing the hearing aid and/or **tinnitus** masker transducer within the mastoid cavity with the elongated coupling rod passing through the aditus ad antrum, and contacting the tip of the elongated coupling rod with the ossicle to be stimulated.

Excerpt(s): The invention relates to a method for coupling an electromechanical transducer of a hearing aid or a **tinnitus** masker to a middle ear ossicle of a hearing impaired person.... Disorders of the inner or middle ear comprise the most common reason for impairments of hearing. In addition thereto, an increasing number of patients complain about a ringing, whistling or buzzing noise in the head which has no external source, a condition known as **tinnitus.** In recent years, it has been found that **tinnitus** may be alleviated or even overcome by providing the patient with a noise signal, for example white narrow band noise, which masks the noise caused by **tinnitus**.... One approach to overcome the above problems is to provide the patient with a hearing aid and/or **tinnitus** masker that is fixed to the external ear. However, this approach has several fundamental disadvantages, amongst which are to be named: (1) stigmatization of the patient; (2) the sound is often found to be unsatisfactory due to the limited frequency range and undesired distortion; (3) in many patients the ear canal fitting device leads to an occlusion effect; (4) acoustic feedback when amplification is high.

Web site: http://www.delphion.com/details?pn=US06077215__

- **Method for treating hyper-excited sensory nerve functions in humans**

    Inventor(s): Leung; Edward (Cary, NC)

    Assignee(s): King Pharmaceuticals Research & Development, Inc. ()

    Patent Number: 6,248,774

    Date filed: September 5, 2000

    Abstract: A method of and a formulation for treating hyper-excited sensory nerve functions are provided. The method comprises administering to a patient in need of treatment thereof a pharmaceutical composition comprising an effective amount of 2-Amino-4,5,6,7-tetrahydrobenzo[b]thiophen-3-yl)(4-chlorophenyl) methanone or a pharmaceutically acceptable salt thereof. The disorder treated include hyperesthesia, dysesthesia, allodynia, hyperalgesia, **tinnitus,** ganglionic dysfunction and combinations thereof. The co-administration of adenosine is not needed. The pharmaceutical preparation is suitable for oral administration. The pharmaceutical preparation is useful in the reduction of neuropathic pain in a conscious human. The use of the pharmaceutical preparation does not result in medically adverse cardiovascular symptoms associated with administration of adenosine.

Excerpt(s): The present invention relates to normalization of a pathologically hyper-excited sensory nerve function in a conscious human subject. In particular, the invention relates to a treatment method for reducing or eliminating hyper-excited sensory symptoms such as neuropathic pain. Some examples of neuropathic pain are diabetic neuropathy, post-herpetic neuralgia (shingles), trigeminal neuralgia, pain associated with AIDS infection and treatment, whip-lash pain, pain due to cancer treatment, phantom limb pain, traumatic injury, complex regional pain syndrome and pain due to peripheral vascular disease.... The development of hyper-excited sensory nerve function has been described by Sollevi 1997 (1). These symptoms are often manifested as neuropathic pain. Neuropathic pain is a persistent, chronic pain usually described as a burning, shooting or lancinating sensation without an obvious cause. These symptoms are often associated with damage to nerves or nerve fibers. Such pain is associated with the transmission of abnormal pain signals from injured peripheral nerves to neurons in the brain and spinal cord. Briefly, the sensory nervous system projects signals to the central nervous system (CNS), mediating information from the periphery to the brain. These comprise signals from sensors in peripheral tissues and other organs, sensitive for qualities like touch, temperature changes, vibration, painful stimuli, pressure, vision, hearing, smell, taste and balance. This sensory nervous system is an important physiological control in the subject's relation to the environment. The sensory nervous system can be damaged by various types of trauma, such as infections and mechanical lesions including whip-lash injury, diseases such as diabetes and HIV infection, cancer or HIV treatments. This can result in disturbance in the signal transmission into the CNS, leading to reduced perception of sensory signals (hypoestesia) as well as hyper-function (more excited signals in the CNS) due to some largely unknown changes in the nerve transmission process (neuropathic damage). The neuropathic condition with hyper-excitation is described as a "wind-up" phenomenon and often involves several of the above mentioned sensory functions. This may therefore be associated with decreased thresholds for touch and temperature (hyperesthesia), discomfort in the perception for touch and temperature (dysesthesia), discomfort or pain with touch, pressure and/or temperature stimulation (allodynia), and hypersensitivity to pain stimuli (hyperalgesia), balance disturbance, disturbance of auditory type (tinnitus) as well as ganglionic dysfunction. These types of hyper-reactive sensory nerves may develop after various types of trauma, and are called chronic when persistent for more than 3-6 months.... Adenosine, administered intravenously or intrathecally, has been proposed as a treatment for this sensory nerve hyper-reactivity (1, 2, 3). The objective of the treatment is to restore a normal perception of pain, as well as other sensory functions, in patients suffering from pathological hyperexcitation due to nerve damage.

Web site: http://www.delphion.com/details?pn=US06248774__

- **Method for treating otic disorders**

    Inventor(s): Donovan; Stephen (Capistrano Beach, CA)

    Assignee(s): Allergan Sales, Inc. (irvine, Ca)

    Patent Number: 6,265,379

    Date filed: October 13, 1999

    Abstract: Methods for treating otic disorders by local administration of a neurotoxin. A botulinum toxin can be administered to myoclonic middle ear muscles and to inner ear efferent and/or afferent nerves to alleviate otic disorders such as **tinnitus,** cochlear nerve dysfunction and Meniere's disease.

    Excerpt(s): The present invention relates to methods for treating otic disorders. In particular the present invention relates to methods for treating otic disorders by local administration of a neurotoxin to a human ear.... The human ear can be divided into an outer ear, a middle ear and an inner ear. The outer ear comprises the auricle (commonly referred to as the ear) and the external acoustic meatus (the auditory canal). The tympanic membrane (commonly called the eardrum) separates the auditory canal from the middle ear (the tympanic cavity). Three small, mobile bones, the incus, malleus and stapes make up an ossicular system which conducts sound through the middle ear to the cochlea. The handle of the malleus is attached to the center of the tympanic membrane. At its opposite end, the malleus is bound to the incus by ligaments, so that movement of the malleus causes the incus to also move. The opposite end of the incus articulates with the stem of the stapes. The faceplate of the stapes rests against the membranous labyrinth in the opening of the oval window, where sound waves are conducted into the inner ear. In the cochlea the sound waves are transduced into coded patterns of impulses transmitted along the afferent cochlear fibers of the vestibulocochlear nerve for analysis in the central auditory pathways of the brain.... The air filled tympanic cavity contains various muscles including the tensor tympani and stapedius muscles. The tensor tympani is a long slender muscle which occupies the bony canal above the osseous pharyngotympanic tube, from which it is separated by a thin bony septum. The tensor tympani muscle receives both motor and proprioceptive innervation. A motor branch derived from the nerve to the medial pterygoid (mandibular division of the V, parasympathetic, trigeminal nerve) passes through the otic (a peripheral, parasympathetic cholinergic) ganglion to the tensor tympani. The stapedius muscle extends from the wall of a conical cavity in the pyramidal eminence, located on the posterior wall of the tympanic cavity. The stapedius is innervated by a branch of the (VII, parasympathetic) facial nerve.

Web site: http://www.delphion.com/details?pn=US06265379__

- **Method for treating severe tinnitus**

    Inventor(s): Hildebrand; Keith Robert (Houlton, WI)

    Assignee(s): Medtronic, Inc. (minneapolis, Mn)

    Patent Number: 6,656,172

    Date filed: September 27, 2002

    Abstract: A method for treating severe **tinnitus** is disclosed. The method of the present invention comprises implanting a catheter into a patient and administering a therapeutic agent intrathecally into the patient's cerebrospinal fluid.

    Excerpt(s): This invention relates to a method for treating severe **tinnitus**.... Tinnitus is the perception of ringing, hissing, or other sounds in the ears or head when no external sound is present. For some people, **tinnitus** is just a nuisance. For others, it is a life-altering condition. According to the American **Tinnitus** Association, over 50 million Americans experience **tinnitus** to some degree and of these, approximately 12 million people have **tinnitus** to a distressing degree.... Approximately 2 million Americans have **tinnitus** to the point where they are so seriously debilitated that they cannot function on a "normal" day-to-day basis and some may commit suicide. Lewis, J. E., S. D. G. Stephens, et al. (1993). "Tinnitus and suicide." Clin Otolaryngol 19: 50-54. It is this severely affected population, which is only poorly managed with therapies available today, that may benefit from intrathecal pharmacotherapy proposed in the current investigation.

    Web site: http://www.delphion.com/details?pn=US06656172__

- **Methods for the treatment of tinnitus and other disorders using R(-)ketoptofen**

    Inventor(s): Jerussi; Thomas P. (Framingham, MA), Rubin; Paul D. (Sudbury, MA)

    Assignee(s): Sepracor, Inc. (marlborough, Ma)

    Patent Number: 6,362,227

    Date filed: February 22, 2000

    Abstract: Methods of treating neuropathic pain, **tinnitus**, and related disorders are disclosed. These methods comprise the administration of optically pure R(-)-ketoprofen. Also disclosed are pharmaceutical compositions useful in the treatment of neuropathic pain and **tinnitus** which comprise optically pure R(-)-ketoprofen.

    Excerpt(s): The invention relates to methods of treating neuropathic pain, **tinnitus,** and other disorders, and to pharmaceutical compositions useful in the treatment of neuropathic pain and **tinnitus**.... Racemic ketoprofen (a mixture of the R(-) and S(+) enantiomers) is sold under the tradenames Orudis.RTM. and Oruvail.RTM. for the treatment of inflammation. Physicians Desk Reference 52.sup.nd Ed., p. 3092 (1998). Generally, ketoprofen is considered to be a nonsteroidal anti-inflammatory agent ("NSAID"). NSAIDs are believed to exhibit activity as COX-1 or COX-2 enzyme inhibitors. Most NSAIDs are believed to cause gastrointestinal irritation.... The S(+) enantiomer of ketoprofen has long been thought to possess most, if not all, of the pharmacological activity of the racemate. See, e.g., Yamaguchi et al., Nippon Yakurigaku Zasshi. 90:295-302 (1987); Abas et al., J. Pharinacol. Exp. Ther., 240:637-641 (1987); and Caldwell et al., Biochem. Pharrnacol. 37:105-114 (1988). Indeed, U.S. Pat. Nos. 4,868,214, 4,962,124, and 4,927,854 each allege that the analgesic activity of ketoprofen resides exclusively in the S(+) enantiomer.

    Web site: http://www.delphion.com/details?pn=US06362227__

- **Minimum energy tinnitus masker**

    Inventor(s): Gooch; Timothy D. (Cordova, TN)

    Assignee(s): Microtek Medical, Inc. (columbus, Ms)

    Patent Number: 5,403,262

    Date filed: March 9, 1993

    Abstract: A **tinnitus** masking device and method for producing a masking signal with a selected center frequency, selected bandwidth, and selected volume is provided. A random noise generator and a clock circuit are employed in conjunction with a switched capacitance filter bank to produce a masking signal with the selected center frequency and selected bandwidth. The masking signal is then received by a volume control unit and then amplified for delivery to the **tinnitus** sufferer's ear or ears by speakers or headphones. Additionally, the **tinnitus** masking device may include a timer and fade out unit.

Excerpt(s): This invention relates to masking devices, and more particularly, but not by way of limitation, to a minimum energy masker for use by sufferers of subjective %+%bold%+%tinnitus.%?%.... Tinnitus describes a perceived sound, e.g., ringing, buzzing, whistling, or roaring, that is experienced by a **tinnitus** sufferer and that does not exist as a physical sound. The condition can be annoying or very painful, and the discomfort caused by **tinnitus** frequently interferes with a sufferer's sleep. **Tinnitus** often occurs at a specific frequency or over a small frequency range and is frequently constant; however, the specific frequency or small frequency range varies from patient to patient.... Most of the relatively recent efforts to treat **tinnitus** have involved attempts to mask the perceived sound. Masking is the interference of one sound on another. Perfect **tinnitus** masking involves providing a masking signal that exactly overrules the perceived sound in terms of psychoacoustics without supplying unnecessary energy to the **tinnitus** sufferer. See e.g., Tinnitus: Diagnosis/Treatment 55 (Abraham Shulman ed. 1991).

Web site: http://www.delphion.com/details?pn=US05403262__

- **Programmable hearing aid operable in a mode for tinnitus therapy**

  Inventor(s): Holube; Inga (Anton Bruckner Str. 43, 91052, Erlangen, DE), Martin; Raimund (Klingenweg 3, 91330, Eggolsheim, DE), Sigwanz; Ullrich (Buckenhofer Weg 39, 91058, Erlangen, DE), Zoels; Fred (Lettenfeldstr. 37, 90592, Altenhann, DE)

  Assignee(s): None Reported

  Patent Number: 6,047,074

  Date filed: June 17, 1997

  Abstract: A digital hearing aid is employable for **tinnitus** therapy, as well as for retraining **tinnitus** therapy, in combination with correction of other hearing impairments of a user of the hearing aid. For this purpose, the hearing aid contains a signal processing chain, between a hearing aid input and a hearing aid output, which is responsible for producing a useful signal by acting on the input signal in a manner to correct the hearing impairment of a user of the hearing aid. The signal processing chain also includes an arrangement for generating a **tinnitus** therapy signal, which is combined in the signal processing chain with the useful signal, dependent on a mode of operation which has been selected or set.

Excerpt(s): The present invention is directed to a programmable hearing aid of the type having at least one acoustoelectrical input transducer, a signal processing chain including a signal converter, an amplifier, a digital signal processor and a memory, and an electroacoustical output transducer.... A hearing aid of this type is disclosed in German Auslegeschrift 27 16 336, corresponding to U.S. Pat. No. 4,187,413. In this hearing aid, a microphone is provided as an input signal source that is connected to an amplifier followed by an analog-to-digital converter that is connected to a digital computer stag. A digital-to-analog converter is connected to the output of the computer stage and supplies an analog signal to an output amplifier to which an earphone is connected as an output transducer. The computer stage of this programmable hearing aid can be a microprocessor with a memory and can be implemented as an integrated module. A number of input signals, for example from a microphone and a pick-up induction coil, can thus be correlated with one another in the processor.... Tinnitus is a condition wherein a person perceives noises in the ear or head for which no external causes exist. This can be extremely uncomfortable and can lead to mental and physical disturbance in serious cases. The possibility of alleviating the **tinnitus** condition by drowning out the **tinnitus** noise with a sound signal supplied to the ear has been investigated for many years in the scientific literature.

Web site: http://www.delphion.com/details?pn=US06047074__

- **Pseudospontaneous neural stimulation system and method**

Inventor(s): Abbas; Paul J. (Iowa City, IA), Brown; Carolyn J. (Iowa City, IA), Rubinstein; Jay T. (Solon, IA), Tyler; Richard S. (West Branch, IA)

Assignee(s): The University of Iowa Research Foundation (iowa City, Ia)

Patent Number: 6,295,472

Date filed: August 13, 1999

Abstract: A system and method for application of pseudospontaneous neural stimulation is provided that can generate stochastic independent activity across an excited nerve or neural population without an additional disadvantageous sensations. High rate pulse trains, for example, can produce random spike patterns in auditory nerve fibers that are statistically similar to those produced by spontaneous activity in the normal ear. This activity is called "pseudospontaneous activity". Varying rates of pseudospontaneous activity can be created by varying the intensity of a fixed amplitude, high rate pulse train stimulus, e.g., 5000 pps. The pseudospontaneous activity can further desynchronize the nerve fiber population as a treatment for **tinnitus** but if indiscriminately applied can generate potentially uncomfortable biological and somatosensory sensations over intervals of time. A method for generating pseudospontaneous activity in an auditory nerve according to the present invention can include generating an electrical signal, and modifying the electrical signal to a sustained effective level while the electrical signal remains substantially physiologically imperceptible to the patient. The applied electrical signal can generate pseudospontaneous activity in the auditory nerve to suppress **tinnitus.**

Excerpt(s): This invention relates generally to an apparatus and method for providing stochastic independent neural stimulation, and in particular, a neural stimulation system and method for initiating pseudospontaneous activity in the auditory nerve, which can be used to treat **tinnitus**.... Fundamental differences currently exist between electrical stimulation and acoustic stimulation of the auditory nerve. Electrical stimulation of the auditory nerve, for example, via a cochlear implant, generally results in more cross-fiber synchrony, less within fiber jitter, and less dynamic range, as compared with acoustic stimulation which occurs in individuals having normal hearing.... Loss of spontaneous activity in the auditory nerve is one proposed mechanism for **tinnitus.** Proposed biological mechanisms for the loss of spontaneous activity in the auditory nerve include loss of hair cells in the cochlea. In addition, the loss of hair cells over time is a proposed mechanism for the loss of auditory neurons likely caused by related activities at synapses connecting the hair cells to the auditory neurons in the cochlea.

Web site: http://www.delphion.com/details?pn=US06295472__

- **Tinnitis masking and suppressor using pulsed ultrasound**

    Inventor(s): Lenhardt; Martin L. (Hayes, VA)

    Assignee(s): Sound Techniques Systems Llc (arlington, Va)

    Patent Number: 6,394,969

    Date filed: October 14, 1999

    Abstract: A system and method for **tinnitus** masking. Ultrasound noise is provided to a head of a patient as a vibration by way of a transducer, to thereby stimulate the auditory cortex. Once stimulated, the auditory cortex will suppress **tinnitus.** The ultrasound noise may be provided as an ultrasound frequency tone or as a range of frequencies that have been multiplied with an audio frequency. Pulsed ultrasound is utilized for ultrasound noise in the MHz range.

Excerpt(s): The present invention relates to a system and method for masking **tinnitus**. In particular, the present invention relates to a system and method for masking **tinnitus** using high frequency signals that affect the cortical auditory neurons in the brain.... Tinnitus is defined as any ringing in the ears for which there is no external source. For example, a ringing, buzzing, whistling, or roaring sound may be heard as a result of **tinnitus. Tinnitus** can be continuous or intermittent, and in either case can be very irritating to one who has such an affliction.... Prior to the present invention, there has been no consistently effective way to counter, or mask, **tinnitus**. Most of the attempts to date have focused on masking the perceived sound. For example, U.S. Pat. No. 4,222,393, issued to Robert Hocks et al., describes a **tinnitus** masker that provides sounds in the range of from 1000 Hz to 5000 Hz, with a peak around 3000 or 4000 Hz. The patient is provided with sounds of varying pitch, one after another, so that the patient can identify the particular external sound having the same pitch as the **tinnitus** that the patient is experiencing. Once this is done, a power operated sound is applied to the ear of the patient, with that sound including a range of frequencies extending in a range above and below the perceived pitch.

Web site: http://www.delphion.com/details?pn=US06394969__

- **Tinnitus masker**

    Inventor(s): Westermann; Soren E. (Hellerup, DK)

    Assignee(s): Topholm & Westermann Aps (vaerloese, Dk)

    Patent Number: 5,325,872

    Date filed: August 31, 1992

    Abstract: The invention relates to a **tinnitus** masker with one or more signal generators, a controllable amplifier (2), one or two electroacoustic transducers (3) for conversion of electrical signals into acoustic signals and a voltage source, whereby at least one of the signal generators (1) generates a continuously repeated, sinusoidal pure tone signal which slowly moves through the audio frequency range and whose cycle duration can be adjusted between 0.1 and 1000 seconds.

    Excerpt(s): The invention relates to a **tinnitus** masker with one or more signal generators, a controllable amplifier section, one or two electroacoustic transducers for conversion of electrical signals into acoustic signals as well as a voltage source.... Such devices are already known in principle.... More than half of the world's population suffers from **tinnitus** in one form or the other. It is a phenomenon which occurs in the hearing system whose causes are still unclear. It may consist of anything from a weak tone which occurs only several times a year up to a continuously audible loud noise, hissing, buzzing or even a very loud tone which is never interrupted.

Web site: http://www.delphion.com/details?pn=US05325872__

- **Tinnitus masker for direct drive hearing devices**

    Inventor(s): Ball; Geoffrey R. (Sunnyvale, CA), Katz; Bob H. (Los Gatos, CA)

    Assignee(s): Symphonix Devices, Inc. (san Jose, Ca)

    Patent Number: 5,795,287

    Date filed: September 30, 1996

    Abstract: Tinnitus maskers for direct drive hearing devices are provided. A circuit generates signals corresponding to sounds to mask **tinnitus** a user perceives. A direct drive hearing device which is coupled to a structure in the user vibrates in response to the signals. The vibrating direct drive hearing device stimulates hearing by vibrating the structure to which it is coupled. A user may select the frequency, intensity and phase of a tone generated. Additionally, a second tone or a background sound may be selected.

    Excerpt(s): The present invention is related to hearing systems and, more particularly, to **tinnitus** masker systems for use with direct drive hearing devices.... Tinnitus is the perception of sound when there is none present. It is most often described as "ringing in the ears" but varies from person to person. Some people hear hissing, buzzing, whistling, roaring, high-pitched screeches, or a sound like steam escaping from a radiator. Still others hear one tone or several tones. Twelve million Americans suffer from a severe case of **tinnitus** and it has been estimated that 20% of the population experiences **tinnitus** at some time in their lives.... Initially, a person suffering from **tinnitus** may be worried or frightened because she is unsure what is wrong or how serious is the condition. Although **tinnitus** itself is not life threatening, some **tinnitus** sufferers describe the constant noise as irritating while others describe it as maddening. The actual medical cause of **tinnitus** is not clear but it is believed that some factors such as exposure to loud noise may produce or worsen **tinnitus.**

    Web site: http://www.delphion.com/details?pn=US05795287__

- **Tinnitus masking using ultrasonic signals**

    Inventor(s): Lippa; Arnold S. (Tucson, AZ), Nunley; James A. (Scottsdale, AZ)

    Assignee(s): Hearing Innovations Incorporated (tucson, Az)

    Patent Number: 6,377,693

    Date filed: June 23, 1994

    Abstract: A method and apparatus for treating tinnitus involves generating a noise signal to mask the ringing or buzzing in the ears caused by tinnitus and transposing the noise signal into the ultrasonic frequency range. As such, the masking signal effectively masks the tinnitus noise without interfering with the subject's perception of normal sounds such as human speech. In an alternative embodiment, human speech is transduced into electrical signals, transposed to the ultrasonic frequency range, and physically applied to the patient while tinnitus masking signals in the auditory range are applied to the patient.

    Excerpt(s): The present invention relates generally to methods and apparatus for improving the hearing sensory response of human subjects and more specifically relates to methods and apparatus for treating the symptoms of tinnitus.... Tinnitus is an affliction of the human sensory system which causes a persistent buzzing, ringing or whistling sound in the ears or head. One possible cause of tinnitus is a defect in the auditory nerve, although all possible causes of tinnitus are not fully known.... In an effort to relieve the annoyance caused by tinnitus, one known treatment is to apply variable preferred bands of white noise to the patient in the auditory range, which serves to mask the tinnitus ringing or buzzing. However, this treatment is usually unsatisfactory because the masking noise can interfere with the patient's normal hearing perception.

    Web site: http://www.delphion.com/details?pn=US06377693__

- **Tinnitus rehabilitation device and method**

    Inventor(s): Davis; Paul Benjamin (Copenhagen, DK)

    Assignee(s): Tinnitech Ltd. (sydney, At)

    Patent Number: 6,682,472

    Date filed: September 17, 2001

    Abstract: A tinnitus method and device for providing relief to a person suffering from the disturbing effects of tinnitus is described. The method can be implemented entirely in software to spectrally modify an audio signal in accordance with a predetermined masking algorithm which modifies the intensity of the audio signal at selected frequencies. A predetermined masking algorithm is described which provides intermittent masking of the **tinnitus** wherein, at a comfortable listening level, during peaks of the audio signal the **tinnitus** is completely obscured, whereas during troughs the perception of the **tinnitus** occasionally emerges. In practice it has been found that such intermittent masking provides an immediate sense of relief, control and relaxation for the person, whilst enabling sufficient perception of the **tinnitus** for habituation and long term treatment to occur. Advantageously the predetermined masking algorithm is specifically tailored to the audiometric configuration of the person. For example, the masking algorithm may be partly tailored to the hearing loss characteristic of the person. A **tinnitus** rehabilitation device used in conjunction with a personal sound reproducing system is also described.

Excerpt(s): The present invention relates to a **tinnitus** rehabilitation device and method for providing relief and treatment to persons suffering from the disturbing effects of **tinnitus** and relates particularly, though not exclusively, to such a method and device that employs intermittent masking of the **tinnitus**.... Tinnitus is the perception of a sound in the absence of any corresponding external sound. It is most commonly perceived as a ringing, buzing, whirring type sound, but can also be perceived as a beating, or pounding sensation. Around one third of people who suffer from **tinnitus** can be quite highly disturbed by it. Continuous perception of **tinnitus** can lead to insomnia, an inability to relax, state and trait anxiety, depression, and even suicide in extreme cases. Often closely associated with **tinnitus** is the perception of hyperacusis, which is a great intolerance to external sounds, even the softer everyday sounds. This distressing condition can even occur as a precursor to **tinnitus,** and is thought to share the same underlying causes. Thus, every reference to **tinnitus** in this document should be construed as including the phenomena of hyperacusis or other types of loudness discomfort.... There are very few effective treatment options available for **tinnitus** sufferers, with the vast majority only being advised that "you'll have to learn to live with it". Most patients find that they can far more readily ignore an external sound than their **tinnitus.** One palliative method has been to use hearing aid-style devices that produce a band of noise to totally mask the perception of the **tinnitus.** This gives a sense of relief and control over the **tinnitus** in around half of patients, but usually has no long-term effect. The prohibitive cost (around A$1500) and aesthetic considerations limits the proportion of sufferers for whom this is a viable measure. The presence of hearing loss for external sounds in the **tinnitus** region often means that the masking noise needs to be unpleasantly loud before the **tinnitus** can be masked, and the noise is often judged to be not much better than the **tinnitus** itself.

Web site: http://www.delphion.com/details?pn=US06682472__

- **Transcanal, transtympanic cochlear implant system for the rehabilitation of deafness and tinnitus**

    Inventor(s): Boylston; Byron Lee (Woodstock, GA), Goldsmith; Miles Manning (Savannah, GA)

    Assignee(s): Microphonics, Inc. (plano, Tx)

    Patent Number: 6,671,559

    Date filed: January 22, 2002

    Abstract: A transcanal, transtympanic cochlear implant system for implantation comprising a molded insert for removable positioning in the auditory canal of the human ear and an insulated receiver coil, preferably in a generally circular or looped form, where the receiver coil receives electromagnetic signals, in a first embodiment, or radio frequency signals, in a second embodiment, through inductive coupling to a solenoid coil within the molded insert.

    Excerpt(s): The present invention is directed to the field of cochlear implants for patients with hearing impairment and/or **tinnitus,** more particularly to a transcanal, transtympanic cochlear implant system that requires a minimum of surgical intrusion that may be performed at a physician's office under local anesthesia.... The present invention relates to a transcanal, transtympanic cochlear implant system ideally suited for those profoundly deaf, where conventional amplifying hearing aids are of limited or no value to those suffering the hearing impairment. That is to say, with maximum gain delivered by the most powerful hearing aids, these profoundly deaf individuals cannot hear sound and hence cannot discriminate and understand speech. In addition, there are an estimated 200-300 million people who have various patterns of severe sensorineural hearing loss, which are imperfectly rehabilitated via hearing aids. An example of such is so called "ski-sloped hearing loss," where there is near normal hearing in the low to middle frequency range, but the hearing drops out dramatically in the higher frequencies. For these types of hearing loss, amplification is ineffective, because the cochlea cannot perform its transductive function of converting the mechanical energy of sound to the electrical current, which is ultimately perceived as sound by the brain. The inner ear structures responsible for this transductive function are known as hair cells, and the electrical currents, which they produce in response to the mechanical stimulation by sound, are known as cochlear microphonics. When these hair cells are sufficiently damaged in the above mentioned scenarios, no amount of amplification will be effective.... The cochlear implant is, in effect, a bionic ear in that it replaces the lost cochlear microphonic with an electrical current that is the precise analog of sound. Current United States Food and Drug Administration ("FDA") approved cochlear implant systems are so-called multichannel long electrode devices, which are expensive, highly complex devices surgically introduced via a complicated and (for the average otolaryngologist) risky procedure under general anesthesia known as the facial recess mastoidectomy. The estimated cost of these cochlear implant systems, including surgical, anesthesia, hospital, and programming fees is currently quite high. The hardware necessary to program these devices adds further to these high costs, and the time to program the first map for these devices averages from four to twelve hours depending upon the age of the patient, among other factors. This prohibitive price and impractical complexity is simply not accessible to the vast majority of the global deaf population. Furthermore, the average otologist in the developing countries of the world typically does not have the sophistication, expertise and equipment to confidently undertake the facial recess mastoidectomy in order to introduce the internal component of the multichannel systems.

Web site: http://www.delphion.com/details?pn=US06671559__

- **Use of DL-(+/-)-.alpha.-lipoic acid, D-(+)-.alpha.-lipoic acid,.alpha.-lipoic acid in reduced or oxidized form or salts for treating circulatory disorders**

    Inventor(s): Conrad; Frank (Frankfurt, DE), Geise; Wolfgang (Dipbach, DE), Henrich; Hermann-August (Wurzburg, DE), Ulrich; Heinz (Niedernberg, DE)

    Assignee(s): Asta Medica Aktiengesellschaft (dresden, De)

    Patent Number: 5,650,429

    Date filed: November 8, 1995

    Abstract: The invention relates to the use of DL-(+/-)-.alpha. lipoic acid, D-(+)-.alpha.-lipoic acid, L-(-)-.alpha.-lipoic acid in reduced or oxidized form or of the metabolites and salts, esters, amides thereof for the preparation of medicines for the treatment of disorders caused by changes or disturbances in the rheological properties of the blood such as blood viscosity, erythrocyte flexibility and the aggregation of erythrocytes, in particular for the treatment of microangiopathy with disturbed microcirculation. It can also be used in the treatment of diabetics and of dialysis patients for protection of the erythrocytes, in central and peripheral circulatory disturbances and in **tinnitus** and hearing loss.

Excerpt(s): In circulatory disturbances therapy using rheologically active substances is gaining in importance, especially when a retrogression of rheological blockages is no longer possible. Rheologically active substances improve the blood flow. If the rheological component predominates as compared with other effects on the circulatory system, these substances which stimulate the circulation are referred to as "rheologica" (Radke et al., 1983). An increased flow capacity increases the flow of blood through the flow paths (microcirculation) and thereby also the oxygen supply to the tissues. This is particularly the case when the blood vessels can no longer continue to be supplied at the pathological initiation site and therefore the vasomotor reserve is exhausted.....alpha.-lipoic acid is referred to chemically as 1,2-dithiolane-3-pentanoic acid, 5-(1,2-dithiolane-3-yl)-valeric acid or 5-3-(1,2-dithioanyl)pentanoic acid..alpha.-lipoic acid possesses a chiral C atom, occurs in two enantiomeric forms and is found physiologically in plants, in bacteria and in the mammalian organism. It has the function of a coenzyme in mitochondrial multienzyme complexes such as, for example, those of pyruvate dehydrogenase, of.alpha.-ketoglutarate dehydrogenase and of the dehydrogenase of the branched-chain amino acids. During metabolism.alpha.-lipoic acid can be converted from the oxidized form (disulphide bridge) to the reduced dihydro form having two free --SH groups. Both forms have a distinct antioxidizing action (for example, Kuklinski et al., 1991; Packer, 1993). The redox pair dihydrolipoic acid/.alpha.-lipoic acid moreover has metal-chelating properties. In the Federal Republic of Germany.alpha.-lipoic acid has been in use since 1966 as a medicine for the treatment of diseases of the liver, in fungal poisoning and in peripheral polyneuropathies. From knowledge of this antioxidizing action, general reference is made in DE-OS 41 38 040 A1 to a compound which catches free radicals and possesses thiol functions. The claim relates to solutions for the perfusion, conservation and reperfusion of organs and does not relate to the present invention, because here a new action in a new application has been found over and above the known antioxidizing property.... The SU Patent 1 769 865 A1 relates to the use of compounds including.alpha.-lipoic acid for the phenomenological improvement of the blood circulation and, more precisely, to the enlargement of the blood stream through the large vessels of the uterus and to the decrease of the volumetric variables in the region of the chorion in placental insufficiency.

Web site: http://www.delphion.com/details?pn=US05650429__

Patent Applications on Tinnitus

As of December 2000, U.S. patent applications are open to public viewing.[24] Applications are patent requests which have yet to be granted (the process to achieve a patent can take several years). The following patent applications have been filed since December 2000 relating to tinnitus:

- **Composition and method for prevention and treatment of health conditions caused by constriction of smooth muscle cells**

    Inventor(s): Rath, Matthias; (Cupertino, CA)

    Correspondence: Kenyon & Kenyon; One Broadway; New York; NY; 10004; US

    Patent Application Number: 20030003162

    Date filed: June 19, 2001

    Abstract: The invention relates to a method of administering to a human subject a composition comprising a vitamin, an amino acid and a trace element for the prevention and treatment of health conditions caused by constriction of smooth muscle cells in organs of the human body like high blood pressure, asthma, glaucoma and **tinnitus**. The composition comprises a vitamin such as ascorbic acid, an amino acid such as arginine, and a trace element such as magnesium.

    Excerpt(s): The present invention relates generally to the prevention and treatment of health conditions caused by constriction of smooth muscle cells in organs of the human body.... The cause of many diseases remains unknown. Among these diseases with unknown origin are most common diseases including high blood pressure, asthma, glaucoma and **tinnitus**. In case of high blood pressure, one of the most renowned textbooks in medicine, Harrison's Principles of Internal Medicine, states that the cause of the disease is unknown in about 90% of the patients. Worldwide several hundred million people suffer from these health conditions and the economic damage to society from not being able to treat these health conditions effectively is immeasurable.... Worldwide several million people suffer from asthma bronchiale (asthma). In its late stages asthma is a debilitating disease leading to the inability to work and to-social isolation. The cause of this disease remains unknown, even though allergens, genetic disposition and psychological factors have been implicated. The common pathomechanism of this disease is an obstruction of the ventilation channels in the lung (bronchioles) and of

---

[24] This has been a common practice outside the United States prior to December 2000.

the passages to the alveoli where the oxygenation takes place. However, the cellular mechanisms that trigger this obstruction, thereby causing asthma, is not yet understood.

Web site: http://appft1.uspto.gov/netahtml/PTO/search-bool.html

- **Composition and method for treating tinnitus**

Inventor(s): Keate, Barry; (Salt Lake City, UT)

Correspondence: Morriss O'bryant Compagni, P.c.; 136 South Main Street; Suite 700; Salt Lake City; UT; 84101; US

Patent Application Number: 20030232098

Date filed: June 11, 2003

Abstract: Therapeutic compositions for the treatment of **tinnitus** are described which contain effective amounts of Ginkgo biloba, garlic and zinc. In formulations containing greater than 50 mg of zinc, the composition may further contain copper. Methods of treating patients having **tinnitus** include prescribing effective daily doses of the therapeutic compositions of the present invention over a sixty to ninety day period to maximize improvement in the condition, followed by a daily regimen of the therapeutic compositions.

Excerpt(s): This is a non-provisional application claiming priority to provisional application Serial No. 60/388,984 filed Jun. 14, 2002.... This invention relates to therapeutic compositions and methods for treating disease conditions, and specifically relates to an improved compositions and methods for treating **tinnitus**.... Tinnitus is a condition of the body which is manifested by a ringing in one or both ears of a person. **Tinnitus** can be intermittent or a constant condition. It can be manifested as a single sound or tone or multiple tones. The perception of volume of the ringing or noise can range from subtle to very loud. The ringing experienced as a result of **tinnitus** can vary among individuals in intensity and timbre of ringing. Nonetheless, many persons who experience **tinnitus** are seriously affected by the constant ringing condition.

Web site: http://appft1.uspto.gov/netahtml/PTO/search-bool.html

- **Cyclic substituted aminomethyl compounds and medicaments comprising these compounds**

  Inventor(s): Koegel, Babette-Yvonne; (Langerwehe-Hamich, DE), Strassburger, Wolfgang Werner Alfred; (Wuerselen, DE), Zimmer, Oswald Karl; (Wuerselen, DE)

  Correspondence: Crowell & Moring Llp; Intellectual Property Group; P.o. Box 14300; Washington; DC; 20044-4300; US

  Patent Application Number: 20030166708

  Date filed: January 10, 2003

  Abstract: Cyclic substituted aminomethyl compounds of general formula IA and IB, methods for production thereof, intermediates in said production methods, a medicament containing at least one of said cyclic substituted aminomethyl compounds, the use of said cyclic substituted aminomethyl compounds for the production of a medicament, pharmaceutical compositions containing said compounds, and methods for the treatment of pain, incontinence, pruritis, **tinnitus** aurium and/or diarrhea using said pharmaceutical compositions.

  Excerpt(s): The present application is a continuation of international patent application no. PCT/EP01/07750, filed Jul. 6, 2001, designating the United States of America and published in German as WO 02/08218, the entire disclosure of which is incorporated herein by reference. Priority is claimed based on Federal Republic of Germany patent application no. 100 33 459.8, filed Jul. 10, 2000.... The present Application relates to cyclic substituted aminomethyl compounds, processes for their preparation, intermediate compounds of these processes, medicaments comprising at least one of the cyclic substituted aminomethyl compounds, the use of the cyclic substituted aminomethyl compounds for the preparation of a medicament for treatment of pain, urinary incontinence, itching, **tinnitus** aurium and/or diarrhea, and pharmaceutical compositions comprising these compounds.... Treatment of chronic and non-chronic states of pain is of great importance in medicine. There is a world-wide need for therapies which have a good action for target-orientated treatment of chronic and non-chronic states of pain appropriate for the patient, by which is to be understood successful and satisfactory pain treatment for the patient.

  Web site: http://appft1.uspto.gov/netahtml/PTO/search-bool.html

- **Dosage forms useful for modifying conditions and functions associated with hearing loss and/or tinnitus**

Inventor(s): Pearson, Don C.; (Lakewood, WA), Richardson, Kenneth T.; (Anchorage, AK)

Correspondence: M. Henry Heines; Townsend and Townsend and Crew Llp; Two Embarcadero Center, 8th Floor; San Francisco; CA; 94111-3834; US

Patent Application Number: 20020061870

Date filed: January 19, 2001

Abstract: The invention defines interdependent biofactors and biomolecules, and clinically useful formulations that are comprised of them. The active agents are demonstrated to be complementary in their physiologic functions especially as these relate to the quenching of free radicals and to the support of endothelial physiology, the reduction of hyperinsulinemia and improvements in vascular health. The active components of the invention are selected for inclusion in precise combinations specifically because they improve these various conditions and physiological functions, and by so doing reduce a variety of risks associated with hearing loss and **tinnitus**. The resulting enhancement of general systemic vascular health, improvement in local VIII.sup.th nerve vascular health, modulation of conditions surrounding blood fluid dynamics, the consequences of hyperinsulinemia, and improvements in free radical defenses, all reduce the potential for cochlear hair cell death and VIII.sup.th nerve atrophy, and the hearing loss and possible deafness that accompany them.

Excerpt(s): This application is related to United States Provisional Patent Application No. 60/178,487, filed Jan. 27, 2000, and claims all benefits legally available therefrom. Provisional Patent Application No. 60/178,487 is hereby incorporated by reference for all purposes capable of being served thereby.... This invention is in the field of pharmacology and relates specifically to the improvement of clinical conditions associated with symptomatic or presymptomatic hearing loss and/or **tinnitus** and the reduction of risks associated with their onset.... The ear of humans consists of three parts: the outer, middle and inner ear. The outer ear consists of the external ear and the auditory canal. The external ear modifies sound waves and the air-filled auditory canal conducts the sound waves to the middle ear, which consists of the tympanic membrane, or eardrum; the eustachian tube; and three tiny bones called the hammer, anvil, and stirrup. Membranes and bone surround the middle ear with the eustachian tube connecting it to the pharynx, equalizing the air pressure between the middle ear and the atmosphere.

Web site: http://appft1.uspto.gov/netahtml/PTO/search-bool.html

- **Method and apparatus for treatment of mono-frequency tinnitus**

  Inventor(s): Choy, Daniel S.J.; (New York, NY)

  Correspondence: Steven L. Nichols; Rader, Fishman & Graver Pllc; 10653 S. River Front Parkway; Suite 150; South Jordan; UT; 84095; US

  Patent Application Number: 20030114728

  Date filed: December 12, 2002

  Abstract: Reciprocal noise cancellation of a patient's mono-frequency **tinnitus** tone is achieved utilizing an externally generated tone which is subjectively defined by a mono-frequency **tinnitus** patient to match his/her **tinnitus** tone in frequency and amplitude. An externally generated sound wave, selectively designated by subjective observations of a patient to match the patient's **tinnitus** tone is first applied to the **tinnitus** patient via earphones or a speaker system and then the same externally generated sound wave is sequentially phase shifted through a plurality of angularly shifted sequence steps to shift or slide the external sound wave through at least a 180 degree phase shift of the generated signal as it is applied to the patient to achieve a series of reductions of the patient's **tinnitus** tone and in one of such shifted steps a reciprocal, canceling relationship with the patient's **tinnitus** tone. The **tinnitus** treatment sequence of an externally generated sound wave and then the phase shifted externally generated tone achieve cancellation of the **tinnitus** tone of the patient as the sequential steps of the generated tone in effect slide across the **tinnitus** sound wave resulting in cancellation of the **tinnitus** tone. By replaying the sequential phase shifted segments of the patient treatment process a patient may utilize the previously recorded sequences in a patient self-treatment process.

  Excerpt(s): This application claims the benefit of the earlier filing date of U.S. Provisional Application No. 60/340,271, filed Dec. 18, 2001 and further relates to U.S. application Ser. No. 10/083,088 filed Mar. 1, 2002. The specification and disclosure of both of these related Applications are incorporated herein in their entirety by this reference.... The present inventions relate to the treatment of **tinnitus** patients and more particularly to improved clinical methods and apparatus for treatment of mono-frequency **tinnitus** patients utilizing phase shift cancellation principles.... Tinnitus is defined as the perception of sound by an individual when no external sound is present, and often takes the form of a hissing, ringing, roaring, chirping or clicking sound which may be intermittent or constant. According to the American **Tinnitus**

Association, **tinnitus** afflicts more than 50 million Americans, and more than 12 million of those suffer so severely from **tinnitus** that they seek medical attention and many cannot function normally on a day-to-day basis.

Web site: http://appft1.uspto.gov/netahtml/PTO/search-bool.html

- **Methods and compositions for the treatment of neuropathic pain, tinnitus, and other disorders using R(-)-ketoprofen**

  Inventor(s): Jerussi, Thomas P.; (Framingham, MA), Rubin, Paul D.; (Sudbury, MA)

  Correspondence: Pennie & Edmonds Llp; 1667 K Street NW; Suite 1000; Washington; DC; 20006

  Patent Application Number: 20020147238

  Date filed: February 5, 2002

  Abstract: Methods of treating neuropathic pain, **tinnitus**, and related disorders are disclosed. These methods comprise the administration of optically pure R(-)-ketoprofen. Also disclosed are pharmaceutical compositions useful in the treatment of neuropathic pain and **tinnitus** which comprise optically pure R(-)-ketoprofen.

  Excerpt(s): The invention relates to methods of treating neuropathic pain, **tinnitus**, and other disorders, and to pharmaceutical compositions useful in the treatment of neuropathic pain and **tinnitus**.... Racemic ketoprofen (a mixture of the R(-) and S(+) enantiomers) is sold under the tradenames Orudis.RTM. and Oruvail.RTM. for the treatment of inflammation. Physicians' Desk Reference 52.sup.nd Ed., p. 3092 (1998). Generally, ketoprofen is considered to be a nonsteroidal anti-inflammatory agent ("NSAID"). NSAIDs are believed to exhibit activity as COX-1 or COX-2 enzyme inhibitors. Most NSAIDs are believed to cause gastrointestinal irritation.... The S(+) enantiomer of ketoprofen has long been thought to possess most, if not all, of the pharmacological activity of the racemate. See, e.g., Yamaguchi et al., Nippon Yakurigaku Zasshi. 90:295-302 (1987); Abas et al., J. Pharinacol. Exp. Ther., 240:637-641 (1987); and Caldwell et al., Biochem. Pharrnacol. 37:105-114 (1988). Indeed, U.S. Pat. Nos. 4,868,214, 4,962,124, and 4,927,854 each allege that the analgesic activity of ketoprofen resides exclusively in the S(+) enantiomer.

  Web site: http://appft1.uspto.gov/netahtml/PTO/search-bool.html

- **Methods of diagnosing and treating small intestinal bacterial overgrowth (SIBO) and SIBO-related conditions**

Inventor(s): Lin, Henry C.; (Manhattan Beach, CA), Pimentel, Mark; (Los Angeles, CA)

Correspondence: Sidley & Austin; 555 West Fifth Street; Los Angeles; CA; 90071-2909; US

Patent Application Number: 20020039599

Date filed: April 17, 2001

Abstract: Disclosed is a method of treating small intestinal bacterial overgrowth (SIBO) or a SIBO-caused condition in a human subject. SIBO-caused conditions include irritable bowel syndrome, fibromyalgia, chronic pelvic pain syndrome, chronic fatigue syndrome, depression, impaired mentation, impaired memory, halitosis, **tinnitus,** sugar craving, autism, attention deficit/hyperactivity disorder, drug sensitivity, an autoimmune disease, and Crohn's disease. Also disclosed are a method of screening for the abnormally likely presence of SIBO in a human subject and a method of detecting SIBO in a human subject. A method of determining the relative severity of SIBO or a SIBO-caused condition in a human subject, in whom small intestinal bacterial overgrowth (SIBO) has been detected, is also disclosed.

Excerpt(s): This application is is a continuation-in-part of U.S. patent application Ser. No. 09/374,142, filed on Aug. 11, 1999. This application is also a continuation-in-part of U.S. patent application Ser. No. 09/546,119, filed on Apr. 10, 2000, which is a continuation-in-part of U.S. patent application Ser. No. 09/420,046, filed Oct. 18, 1999, which is a continuation-in-part of U.S. patent application Ser. No. 09/359,583, filed on Jul. 22, 1999, abandoned, which was a continuation of U.S. patent application Ser. No. 08/832,307, filed on Apr. 3, 1997 and issued as U.S. Pat. No. 5,977,175 on Nov. 2, 1999, which was a continuation of U.S. patent application Ser. No. 08/442,843, filed on May 17,1995, abandoned.... Throughout this application various publications are referenced within parentheses. The disclosures of these publications in their entireties are hereby incorporated by reference in this application in order to more fully describe the state of the art to which, this invention pertains.... Small intestinal bacterial overgrowth (SIBO), also known as small bowel bacterial overgrowth (SBBO), is an abnormal condition in which aerobic and anaerobic enteric bacteria from the colon proliferate in the small intestine, which is normally relatively free of bacterial contamination. SIBO is defined as greater than 10^6 CFU/mL small intestinal effluent (R. M. Donaldson, Jr., Normal bacterial populations of the intestine and their relation to intestinal function, N. Engl. J. Med.

270:938-45 [1964]). Typically, the symptoms include abdominal pain, bloating, gas and alteration in bowel habits, such as constipation and diarrhea.

Web site: http://appft1.uspto.gov/netahtml/PTO/search-bool.html

- **Neurotoxin therapy for inner ear disorders**

  Inventor(s): Donovan, Stephen; (Capistrano Beach, CA)

  Correspondence: Stephen Donovan; Allergan, Inc. T2-7h; 2525 Dupont Drive; Irvine; CA; 92612; US

  Patent Application Number: 20010025024

  Date filed: May 24, 2001

  Abstract: Methods for treating otic disorders by local administration of a neurotoxin. A botulinum toxin can be administered to myoclonic middle ear muscles and to inner ear efferent and/or afferent nerves to alleviate otic disorders such as **tinnitus,** cochlear nerve dysfunction and Meniere's disease.

  Excerpt(s): The present invention relates to methods for treating otic disorders. In particular the present invention relates to methods for treating otic disorders by local administration of a neurotoxin to a human ear.... The human ear can be divided into an outer ear, a middle ear and an inner ear. The outer ear comprises the auricle (commonly referred to as the ear) and the external acoustic meatus (the auditory canal). The tympanic membrane (commonly called the eardrum) separates the auditory canal from the middle ear (the tympanic cavity). Three small, mobile bones, the incus, malleus and stapes make up an ossicular system which conducts sound through the middle ear to the cochlea. The handle of the malleus is attached to the center of the tympanic membrane. At its opposite end, the malleus is bound to the incus by ligaments, so that movement of the malleus causes the incus to also move. The opposite end of the incus articulates with the stem of the stapes. The faceplate of the stapes rests against the membranous labyrinth in the opening of the oval window, where sound waves are conducted into the inner ear. In the cochlea the sound waves are transduced into coded patterns of impulses transmitted along the afferent cochlear fibers of the vestibulocochlear nerve for analysis in the central auditory pathways of the brain.... The air filled tympanic cavity contains various muscles including the tensor tympani and stapedius muscles. The tensor tympani is a long slender muscle which occupies the bony canal above the osseous pharyngotympanic tube, from which it is separated by a thin bony septum. The tensor tympani muscle receives both motor and proprioceptive innervation. A motor branch derived from the nerve to the medial pterygoid (mandibular division of the V, parasympathetic, trigeminal nerve) passes through the otic (a peripheral, parasympathetic cholinergic) ganglion to the tensor tympani. The stapedius muscle extends from the wall of a conical cavity in the pyramidal eminence, located on the posterior wall of the tympanic cavity. The stapedius is innervated by a branch of the (VII, parasympathetic) facial nerve.

Web site: http://appft1.uspto.gov/netahtml/PTO/search-bool.html

- **Novel method and compositions for local treatment of meniere's disease, tinnitus and/or hearing loss**

Inventor(s): Rask-Andersen, Helge; (Uppsala, SE), Stjernschantz, Johan; (Uppsala, SE)

Correspondence: Dinsmore & Shohl, Llp; 1900 Chemed Center; 255 East Fifth Street; Cincinnati; OH; 45202; US

Patent Application Number: 20040029970

Date filed: June 5, 2003

Abstract: A novel method and compositions for the local treatment of Meniere's disease, **tinnitus** and hearing loss are described. The treatment is based on the administration of a therapeutically effective amount of a prostaglandin of the F-type to the inner ear. The treatment can be either continuous or intermittent and may invlove the use of pumps, gels, or slow release drug inserts.

Excerpt(s): The present invention concerns a novel method and composition for the treatment of Meniere's disease, hearing loss and **tinnitus**.... Meniere's disease, a disorder of the inner ear, afflicts around 0.1-0.5% of the adult population. The disease is characterized by vertigo, hearing loss and **tinnitus,** and usually begins in the middle life, although it may manifest itself even at lower age. The disease occurs in both sexes at about the same rate. It typically occurs in episodes of marked vertigo, hearing loss and **tinnitus,** lasting for hours up to a few days, but also during the intermittent time periods the patients may suffer from **tinnitus** and hearing loss. Usually Meniere's disease is unilateral, but with time both ears may become involved, and an estimated 12 percent have bilateral disease.... Although the disease tends to be episodic with severe vertigo, nausea and hearing loss and subsequent remissions, with time patients usually suffer from general hearing loss and **tinnitus.** The remissions may last from a day to several years, but most commonly they last for a few weeks to months. Not uncommonly speech perception is reduced during the attacks. Complete deafness in the affected ear has been reported to occur at a rate of about 10 percent. The individual symptoms of Meniere's disease may vary greatly between patients as may the duration of the remissions, but the disease typically is chronic lasting the whole remaining life from its onset. The disease may impair the working ability and social life of the patients leading to psychological and mental disturbances, and in severe cases patients have even committed suicide because of the disease.

Web site: http://appft1.uspto.gov/netahtml/PTO/search-bool.html

- **Pharmaceutical compositions containing triazolones and methods of treating neurodegenerative disease using triazolones**

  Inventor(s): Bechtel, Wolf-Dietrich; (Appenheim, DE), Brenner, Michael; (Bingen, DE), Palluk, Rainer; (Bingen, DE), Weiser, Thomas; (Nieder-Olm, DE), Wienrich, Marion; (Weiterstadt, DE)

  Correspondence: Boehringer Ingelheim Corporation; 900 Ridgebury Road; P. O. Box 368; Ridgefield; CT; 06877; US

  Patent Application Number: 20020045651

  Date filed: April 23, 2001

  Abstract: A method for treating a neurodegenerative disease or cerebral ischemia arising from conditions selected from the group consisting of Status epilepticus, hypoglycaemia, hypoxia, anoxia, brain trauma, brain oedema, amyotropic lateral sclerosis, Huntington's disease, Alzheimer's disease, hypotonia, cardiac infarction, brain pressure (elevated intracranial pressure), ischaemic and haemorrhagic stroke, global cerebral ischaemia with heart stoppage, diabetic polyneuropathy, **tinnitus**, perinatal asphyxia, psychosis, schizophrenia, depression, and Parkinson's disease, the method of treatment comprising administering to a host in need of such treatment a therapeutic amount of a compound of formula (I) 1wherein R.sup.1, R.sup.2, R.sup.3, R.sup.4, R.sup.5, R.sup.6, and R.sup.7 are as defined herein, or a pharmaceutically acceptable salt thereof, and pharmaceutical compositions containing a compound of formula (I).

  Excerpt(s): The invention relates to the use of triazolones as pharmaceutical compositions, particularly pharmaceutical compositions with a neuroprotective activity, as well as new triazolones and processes for preparing them.... Triazolones are known from the prior art and are disclosed, for example, by published German applications DE 19521162 and DE 3631511 and also by European Patent applications EP 270 061 and EP 208 321. The compounds disclosed therein are effective pesticides and may be used in particular as insecticides and acaricides.... The present invention, by contrast, discloses triazolones which can be used as pharmaceuticals, particularly pharmaceutical compositions with a neuroprotective activity. Surprisingly, it has been found that the compounds according to the invention have an affinity for or an effect on various types of receptors and exhibit a neuroprotective activity.

Web site: http://appft1.uspto.gov/netahtml/PTO/search-bool.html

- **Salts of bicyclic, N-acylated imidazo-3-amines and imidazo-5-amines**

  Inventor(s): Gerlach, Matthias; (Brachttal, DE), Sundermann, Corinna; (Aachen, DE)

  Correspondence: Crowell & Moring Llp; Intellectual Property Group; P.o. Box 14300; Washington; DC; 20044-4300; US

  Patent Application Number: 20030119842

  Date filed: October 18, 2002

  Abstract: Salts of a bicyclic, N-acylated imidazo-3-amine or an imidazo-5-amine of the formula: 1addition products thereof with acids, and methods for preparing the salts and addition products. Also disclosed are pharmaceutical compositions comprising the same and methods using the pharmaceutical compositions for the treatment or prophylaxis of pain, drug or alcohol abuse, diarrhoea, gastritis, ulcers, urinary incontinence, depression, narcolepsy, overweight, asthma, glaucoma, **tinnitus,** itching, hyperkinetic syndrome, epilepsy, or schizophrenia, for inducing anesthesia, and for anxiolysis.

  Excerpt(s): The present application is a continuation of international patent application no. PCT/EP01/03772, filed Apr. 3, 2001, designating the United States of America, and published in German as WO 01/81344, the entire disclosure of which is incorporated herein by reference. Priority is claimed based on Federal Republic of Germany patent application no. 100 19 714.0, filed Apr. 20, 2000.... The present invention relates to salts of bicyclic, N-acylated imidazo-3-amines and imidazo-5-amines, to a process for producing them, to their use for producing pharmaceutical compositions and to pharmaceutical compositions containing these compounds.... Individual compounds from the category of non-acylated bicyclic imidazo-3-amines and imidazo-5-amines which form the basis of the compounds according to the present invention are known to have interesting pharmacological properties. Thus, certain imidazo[1,2-a]pyridines are described as blood pressure-reducing active ingredients (GB-B-1,135,893), as anthelmintics and antimycotics (J. Med. Chem. 1972, 15, 982-985) and as anti-secretory active ingredients for the treatment of inflammatory diseases (EP-A-0 068 378). EP-A-0 266 890 and J. Med. Chem. 1987, 30, 2031-2046 also describe an effect of individual imidazopyridines against inflammatory diseases, in particular of the stomach. Further pharmacological effects described for individual representatives of the category of non-acylated imidazo-3-amines and imidazo-5-amines are antibacterial properties (Chem. Pharm. Bull. 1992, 40, 1170), antiviral properties (J. Med. Chem. 1998, 41 5108-5112) and the effect as benzodiazepine-receptor antagonist (J. Heterocyclic Chem. 1998, 35, 1205-1217).

Web site: http://appft1.uspto.gov/netahtml/PTO/search-bool.html

- **Substituted 3,4-dihydropyrido[1,2-a]pyrimidines**

Inventor(s): Gerlach, Matthias; (Brachttal, DE), Jagusch, Utz-Peter; (Aachen, DE), Maul, Corinna; (Aachen, DE)

Correspondence: Crowell & Moring Llp; Intellectual Property Group; P.o. Box 14300; Washington; DC; 20044-4300; US

Patent Application Number: 20030229104

Date filed: April 11, 2003

Abstract: Substituted 3,4-dihydropyrido[1,2-a]pyrimidines of formula I 1and processes for the production thereof Also disclosed are substance libraries and pharmaceutical compositions containing the compound, and methods of treatment for pain, urinary incontinence, pruritus, **tinnitus** and/or diarrhoea using the pharmaceutical composition.

Excerpt(s): The present application is a continuation of International Patent Application No. PCT/EP01/11700, filed Oct. 10, 2001, designating the United States of America and published in German as WO 02/30933 A1, the entire disclosure of which is incorporated herein by reference. Priority is claimed based on Federal Republic of Germany Patent Application No. 100 50 662.3, filed Oct. 13, 2000.... The present application relates to substituted 3,4-dihydropyrido[1,2-a]pyrimidines, to processes for the production thereof, to substance libraries containing them, to pharmaceutical preparations containing these compounds, to the use of these compounds for the production of pharmaceutical preparations, and methods for the treatment of pain, urinary incontinence, pruritus, **tinnitus** and/or diarrhea and to pharmaceutical compositions containing these compounds.... The treatment of chronic and non-chronic pain is of great significance in medicine. There is a worldwide requirement for effective therapeutic methods for providing tailored and targeted treatment of chronic and non-chronic pain, especially effective and satisfactory pain treatment from the patient's standpoint.

Web site: http://appft1.uspto.gov/netahtml/PTO/search-bool.html

- **System and method for diagnosing and/or reducing tinnitus**

    Inventor(s): Brown, Carolyn J.; (Iowa City, IA), Rubinstein, Jay T.; (Solon, IA), Tyler, Richard S.; (West Branch, IA)

    Correspondence: Fleshner & Kim, Llp; P.o. Box 221200; Chantilly; VA; 20153-1200; US

    Patent Application Number: 20020091423

    Date filed: September 25, 2001

    Abstract: A system and method for application of pseudospontaneous neural stimulation is provided that can generate stochastic independent activity across an excited nerve or neural population without an additional disadvantageous sensations. High rate pulse trains, for example, can produce random spike patterns in auditory nerve fibers that are statistically similar to those produced by spontaneous activity in the normal ear. This activity is called "pseudospontaneous activity". Varying rates of pseudospontaneous activity can be created by varying the intensity of a fixed amplitude, high rate pulse train stimulus, e.g., 5000 pps. A method and apparatus for diagnosing treatment for **tinnitus** with neural prosthetic devices according to the present invention that can use, for example, physiological responses to pseudospontaneous activity in an auditory nerve prior to the implementation of the neural prosthetic. Monitored patient response to the generated pseudospontaneous activity in the auditory nerve, even if temporary, can produce successful reduction or elimination in perceived **tinnitus** by subsequent treatment.

    Excerpt(s): This application is a continuation-in-part application of U.S. Pat. No. 6,295,472 that issued on Sep. 25, 2001, which is a continuation-in-part application of U.S. Pat. No. 6,078,838 that issued on Jun. 20, 2000, and claims priority to U.S. Provisional Application, Attorney Docket No. UIOWA-0045PR, filed Sep. 24, 2001, the entire disclosure of each is incorporated herein by reference.... This invention relates generally to an apparatus and method for providing stochastic independent neural stimulation, and in particular, a neural stimulation system and method for identifying candidates for intervention and treatment of **tinnitus** by initiating pseudospontaneous activity in the auditory nerve.... Fundamental differences currently exist between electrical stimulation and acoustic stimulation of the auditory nerve. Electrical stimulation of the auditory nerve, for example, via a cochlear implant, generally results in more cross-fiber synchrony, less within fiber jitter, and less dynamic range, as compared with acoustic stimulation which occurs in individuals having normal hearing.

    Web site: http://appft1.uspto.gov/netahtml/PTO/search-bool.html

- **Tinnitus masker/suppressor**

  Inventor(s): Lenhardt, Martin L.; (Hayes, VA)

  Correspondence: George E. Quillin; Foley & Lardner; Washington Harbour; 3000 K Street, Nw., Suite 500; Washington; DC; 20007-5109; US

  Patent Application Number: 20010051776

  Date filed: April 2, 2001

  Abstract: A system and method for **tinnitus** masking or suppression. At least one upper audio frequency is provided to a head of a patient, to thereby stimulate the auditory cortex. The upper audio frequency is preferably applied by way of air conduction. At least one ultrasound frequencies can also be applied by way of bone conduction. Once stimulated, the auditory cortex will mask or suppress **tinnitus.**

  Excerpt(s): This application is a continuation in part of U.S. patent application Ser. No. 09/417,772, filed Oct. 14, 1999 which itself claims priority to U.S. provisional patent application Ser. No. 60/104,233, filed Oct. 14, 1998, both of which are incorporated in their entirety herein by reference.... The present invention relates to a system and method for masking or suppressing **tinnitus.** In particular, the present invention relates to a system and method for masking or suppressing **tinnitus** using high frequency signals, such as upper audio signals in one embodiment and ultrasound and higher range signals in other embodiments, that affect the cortical auditory and other neurons in the brain.... Tinnitus is defined as any ringing in the ears for which there is no external source. **Tinnitus** is considered a phantom sound, which arises in the brain and not actually in the ears as it appears to subjectively. For example, a ringing, buzzing, whistling, or roaring sound may be perceived as **tinnitus. Tinnitus** can be continuous or intermittent, and in either case can be very irritating to one who has such an affliction.

  Web site: http://appft1.uspto.gov/netahtml/PTO/search-bool.html

- **Topical application of muscarinic and opioid agents for treatment of tinnitus**

  Inventor(s): El Khoury, George F.; (Long Beach, CA)

  Correspondence: Millen, White, Zelano & Branigan, P.c.; 2200 Clarendon Blvd.; Suite 1400; Arlington; VA; 22201; US

  Patent Application Number: 20020010191

  Date filed: July 17, 2001

Abstract: The present invention relates to a compositions and methods for treating **tinnitus.** In preferred embodiments of the invention, muscurinic and/or opioid agents are administered to the affected ear in amount effective to relieve one or more **tinnitus** symptoms. A preferred agent is an anticholinesterase inhibitor, such as neoostigmine.

Excerpt(s): This application is a continuation-in-part of application Ser. No. 09/318,573, filed May 27, 1999, which is hereby incorporated by reference in its entirety.... The present invention relates to compositions and methods for treating **tinnitus. Tinnitus** can be described as "ringing" and other head noises that are perceived in the absence of any external noise source. It is estimated that 1 out of every 5 people experience some degree of **tinnitus....** Tinnitus can be classified into two forms: objective and subjective. Objective **tinnitus,** the rarer form, consists of head noises audible to other people in addition to the sufferer. The noises are usually caused by vascular anomalies, repetitive muscle contractions, or inner ear structural defects. The sounds are heard by the sufferer and are generally external to the auditory system. This form of **tinnitus** means that an examiner can hear the sound heard by the sufferer by using a stethoscope. Benign causes, such as noise from TMJ, openings of the eustachian tubes, or repetitive muscle contractions may be the cause of objective **tinnitus.** The sufferer might hear the pulsatile flow of the carotid artery or the continuous hum of normal venous outflow through the jugular vein when in a quiet setting. It can also be an early sign of increased intra cranial pressure and is often overshadowed by other neurologic abnormalities. The sounds may arise from a turbulent flow through compressed venous structures at the base of the brain.

Web site: http://appft1.uspto.gov/netahtml/PTO/search-bool.html

- **Use of a composition**

Inventor(s): Gidlund, Bo; (Uppsala, SE)

Correspondence: Browdy and Neimark, P.l.l.c.; 624 Ninth Street, NW; Suite 300; Washington; DC; 20001-5303; US

Patent Application Number: 20010033871

Date filed: March 2, 2001

Abstract: Use of an extract derived from the fruits, the leaves, the bark or the roots of Morinda citrifolia L. for the manufacture of a medicament for the treatment of a mammal suffering from **tinnitus.** The extract may be a liquid present in the medicament in an amount such as to give a daily dosage of 0.1-2 ml, or 0.2-1 ml, e.g. 0.4-0.7 ml, per kg body weight of the patient. The extract also may be a solid present in the medicament in an amount such as to give a daily dosage of 5-200 mg, or 10-100 mg, e.g. 20-70 mg, per kg body weight of the patient. Optionally, the medicament also may comprise lycopene, vitamine C, coenyme Q10 and an extract from the leaves of Ginkgo biloba. The medicament may be given e.g. by oral, rectal, transdermal or inhalation administration.

Excerpt(s): The present invention relates to the manufacture of a medicament for the treatment of a mammal suffering from **tinnitus**.... More specifically the present invention relates to the use of a composition comprising an extract from Morinda citrifolia L. (Rubiaceae) for the manufacture of such a medicament.... Morinda citrifolia L. (Rubiaceae), the Indian mulberry, also called noni, is an evergreen shrub tree which is native to Asia, Australia and some Pacific Islands. Its botanical description is given e.g. in Levand O. (Part I Some chemical constituents of Morinda citrifolia L (noni), thesis, University of Hawaii, 1963). The roots, bark, stem, leaves and fruits thereof have traditionally been used in medicine, in food and as a dye in different cultures, e.g. on Hawaii and in the French Polynesia. As an example, a plurality of indications of use is reported in the indigenous Samoan medicine, (Dittmar A."Morinda citrifolia L.--Use in Indigenous Samoan Medicine", J. of Herbs, Spices & Medicinal Plants, Vol. 1(3) pp 77-91 (1993)), covering a wide range of ailments, such as tooth ache (roots), septicemia (leaf), diarrhea of infants (bark) and eye complaints (fruit)... just to mention a few.

Web site: http://appft1.uspto.gov/netahtml/PTO/search-bool.html

- **Use of benzopyranols to treat neurological disorders**

   Inventor(s): Evans, John Morris; (Roydon, GB), Parsons, Andrew; (Arlesey, GB), Thompson, Mervyn; (Harlow, GB), Upton, Neil; (Harlow, GB)

   Correspondence: Glaxosmithkline; Corporate Intellectual Property - Uw2220; P.o. Box 1539; King of Prussia; PA; 19406-0939; US

   Patent Application Number: 20020010209

   Date filed: July 19, 2001

   Abstract: Benzopyran derivatives and analogs are disclosed as useful for the treatment and/or prophylaxis of degenerative diseases such as Huntingdon's chorea, schizophrenia, neurological deficits associated with AIDS, sleep disorders (including circadian rhythm disorders, insomnia and narcolepsy), tics (e.g. Giles de la Tourette's syndrome), traumatic brain injury, **tinnitus**, neuralgia, especially trigeminal neuralgia, neuropathic pain, dental pain, cancer pain, inappropriate neuronal activity resulting in neurodysthesias in diseases such as diabetes, MS and motor neurone disease, ataxias, muscular rigidity (spasticity), temporomandibular joint dysfunction.

Excerpt(s): This invention relates to a novel method of treatment.... EP-A-0 126 311 discloses substituted benzopyran compounds having blood pressure lowering activity, including 6-acetyl-trans-4-(4-fluorobenzoylamino)-3,4-dihydro-2,2-dimethyl-2H-1-benzopyran-3-ol.... Also EP-A-0 376 524, EP-A-0 205 292, EP-A-0 250 077, EP-A-0 093 535, EP-A-0 150 202, EP-A-0 076 075 and WO/89/05808 (Beecham Group plc) describe certain benzopyran derivatives which possess anti-hypertensive activity.

Web site: http://appft1.uspto.gov/netahtml/PTO/search-bool.html

- **USE OF MORPHINE DERIVATIVES AS MEDICAMENTS FOR THE TREATMENT OF NEUROPATHIC PROBLEMS**

Inventor(s): Buschmann, Helmut; (Aachen, DE), Krueger, Thomas; (Langerwehe-Schlich, DE), Reiss-Mueller, Elke; (Bielefeld, DE), Strassburger, Wolfgang; (Wuerselen, DE), Wnendt, Stephan; (Aachen, DE)

Correspondence: Crowell & Moring Llp; Intellectual Property Group; P.o. Box 14300; Washington; DC; 20044-4300; US

Patent Application Number: 20020165247

Date filed: February 15, 2002

Abstract: A method for agonizing or antagonizing the ORL1 (opioid receptor-like) receptor of the nociceptin/orphanin FQ ligand ORL1 receptor system using a morphinan compound of the general formula I or derivatives thereof. Also disclosed are methods for treating neuropathic pain and/or anxiolysis and/or depression and/or diuresis and/or urinary incontinence and/or hypotension and or hypertension and/or senile dementia and/or Alzheimer's disease and/or general cognitive dysfunctions and/or **tinnitus** and/or impaired hearing and/or epilepsy and/or obesity and/or cachexia.

Excerpt(s): The present application is a continuation of international patent application no. PCT/EP00/07585, filed Aug. 4, 2000, designating the United States of America, the entire disclosure of which is incorporated herein by reference. Priority is claimed based on Federal Republic of Germany patent application no. 199 39 044.4, filed Aug. 18, 1999.... The present invention relates to the use of morphinan derivatives as well as their bases or salts of physiologically compatible acids as regulators for the nociceptin/orphanin FQ ligand ORL1 receptor system and for the production of a medicament.... The heptadecapeptide nociceptin/orphanin FQ is an endogenous ligand of the ORL1 (opioid receptor-like) receptor (Meunier et al., Nature 377, 1995, pp. 532-535) that belongs to the family of opioid receptors and can be found in many regions of the brain and spinal cord (Mollereau et al., FEBS Letters, 341, 1994, pp. 33-38, Darland et al., Trends in Neurosciences, 21, 1998, pp. 215-221). The peptide is characterised by a high affinity, with a K.sub.d value of around 56 pM (Ardati et al., Mol. Pharmacol. 51, pp. 816-824), and by a high selectivity for the ORL1 receptor. The ORL1 receptor is homologous to the.mu.,.kappa. and.delta. opioid receptors, and the amino acid sequence of the nociceptin/orphanin FQ peptide has a strong similarity to those of the known opioid peptides. The activation of the receptor induced by nociceptin/orphanin FQ leads via the coupling with G.sub.i/o proteins to an inhibition of adenylate cyclase (Meunier et al., Nature 377, 1995, pp. 532-535) Also, at the cellular level there are functional similarities between the.mu.,.kappa. and.delta. opioid receptors and the ORL1 receptor as regards the activation of the potassium channel (Matthes et al., Mo. Pharmacol. 50, 1996, pp. 447-450; Vaughan et al., Br. J. Pharmacol. 117, 1996, pp. 1609-1611) and the inhibition of the L, N and P/Q type calcium channels (Conner et al., Br. J. Pharmacol. 118, 1996, pp. 205-207; Knoflach et al., J. Neuroscience 16, 1996, pp. 6657-6664).

Web site: http://appft1.uspto.gov/netahtml/PTO/search-bool.html

- **Use of riluzole in the treating acoustic traumas**

    Inventor(s): Randle, John; (Brookline, MA), Stutzmann, Jean-Marie; (Villecresnes, FR)

    Correspondence: Aventis Pharmaceuticals, Inc.; Patents Department; Route 202-206, P.o. Box 6800; Bridgewater; NJ; 08807-0800; US

    Patent Application Number: 20020004516

    Date filed: June 15, 2001

    Abstract: The invention concerns the use of riluzole or one of its pharmaceutically acceptable salts for preventing and/or treating acoustic traumas and, in particular, different types of deafness and **tinnitus.**

    Excerpt(s): This application is a continuation of International application No. PCT/FR99/03,108, filed Dec. 13, 1999; which claims the benefit of priority of French Patent Application No. 98/15,834, filed Dec. 15, 1998.... The present invention relates to the use of riluzole or one of its pharmaceutically acceptable salts in the prevention and/or treatment of acoustic traumas and, in particular, of deafness and of **tinnitus.**... Riluzole (2-amino-6-trifluoromethoxy-benzothiazole) is marketed for the treatment of amyotrophic lateral sclerosis. This compound is also useful as an anticonvulsant, an anxiolytic and a hypnotic (EP 50551), in the treatment of schizophrenia (EP 305276), in the treatment of sleep disorders and of depression (EP 305277), in the treatment of cerebrovascular disorders and as an anesthetic (EP 282971), in the treatment of spinal, cranial and craniospinal traumas (WO 94/13288), as a radio restorative (WO 94/15600), in the treatment of Parkinson's disease (WO 94/15601), in the treatment of neuro-AIDS (WO 94/20103), in the treatment of mitochondrial diseases (WO 95/19170). All of these references are herein incorporated by reference in their entirety.

Web site: http://appft1.uspto.gov/netahtml/PTO/search-bool.html

Keeping Current

In order to stay informed about patents and patent applications dealing with tinnitus, you can access the U.S. Patent Office archive via the Internet at the following Web address: **http://www.uspto.gov/patft/index.html**. You will see two broad options: (1) Issued Patent, and (2) Published Applications. To see a list of issued patents, perform the following steps: Under "Issued Patents," click "Quick Search." Then, type "tinnitus" (or synonyms) into the "Term 1" box. After clicking on the search button, scroll down to see the various patents which have been granted to date on tinnitus.

You can also use this procedure to view pending patent applications concerning tinnitus. Simply go back to **http://www.uspto.gov/patft/index.html**. Select "Quick Search" under "Published Applications." Then proceed with the steps listed above.

Vocabulary Builder

Circadian: Repeated more or less daily, i. e. on a 23- to 25-hour cycle. [NIH]

Dermatitis: Inflammation of the skin. [NIH]

Dimethyl: A volatile metabolite of the amino acid methionine. [NIH]

Disulphide: A covalent bridge formed by the oxidation of two cysteine residues to a cystine residue. The-S-S-bond is very strong and its presence confers additional stability. [NIH]

Electrode: Component of the pacing system which is at the distal end of the lead. It is the interface with living cardiac tissue across which the stimulus is transmitted. [NIH]

Enhancer: Transcriptional element in the virus genome. [NIH]

Epilepticus: Repeated and prolonged epileptic seizures without recovery of consciousness between attacks. [NIH]

Fatigue: The feeling of weariness of mind and body. [NIH]

Involuntary: Reaction occurring without intention or volition. [NIH]

Labyrinthine: A vestibular nystagmus resulting from stimulation, injury, or disease of the labyrinth. [NIH]

Meatus: A canal running from the internal auditory foramen through the petrous portion of the temporal bone. It gives passage to the facial and auditory nerves together with the auditory branch of the basilar artery and the internal auditory veins. [NIH]

Narcolepsy: A condition of unknown cause characterized by a periodic uncontrollable tendency to fall asleep. [NIH]

Nystagmus: Rhythmical oscillation of the eyeballs, either pendular or jerky. [NIH]

Pterygoid: A canal in the sphenoid bone for the vidian nerve. [NIH]

Racemic: Optically inactive but resolvable in the way of all racemic compounds. [NIH]

Radiological: Pertaining to radiodiagnostic and radiotherapeutic procedures, and interventional radiology or other planning and guiding medical radiology. [NIH]

Retrogression: A reversion to some earlier stage of succession consequent on the introduction of an adverse factor, commonly soil degradation. [NIH]

Secretory: Secreting; relating to or influencing secretion or the secretions. [NIH]

Senile: Relating or belonging to old age; characteristic of old age; resulting from infirmity of old age. [NIH]

Spike: The activation of synapses causes changes in the permeability of the dendritic membrane leading to changes in the membrane potential. This difference of the potential travels along the axon of the neuron and is called spike. [NIH]

Stethoscope: An instrument used for the detection and study of sounds within the body that conveyed to the ears of the observer through rubber tubing. [NIH]

Synchrony: The normal physiologic sequencing of atrial and ventricular activation and contraction. [NIH]

Ulcer: A localized necrotic lesion of the skin or a mucous surface. [NIH]

CHAPTER 6. BOOKS ON TINNITUS

Overview

This chapter provides bibliographic book references relating to tinnitus. You have many options to locate books on tinnitus. The simplest method is to go to your local bookseller and inquire about titles that they have in stock or can special order for you. Some patients, however, feel uncomfortable approaching their local booksellers and prefer online sources (e.g. **www.amazon.com** and **www.bn.com**). In addition to online booksellers, excellent sources for book titles on tinnitus include the Combined Health Information Database and the National Library of Medicine. Once you have found a title that interests you, visit your local public or medical library to see if it is available for loan.

Book Summaries: Federal Agencies

The Combined Health Information Database collects various book abstracts from a variety of healthcare institutions and federal agencies. To access these summaries, go directly to the following hyperlink: **http://chid.nih.gov/detail/detail.html**. You will need to use the "Detailed Search" option. To find book summaries, use the drop boxes at the bottom of the search page where "You may refine your search by." Select the dates and language you prefer. For the format option, select "Monograph/Book." Now type "tinnitus" (or synonyms) into the "For these words:" box. You will only receive results on books. You should check back periodically with this database which is updated every 3 months. The following is a typical result when searching for books on tinnitus:

- **Tinnitus Handbook**

    Source: San Diego, CA: Singular Publishing Group. 2000. 477 p.

    Contact: Available from Singular-Thomson Learning. P.O. Box 6904, Florence, KY 41022. (800) 477-3692. Fax (606) 647-5963. Website: www.singpub.com. PRICE: $65.95 plus shipping and handling. ISBN: 1565939220.

    Summary: This audiology textbook offers clinicians and recent graduates information on tinnitus (ringing or other sounds in the ears). The author includes information on tinnitus, insomnia, physiological mechanisms and neural models, medical and surgical evaluation and management, tinnitus and children, and an historical perspective on tinnitus. Specific topics include psychoacoustical measurement, spontaneous otoacoustic emissions and tinnitus, and the psychological measurement of tinnitus. The author reviews the options for therapy and treatment, including hearing aids, maskers, cognitive behavior modification, electrical stimulation, habituation therapy, counseling, and biofeedback. Additional chapters address the medicolegal issues of tinnitus and resources including the American Tinnitus Association and self help groups. Each chapter includes a list of references and the textbook concludes with a subject index.

- **Tinnitus: What is That Noise in My Head?**

    Source: Auckland, New Zealand: Sandalwood Enterprises. 1994. 104 p.

    Contact: Available from American Tinnitus Association (ATA). P.O. Box 5, Portland, OR 97207-0005. (800) 634-8978 or (503) 248-9985. Fax (503) 248-0024. E-mail: tinnitus@ata.org. Website: www.ata.org. PRICE: $14.50 for members; $18.00 for nonmembers. ISBN: 0473015625.

    Summary: This book familiarizes readers with the common causes and symptoms of tinnitus and explains how people with tinnitus can take steps toward relieving the condition. Written in non-technical language, the book features eight chapters covering a definition of tinnitus, pathology of the ear, medical treatments, non-medical treatments, the role of stress, the role of nutrition, self-help groups, and research and future trends. The book includes a bibliography, glossary of terms, and addresses for resource organizations (primarily in New Zealand and Australia). 15 references.

- **Tinnitus: Advances in Diagnosis and Management**

    Source: Alexandria, VA: American Academy of Otolaryngology-Head and Neck Surgery Foundation, Inc. 1999. 34 p.

Contact: Available from American Academy of Otolaryngology-Head and Neck Surgery. One Prince Street, Alexandria, VA 22314-3357. (703) 836-4444. Fax (703) 683-5100. E-mail: orders@entnet.org. Website: www.entnet.org. PRICE: $12.00 plus shipping and handling for members; $15.00 plus shipping and handling for nonmembers. ISBN: 1567720269.

Summary: This educational booklet offers otolaryngologists an update on the diagnosis and management of tinnitus (ringing or other noises in the ears). The author notes that, in the past, because of poor understanding of tinnitus, many patients had been condemned to live with this very disturbing symptom for the rest of their lives. Recent developments in tinnitus research, however, have led to a more optimistic approach for the management of these patients. The booklet separates tinnitus into nonpulsatile (subjective) and pulsatile categories. Topics in the first section including pathophysiology; components of evaluation, including patient history, neurootologic examination, audiologic evaluation, electrophysiologic testing, radiologic evaluation, metabolic and allergy testing, and tinnitus analysis (pitch matching, loudness matching, minimum masking level, residual inhibition); and management issues, including masking, habituation technique, electrical stimulation, biofeedback, medical treatment, and surgical treatment. In the section on pulsatile tinnitus, the author discusses pathophysiology and classification; arterial etiologies, including atherosclerotic carotid artery disease, venous etiologies (idiopathic intracranial hypertension syndrome), nonvascular etiologies (palatal, stapedial, and tensor tympani muscle myoclonus), patient evaluation, radiologic evaluation, and patient management. 3 figures. 11 tables. 144 references.

- **Proceedings of the Fifth International Tinnitus Seminar**

    Source: Portland, OR: American Tinnitus Association (ATA). 1996. 668 p.

    Contact: Available from American Tinnitus Association (ATA). P.O. Box 5, Portland, OR 97207-0005. (800) 634-8978 or (503) 248-9985. Fax (503) 248-0024. E-mail: tinnitus@ata.org. Website: www.ata.org. PRICE: $10.00 plus shipping and handling.

    Summary: This lengthy document presents the proceedings of the 5th Annual Tinnitus Seminar, held in 1995 in Portland, Oregon. The book, a compilation of the papers, posters, and workshops that were part of the Seminar, presents both scientific information and personal viewpoints from a broad spectrum of people interested in tinnitus. After a reprinting of the Special Speakers' presentations, the book categorizes the proceedings into 13 sections: etiology, alternative treatments, animal models and object measures, assessment measures, drugs, epidemiology and demographics, instrumentation, legal and noise issues, mechanisms, medical and clinical considerations, psychological and rehabilitation issues, the role of self-help, and temporomandibular joint disorders. Most presentations include references. (AA-M).

- **Tinnitus. A Self-Management Guide for the Ringing in Your Ears**

Source: Boston, MA: Allyn & Bacon. 2002. 209 p.

Contact: Available from Allyn & Bacon, Publisher. Web site: www.ablongman.com. PRICE: $29.00 plus shipping, tax, and handling. Available in softcover.

Summary: This self-help book for people with tinnitus describes practical strategies for coping with the condition. Step-by-step guidelines are provided for psychological techniques such as relaxation, stress management, and attentional control. Emphasis is placed on the effect of attitude on the perception of tinnitus as a problem. The text reviews the causes of tinnitus, typical medical and audiological treatments, and common problems related to tinnitus. Self-assessment exercises are provided throughout discussions about the impact of tinnitus on daily activities, emotional reactions, the control of negative thought processes, problem-solving, and preparation for high-risk situations. Lifestyle modifications, distress, anger, sleep problems, and coping techniques in quiet and noisy environments are addressed.

- **Tinnitus: New Hope for a Cure**

Source: Seal Beach, CA: Mr. Paul VanValkenburgh. 1995. 127 p.

Contact: Available from Mr. Paul VanValkenburgh. Box 3611, Seal Beach, CA 90740. PRICE: $15.00 each. ISBN: 0961742526.

Summary: This self-published book provides information on tinnitus, its causes, and how to manage the condition. The author writes in a casual style, but uses technical language. He cites passages from medical journals and responds to these passages with his own comments and speculations. Topics covered include the dynamics of perception and the importance of psychosocial factors and attitude; the filter-bank theory and how the cochlea works; everyday sub-conscious causes of ringing sounds; filter overload; biological ear defenses; the physiology of the ear and the jaw bone; middle ear anatomy and resonance; the olivo-cochlear crossover; the blood supply of the cochlea; human filter dynamics; and future developments, including in hearing aids, maskers, hair cell regeneration, and treating the cause, not the symptoms. The book is illustrated with diagrams and black and white photographs and concludes with a subject index. 31 figures. 56 references. (AA-M).

- **Dizziness, Hearing Loss, and Tinnitus**

    Source: Philadelphia, PA: F.A. Davis Company. 1998. 240 p.

    Contact: Available from Oxford University Press, Inc. Business Office, 2001 Evans Road, Cary, NC 27513. (800) 451-7556 or (919) 677-0977. Fax (919) 677-1303. PRICE: $65.00 plus shipping and handling.

    Summary: This textbook presents a concise approach to evaluating patients with dizziness, hearing loss, and tinnitus. In the first section, the author briefly reviews clinically relevant anatomy and physiology to provide a framework for understanding the pathophysiology of vestibular and auditory symptoms. The second section outlines the important features in the patient's history and examination that determine the probable site of a lesion. Separate chapters provide a systematic approach to evaluating patients with different types of dizziness and tinnitus. Numerous tables and flowcharts guide the reader through the diagnostic workup. The section on diagnosis and treatment covers the key differential diagnosis points that help the clinician decide the cause of the patient's problem and how to treat it. The description of each disease begins with an outline of symptoms, signs, laboratory findings, and treatment options. Each chapter includes references and a subject index concludes the volume.

Book Summaries: Online Booksellers

Commercial Internet-based booksellers, such as Amazon.com and Barnes & Noble.com, offer summaries which have been supplied by each title's publisher. Some summaries also include customer reviews. Your local bookseller may have access to in-house and commercial databases that index all published books (e.g. Books in Print®). The following have been recently listed with online booksellers as relating to tinnitus (sorted alphabetically by title; follow the hyperlink to view more details at Amazon.com):

- **Dizziness, Hearing Loss, and Tinnitus** by Robert W., Md. Baloh; ISBN: 0803603304;
    http://www.amazon.com/exec/obidos/ASIN/0803603304/icongroupinterna

- **Dizziness, Hearing Loss, and Tinnitus: The Essentials of Neurotology** by Robert W. Baloh; ISBN: 0803605811;
    http://www.amazon.com/exec/obidos/ASIN/0803605811/icongroupinterna

- **Ear Clinics International Sensorineural Hearing Loss, Vertigo and Tinnitus** by Michael Paparella; ISBN: 0686777689;
http://www.amazon.com/exec/obidos/ASIN/0686777689/icongroupinterna

- **Ear, Nose, and Throat Disorders Sourcebook: Basic Information About Disorders of the Ears, Nose, Sinus Cavities, Pharynx, and Larynx Including Ear Infections, Tinnitus, Vestibular Disorders (Health Reference Series, Vol 37)** by Linda M. Shin (Editor), et al; ISBN: 0780802063;
http://www.amazon.com/exec/obidos/ASIN/0780802063/icongroupinterna

- **Hearing Loss & Tinnitus (Ward Lock Family Health Guide)** by Lorraine Jeffrey; ISBN: 0706373960;
http://www.amazon.com/exec/obidos/ASIN/0706373960/icongroupinterna

- **How to Cope With Tinnitus and Hearing Loss [LARGE PRINT]** by Robert Youngson; ISBN: 1850895252;
http://www.amazon.com/exec/obidos/ASIN/1850895252/icongroupinterna

- **Layman's Guide to Tinnitus** by Robert Slater; ISBN: 0900634405;
http://www.amazon.com/exec/obidos/ASIN/0900634405/icongroupinterna

- **Leben mit Tinnitus.** by Richard Hallam (Author); ISBN: 3820817158;
http://www.amazon.com/exec/obidos/ASIN/3820817158/icongroupinterna

- **Lesungen mit Tinnitus. Gedichte 1980 - 1985.** by Oskar Pastior (Author); ISBN: 3446145303;
http://www.amazon.com/exec/obidos/ASIN/3446145303/icongroupinterna

- **Living With Tinnitus (Living With Series)** by David W. Rees, Simon W. Smith; ISBN: 0719033675;
http://www.amazon.com/exec/obidos/ASIN/0719033675/icongroupinterna

- **Mechanisms of Tinnitus** by Jack A. Vernon (Author), Aage R. Moller (Author); ISBN: 0205140831;
http://www.amazon.com/exec/obidos/ASIN/0205140831/icongroupinterna

- **Natural Relief from Tinnitus** by Paul, Jr. Yanick, Paul Yannick; ISBN: 0879836555;

http://www.amazon.com/exec/obidos/ASIN/0879836555/icongroupinterna

- **New Self Help Series Tinnitus and Catarrhal Deafness** by Arthur White; ISBN: 0722513054; http://www.amazon.com/exec/obidos/ASIN/0722513054/icongroupinterna

- **Psychological Management of Chronic Tinnitus, The: A Cognitive-Behavioral Approach** by Jane L. Henry (Author), Peter H. Wilson (Author); ISBN: 0205313655; http://www.amazon.com/exec/obidos/ASIN/0205313655/icongroupinterna

- **Psychologische Behandlung des chronischen Tinnitus** by Birgit. Krä¶ner-Herwig (Author); ISBN: 3621273794; http://www.amazon.com/exec/obidos/ASIN/3621273794/icongroupinterna

- **Psychotherapie bei Tinnitus. Ein Einstieg zu einem therapeutischen Zugang.** by Helm Schaaf (Author), Hedwig Holtmann (Author); ISBN: 3794521552; http://www.amazon.com/exec/obidos/ASIN/3794521552/icongroupinterna

- **Sensorineural Hearing Loss, Vertigo, and Tinnitus** by Meyerhof; ISBN: 0683067508; http://www.amazon.com/exec/obidos/ASIN/0683067508/icongroupinterna

- **SOS aus dem Innenohr. Hilfe bei Tinnitus.** by Michele Markus (Author), Alexander Hoffmann (Author); ISBN: 3431035574; http://www.amazon.com/exec/obidos/ASIN/3431035574/icongroupinterna

- **Stop Your Tinnitus: Causes, Preventatives, and Alternatives** by Phyllis Avery; ISBN: 1880598221; http://www.amazon.com/exec/obidos/ASIN/1880598221/icongroupinterna

- **Terror Tinnitus. Die neue, individuelle Therapie.** by Hans-Jã¼rgen Heinrichs (Author); ISBN: 3530401528; http://www.amazon.com/exec/obidos/ASIN/3530401528/icongroupinterna

- **The Tinnitus Handbook: A Self Help Guide** by Bill Habets, et al; ISBN: 1887053069; http://www.amazon.com/exec/obidos/ASIN/1887053069/icongroupinterna

- **Tinnitus** by Richard Hallam; ISBN: 0722518013; http://www.amazon.com/exec/obidos/ASIN/0722518013/icongroupinterna

- **Tinnitus** by Jonathan W.P. Hazell (Editor); ISBN: 0443021562; http://www.amazon.com/exec/obidos/ASIN/0443021562/icongroupinterna

- **Tinnitus**; ISBN: 999801199X; http://www.amazon.com/exec/obidos/ASIN/999801199X/icongroupinterna

- **Tinnitus (Human Horizons Series)**; ISBN: 0285632833; http://www.amazon.com/exec/obidos/ASIN/0285632833/icongroupinterna

- **Tinnitus 85**; ISBN: 0272796395; http://www.amazon.com/exec/obidos/ASIN/0272796395/icongroupinterna

- **Tinnitus 91** by J. M. Aran (Editor); ISBN: 9062990878; http://www.amazon.com/exec/obidos/ASIN/9062990878/icongroupinterna

- **Tinnitus and Its Management: A Clinical Text for Audiologists** by John Greer Clark, Paul Yanick (Editor); ISBN: 0398050430; http://www.amazon.com/exec/obidos/ASIN/0398050430/icongroupinterna

- **Tinnitus Handbook (Singular Audiology Text,)** by Richard Tyler (Editor); ISBN: 1565939220; http://www.amazon.com/exec/obidos/ASIN/1565939220/icongroupinterna

- **Tinnitus- Hilfe.** by Bernhard Kellerhals (Author), Regula Zogg (Author); ISBN: 3805571275; http://www.amazon.com/exec/obidos/ASIN/3805571275/icongroupinterna

- **Tinnitus lindern.** by Maria Holl (Author); ISBN: 3035050058; http://www.amazon.com/exec/obidos/ASIN/3035050058/icongroupinterna

- **Tinnitus New Hope for a Cure** by Paul V. Valkenburgh, Paul Van Valkenburgh; ISBN: 0961742526; http://www.amazon.com/exec/obidos/ASIN/0961742526/icongroupinterna

- **Tinnitus Rehabilitation by Retraining: A Workbook for Sufferers, Their Doctors, and Other Health Care Professionals** by Bernhard

Kellerhals, Regula Zogg; ISBN: 3805569300;
http://www.amazon.com/exec/obidos/ASIN/3805569300/icongroupinterna

- **Tinnitus Retraining Therapy : Neurophysiological Model** by Pawel J. Jastreboff (Author), Jonathan W. P. Hazell (Author); ISBN: 0521592569;
http://www.amazon.com/exec/obidos/ASIN/0521592569/icongroupinterna

- **Tinnitus und Hyperakusis. Fortschritte der Psychotherapie.** by Gerhard Goebel (Author); ISBN: 380171117X;
http://www.amazon.com/exec/obidos/ASIN/380171117X/icongroupinterna

- **Tinnitus. Ein Manual zur Tinnitus- Retrainingtherapie.** by Wolfgang Delb (Author), et al; ISBN: 3801713792;
http://www.amazon.com/exec/obidos/ASIN/3801713792/icongroupinterna

- **Tinnitus: A Guide for Sufferers and Professionals** by Robert Slater, et al; ISBN: 070993338X;
http://www.amazon.com/exec/obidos/ASIN/070993338X/icongroupinterna

- **Tinnitus: A Self-Management Guide for the Ringing in Your Ears** by Jane L. Henry (Author), Peter H. Wilson (Author); ISBN: 0205315372;
http://www.amazon.com/exec/obidos/ASIN/0205315372/icongroupinterna

- **Tinnitus: Advances in Diagnosis and Management** by Aristides Sismanis; ISBN: 1567720269;
http://www.amazon.com/exec/obidos/ASIN/1567720269/icongroupinterna

- **Tinnitus: Diagnosis/Treatment** by Abraham, Md. Shulman, Barbara, Ph.D. Goldstein; ISBN: 0769300227;
http://www.amazon.com/exec/obidos/ASIN/0769300227/icongroupinterna

- **Tinnitus: Facts, Theories and Treatments** by Dennis McFadden (Editor); ISBN: 0309033284;
http://www.amazon.com/exec/obidos/ASIN/0309033284/icongroupinterna

- **Tinnitus: Help and Hope** by Terri E. Clancy; ISBN: 1414001339;
http://www.amazon.com/exec/obidos/ASIN/1414001339/icongroupinterna

- **Tinnitus: Learning to Live With It** by Leslie Sheppard, Audrey Hawkridge (Contributor); ISBN: 0906798809;
  http://www.amazon.com/exec/obidos/ASIN/0906798809/icongroupinterna

- **Tinnitus: Living With the Ringing in Your Ears** by Richard Hallam; ISBN: 0722529406;
  http://www.amazon.com/exec/obidos/ASIN/0722529406/icongroupinterna

- **Tinnitus: Pathophysiology and Management** by Masaaki Kitahara (Editor); ISBN: 0318400790;
  http://www.amazon.com/exec/obidos/ASIN/0318400790/icongroupinterna

- **Tinnitus: Questions and Answers** by Jack A. Vernon (Author), Barbara Tabachnick Sanders (Author); ISBN: 0205326854;
  http://www.amazon.com/exec/obidos/ASIN/0205326854/icongroupinterna

- **Tinnitus: Theory and Management** by Snow; ISBN: 155009243X;
  http://www.amazon.com/exec/obidos/ASIN/155009243X/icongroupinterna

- **Tinnitus: Treatment and Relief** by Jack A. Vernon; ISBN: 0205182690;
  http://www.amazon.com/exec/obidos/ASIN/0205182690/icongroupinterna

- **Tinnitus: Turning the Volume Down (Revised Edition)** by Kevin Hogan; ISBN: 097093212X;
  http://www.amazon.com/exec/obidos/ASIN/097093212X/icongroupinterna

- **Vertigo, Nausea, Tinnitus and Hearing Loss in Cardiovascular Diseases: Proceedings of the Neurootological and Equilibriometric Society: Vertigo in** by C.F. Claussen; ISBN: 0444808256;
  http://www.amazon.com/exec/obidos/ASIN/0444808256/icongroupinterna

- **Vertigo, Nausea, Tinnitus and Hearing Loss in Central and Peripheral Vestibular Diseases** by Neurootological and Equilibriometric Society Scientific Meeting 1995, et al; ISBN: 0444821937;
  http://www.amazon.com/exec/obidos/ASIN/0444821937/icongroupinterna

- **Vertigo, Nausea, Tinnitus, and Hypoacusia Due to Head and Neck Trauma: Proceedings of the Xviith Scientific Meeting of the Neurootological and Equil** by Claus-Frenz Claussen, Milind V. Kirtane (Editor); ISBN: 0444811508;

http://www.amazon.com/exec/obidos/ASIN/0444811508/icongroupinterna

- **Vertigo, Nausea, Tinnitus, and Hypoacusia in Metabolic Disorders: Proceedings (International Congress Series, No 791)** by Claus-Frenz Claussen, et al; ISBN: 0444810242;
http://www.amazon.com/exec/obidos/ASIN/0444810242/icongroupinterna

Chapters on Tinnitus

Frequently, tinnitus will be discussed within a book, perhaps within a specific chapter. In order to find chapters that are specifically dealing with tinnitus, an excellent source of abstracts is the Combined Health Information Database. You will need to limit your search to book chapters and tinnitus using the "Detailed Search" option. Go directly to the following hyperlink: **http://chid.nih.gov/detail/detail.html**. To find book chapters, use the drop boxes at the bottom of the search page where "You may refine your search by." Select the dates and language you prefer, and the format option "Book Chapter." By making these selections and typing in "tinnitus" (or synonyms) into the "For these words:" box, you will only receive results on chapters in books. The following is a typical result when searching for book chapters on tinnitus:

- **Tinnitus After Acute Acoustic Trauma**

    Source: in Hazell, J., ed. Proceedings of the Sixth International Tinnitus Seminar. London, England: Tinnitus and Hyperacusis Centre. 1999. p. 565-566.

    Contact: Available from Tinnitus and Hyperacusis Centre. 32 Devonshire Place, London, W1N 1PE, United Kingdom. Fax 44 + (0) 207 486 2218. E-mail: thc@dr.com. Website: www.tinnitus.org. PRICE: Contact publisher for price. ISBN: 0953695700. Also available on CD-ROM.

    Summary: Acute acoustic trauma (AAT) from firearm shooting is a common cause of tinnitus. The natural history and long term effects of AAT induced tinnitus are not well known. This article reports on a study undertaken to investigate the duration and long term annoyance of AAT induced tinnitus in 418 conscripts who had suffered AAT during their service in the Finnish Defense Forces 11 to 15 years earlier. The article is from a lengthy document that reprints the proceedings of the Sixth International Tinnitus Seminar, held in Cambridge, United Kingdom, in September 1999 and hosted by the British Society of Audiology. Results showed that tinnitus was a prominent symptom immediately after AAT in all cases. In most cases, it disappeared or was attenuated to an undisturbing level within a few weeks following trauma so that in more than two thirds of the cases, tinnitus was no longer present three months after the AAT. Thirty percent of the patients (122 conscripts) stated that they still had tinnitus when they finished their military service. The authors contacted this group of patients for a long term follow up, successfully reaching 101 cases (83 percent). Of these 101 patients, 42 claimed that they still suffered considerably from tinnitus (11 to 15 years after the AAT) and were interested in any new treatment possibility if available. 4 tables.

- **Tinnitus in Children**

    Source: in Tyler, R.S., ed. Tinnitus Handbook. San Diego, CA: Singular Publishing Group. 2000. p. 243-261.

    Contact: Available from Singular-Thomson Learning. P.O. Box 6904, Florence, KY 41022. (800) 477-3692. Fax (606) 647-5963. Website: www.singpub.com. PRICE: $65.95 plus shipping and handling. ISBN: 1565939220.

    Summary: Children rarely complain of tinnitus, and when they do it does not appear to have the debilitating effects it has on adults. However, when children do complain of tinnitus, they should be taken seriously. This chapter on tinnitus in children is from an audiology textbook that offers clinicians and recent graduates information on tinnitus (ringing or other sounds in the ears). In the chapter, the authors discuss tinnitus in children with normal hearing; tinnitus in children with different levels of hearing loss; differences between the tinnitus experienced by children and adults; the etiology of sensorineural tinnitus in children, including ototoxic drugs, Meniere's disease, perilymph fistula, noise exposure, and pharmacologic agents; more rare causes of tinnitus in children, including acoustic neuromas, congenital neurosyphilis, blood dyscrasias, middle ear tinnitus, venous hums, transmitted bruit (vascular abnormalities), glomus tumors (a growth in the middle ear), and hydrocephalus (increased intracranial pressure); vascular malformations of the middle ear, including dural arteriovenous fistulae, dehiscent jugular bulb, aberrant carotid artery, and persistent stapedial artery; the causes of nonpulsatile middle ear tinnitus, including palatal myoclonus (rhythmic, involuntary contractions of the soft palate), middle ear myoclonus, patulous Eustachian tube, temporomandibular joint disorders, and familial tinnitus; and the evaluation of the child with complaints of tinnitus, including history, physical examination, audiologic evaluation, radiologic evaluation, and counseling and treatment options for children.

The authors stress that since tinnitus is most often a symptom of an underlying disease, an accurate diagnosis must first be established before attempting treatment. 1 figure. 1 table. 102 references.

- **Hyperacusis Assessment: Relationships with Tinnitus**

    Source: in Hazell, J., ed. Proceedings of the Sixth International Tinnitus Seminar. London, England: Tinnitus and Hyperacusis Centre. 1999. p. 128-132.

    Contact: Available from Tinnitus and Hyperacusis Centre. 32 Devonshire Place, London, W1N 1PE, United Kingdom. Fax 44 + (0) 207 486 2218. E-mail: thc@dr.com. Website: www.tinnitus.org. PRICE: Contact publisher for price. ISBN: 0953695700. Also available on CD-ROM.

    Summary: Clinical hyperacusis consists of a marked intolerance to ordinary environmental sounds while hearing thresholds are normal. This article on the interrelationship between hyperacusis and tinnitus is from a lengthy document that reprints the proceedings of the Sixth International Tinnitus Seminar, held in Cambridge, United Kingdom, in September 1999 and hosted by the British Society of Audiology. In this article, the authors note that the incidence of hyperacusis in individuals with tinnitus has been reported to be as high as 40 to 45 percent. Moreover, it seems that a peripheral auditory system, the medial-olivo cochlear system, is less efficient among patients with tinnitus. The authors report on a study undertaken to explore this efferent system functioning in hyperacusic patients with no other pathology (like tinnitus) to study the involvement of those fibers in auditory hypersensitivity itself. Hyperacusic individuals tend to isolate themselves (according to patient self report). The authors performed psychoacoustical tests, including loudness discomfort level measurements and loudness growth assessments, to quantify the auditory hypersensitivity of these patients. Results showed that the auditory dynamic ranges were lower in hyperacusic persons compared to control subjects. The medial-olivo cochlear system appeared to be more efficient in control than in hyperacusic subjects, but this tendency was not systematic. 4 figures. 23 references.

- **Patterns of Audiologic Findings for Tinnitus Patients**

    Source: in Hazell, J., ed. Proceedings of the Sixth International Tinnitus Seminar. London, England: Tinnitus and Hyperacusis Centre. 1999. p. 442-445.

    Contact: Available from Tinnitus and Hyperacusis Centre. 32 Devonshire Place, London, W1N 1PE, United Kingdom. Fax 44 + (0) 207 486 2218. E-

mail: thc@dr.com. Website: www.tinnitus.org. PRICE: Contact publisher for price. ISBN: 0953695700. Also available on CD-ROM.

Summary: Comprehensive diagnostic audiologic assessment is a critical step in the professional management of tinnitus patients. Within recent years, otoacoustic emissions (OAEs) have assumed an important role in the diagnostic audiologic test battery. OAEs offer an objective and highly sensitive clinical measure of cochlear (outer hair cell) function. The article on patterns of audiologic findings for tinnitus patients is from a lengthy document that reprints the proceedings of the Sixth International Tinnitus Seminar, held in Cambridge, United Kingdom, in September 1999 and hosted by the British Society of Audiology. In this study, the authors report audiologic findings for a series of 225 patients presenting to a medical center audiology clinic with the complaint of tinnitus. In addition to OAEs, the audiologic test battery included measurement of aural immittance, pure tone hearing thresholds, word recognition scores, loudness discomfort levels (LDLs) and, in selected patients, ultra high frequency pure tone audiometry. Tinnitus pitch, loudness, and maskability were also determined for all patients. Findings from a comprehensive diagnostic audiologic test battery not only serve to confirm cochlear hearing loss, they also contribute to patient counseling and education and thus constitute a definitive step toward successful management of tinnitus. One figure offers a simplified patient care algorithm for tinnitus assessment and management. 3 figures.

- **Musicians and Tinnitus**

Source: in Hazell, J., ed. Proceedings of the Sixth International Tinnitus Seminar. London, England: Tinnitus and Hyperacusis Centre. 1999. p. 232-240.

Contact: Available from Tinnitus and Hyperacusis Centre. 32 Devonshire Place, London, W1N 1PE, United Kingdom. Fax 44 + (0) 207 486 2218. E-mail: thc@dr.com. Website: www.tinnitus.org. PRICE: Contact publisher for price. ISBN: 0953695700. Also available on CD-ROM.

Summary: Legislation concerning noise-exposed workers may exclude musicians. As a group, they are not often considered as noise-exposed workers. However, as trained listeners exposed to high levels of noise and dependent on hearing for the performance and enjoyment of their profession, musicians represent a unique noise-exposed group. This article on musicians and tinnitus is from a lengthy document that reprints the proceedings of the Sixth International Tinnitus Seminar, held in Cambridge, United Kingdom, in September 1999 and hosted by the British Society of Audiology. In this article, the author describes a study covering a five year period of a group of symphony orchestra players.

Hearing loss, tinnitus, and hearing protection of musicians are discussed. The author concludes that Distortion Product Otoacoustic Emissions (DPOAEs) are a useful screening tool, that tinnitus can be an early indicator of hearing problems, and that using an industrial hearing conservation framework may be inadequate for the performing arts. Otoacoustic emissions should be part of regular hearing screening for musicians and hearing screening should take place more frequently than in industry. 18 figures. 13 references.

- **Local Drug Delivery Systems for the Treatment of Tinnitus: Principles, Surgical Techniques and Results**

  Source: in Hazell, J., ed. Proceedings of the Sixth International Tinnitus Seminar. London, England: Tinnitus and Hyperacusis Centre. 1999. p. 73-75.

  Contact: Available from Tinnitus and Hyperacusis Centre. 32 Devonshire Place, London, W1N 1PE, United Kingdom. Fax 44 + (0) 207 486 2218. E-mail: thc@dr.com. Website: www.tinnitus.org. PRICE: Contact publisher for price. ISBN: 0953695700. Also available on CD-ROM.

  Summary: Local treatment of inner ear diseases involves the direct application of pharmacological substances and or electrical stimulation of the inner ear structures. This article on local drug delivery systems for the treatment of tinnitus is from a lengthy document that reprints the proceedings of the Sixth International Tinnitus Seminar, held in Cambridge, United Kingdom, in September 1999 and hosted by the British Society of Audiology. In this article, the authors note that, in contrast to systemic pharmacotherapy, these local delivery systems present no dosage problems, result in no systemic side effects, and bypass the blood cochlea barrier. The round window membrane is the preferred access. The basic precondition is a stable coupling element, which allows a controlled drug release into the perilymphatic space. While technical difficulties do not allow direct access to the perilymphatic space, a catheter possessing a certain shape may be inserted into the round window niche. Among the disadvantages of these local drug delivery systems are the necessity of a surgical procedure, local side effects in the inner ear, only short term benefits from treatment, and the lack of coupling elements and implantable microdosage systems. The authors report on their clinical experiences using this type of local drug delivery system with lidocaine, glutamate, glutamic acid, diethylaesther, caroverine, and gentamycin. 8 references.

- **Outcome for Tinnitus Patients After Consultation with an Audiologist**

Source: in Hazell, J., ed. Proceedings of the Sixth International Tinnitus Seminar. London, England: Tinnitus and Hyperacusis Centre. 1999. p. 378-380.

Contact: Available from Tinnitus and Hyperacusis Centre. 32 Devonshire Place, London, W1N 1PE, United Kingdom. Fax 44 + (0) 207 486 2218. E-mail: thc@dr.com. Website: www.tinnitus.org. PRICE: Contact publisher for price. ISBN: 0953695700. Also available on CD-ROM.

Summary: Patients seeking professional care for tinnitus naturally expect the initial consultation to be the first step toward successful management of their health problem. Unfortunately, they are often rather quickly dismissed with an inaccurate summary of their audiologic status, a poor prognosis for tinnitus treatment, or inappropriate professional guidance. This article reports outcome for an unselected series of over 200 patients presenting to a medical center audiology clinic for a formal tinnitus consultation by an audiologist with more than 20 years of clinical experience. The article is from a lengthy document that reprints the proceedings of the Sixth International Tinnitus Seminar, held in Cambridge, United Kingdom, in September 1999 and hosted by the British Society of Audiology. The data showed that more the 90 percent of the patients had previously sought, without success, medical treatment for their tinnitus. Prior to the tinnitus consultation, patients completed the Tinnitus Handicap Inventory (THI) and a comprehensive survey questioning the nature of their tinnitus and the effect it had on their daily activities. During an hour consultation, patients were given detailed, current information on the causes of and treatments for tinnitus. Patients also had ample opportunity to ask questions about tinnitus and discuss their problem with the audiologist. The initial group was subsequently subdivided into patients who declined management following the consultation versus those who chose to pursue a formal treatment plan, such as Tinnitus Retraining Therapy (TRT). Then, 6 to 18 months after the initial consultation, outcome for all patients was measured using the THI and baseline survey. The majority of patients declined formal tinnitus management. This decision was inversely related to tinnitus severity. Outcome for this subgroup was significantly improved by the consultation. The authors conclude that either the consultation itself, and or the patient's compliance with simple recommendations made during this visit can improve outcome and minimize the requirement for extended tinnitus treatment. 3 figures. 1 table.

- **Tinnitus and Insomnia**

    Source: in Tyler, R.S., ed. Tinnitus Handbook. San Diego, CA: Singular Publishing Group. 2000. p. 59-84.

    Contact: Available from Singular-Thomson Learning. P.O. Box 6904, Florence, KY 41022. (800) 477-3692. Fax (606) 647-5963. Website: www.singpub.com. PRICE: $65.95 plus shipping and handling. ISBN: 1565939220.

    Summary: Sleep disturbance is a frequent complaint of people with tinnitus; indeed some patients regard it as an integral element of the experience of tinnitus. This chapter on tinnitus and insomnia is from an audiology textbook that offers clinicians and recent graduates information on tinnitus (ringing or other sounds in the ears). In the chapter, the author discusses the prevalence and definitions of insomnia (a range of sleep related complaints, including sleep of insufficient duration, of poor quality or effectiveness); the nature and function of sleep; the characteristics of insomnia; the extent of the problem of tinnitus related insomnia; assessment methods, including clinical interview, sleep diaries, assessment of mood, sleep questionnaires, polysomnographic recordings, and other behavioral assessments; models of insomnia; the mechanisms of tinnitus related insomnia; the management of insomnia, including medication, behavioral treatment, relaxation therapy, stimulus control techniques, paradoxical intention, sleep restriction, and approaches to the management of intrusive cognition (thoughts); and the management of tinnitus related insomnia. The author concludes that the high prevalence of sleep disorders in populations with tinnitus, and vice versa, requires that researchers and clinicians in the tinnitus field have a responsibility to investigate tinnitus related insomnia more carefully and to seek solutions to the problem. 1 figure. 73 references.

- **Subjective Tinnitus: Its Mechanisms and Treatment**

    Source: in Valente, M.; Hosford-Dunn, H.; Roeser, R.J., eds. Audiology: Treatment. New York, NY: Thieme. 2000. p. 691-714.

    Contact: Available from Thieme. 333 Seventh Avenue, New York, NY 10001. (800) 782-3488. Fax (212) 947-0108. E-mail: custserv@thieme.com. PRICE: $69.00 plus shipping and handling. ISBN: 0865778590.

    Summary: Subjective tinnitus is defined as the perception of an acoustic like sensation (sounds) for which no external generation can be found; tinnitus can include buzzing or ringing in the ears or head, or other types of noise sensations. This chapter on the mechanisms and treatment of subjective tinnitus is from a textbook that provides a comprehensive overview of the numerous treatment options available to help patients relieve the clinical symptoms seen in an audiology practice. Topics include an historical overview of tinnitus; the cause and prevalence of tinnitus; sounds of tinnitus; mechanisms of tinnitus; the assessment and evaluation of tinnitus, including medical evaluation and case history, audiometric evaluation, pitch matching, loudness matching, minimum masking level, residual inhibition, loudness discomfort level, and subjective assessment; treatment modalities, including drug therapy, antianxiety drugs, antidepression drugs, laser therapy, psychological intervention, biofeedback, masker therapy, and habituation therapy (Tinnitus Retraining Therapy); other therapeutic approaches; and hyperacusis (heightened sensitivity to sound). The chapter includes an outline of the topic covered, a list of references, a summary outline of the related preferred practice guidelines, and various 'pearls and pitfalls' offering practical advice to the reader. 2 figures. 57 references.

- **Quality Management in the Therapy of Chronic Tinnitus**

  Source: in Hazell, J., ed. Proceedings of the Sixth International Tinnitus Seminar. London, England: Tinnitus and Hyperacusis Centre. 1999. p. 357-363.

  Contact: Available from Tinnitus and Hyperacusis Centre. 32 Devonshire Place, London, W1N 1PE, United Kingdom. Fax 44 + (0) 207 486 2218. E-mail: thc@dr.com. Website: www.tinnitus.org. PRICE: Contact publisher for price. ISBN: 0953695700. Also available on CD-ROM.

  Summary: The assessment of psychological complaint patterns has become increasingly important during the past years for studies of chronic tinnitus patients. Unlike research in the area of chronic pain, only about nine scientifically relevant questionnaires designed to evaluate the degree of tinnitus severity exist world wide. This article on quality management in the therapy of chronic tinnitus is from a lengthy document that reprints the proceedings of the Sixth International Tinnitus Seminar, held in Cambridge, United Kingdom, in September 1999 and hosted by the British Society of Audiology. In this article, all available questionnaires for the assessment of psychological tinnitus severity are summarized, and their individual advantages and disadvantages are compared and discussed critically. The authors found an acceptable psychometric stability only in four questionnaires. The authors conclude that tinnitus questionnaires are important diagnostic instruments for assessing various complaints from different fields of life in connection with tinnitus. By distribution and growing acceptance of valid instruments in science, in medical appraisals, and in certain therapeutic areas, the problems associated with tinnitus will become clearer, and clinicians will be able to guide patients to individually suitable therapeutic options with more efficiency. The authors make their conclusions based on experiences collected in German speaking countries. 4 tables. 34 references.

- **Tinnitus in the Federal Republic of Germany: A Representative Epidemiological Study**

    Source: in Hazell, J., ed. Proceedings of the Sixth International Tinnitus Seminar. London, England: Tinnitus and Hyperacusis Centre. 1999. p. 64-67.

    Contact: Available from Tinnitus and Hyperacusis Centre. 32 Devonshire Place, London, W1N 1PE, United Kingdom. Fax 44 + (0) 207 486 2218. E-mail: thc@dr.com. Website: www.tinnitus.org. PRICE: Contact publisher for price. ISBN: 0953695700. Also available on CD-ROM.

    Summary: This article is from a lengthy document that reprints the proceedings of the Sixth International Tinnitus Seminar, held in Cambridge, United Kingdom, in September 1999 and hosted by the British Society of Audiology. In this article, the authors report on their epidemiological study on tinnitus in Germany, which evaluated the prevalence and incidence rate of the symptom. In a random sample of persons aged more than ten years, 3,049 telephone interviews were performed. The sample was stratified by the state in order to realize an exhaustive reflection of the country. The main results showed that 18.7 million citizens (24.9 percent of the population) have or have once had noise in the ear; 2.9 million citizens (3.9 percent of the population) had noise in the ear at the time of the study; and 2.7 million citizens (3.6 percent of the population) have ear noise that has lasted longer than one month. Each year there are 250,000 citizens (0.33 percent of the population) as new chronic patients. Of patients with chronic tinnitus, 53 percent report a hearing impairment, but only 7.5 percent of these patients have been supplied with a hearing aid. Thirteen percent of the patients regarded the medical assistance as very helpful; 20 percent as completely inadequate. Fifty-five percent of patients replied that no therapy had helped. The authors list many other results in this article. 10 references.

- **Neurophysiological Model of Tinnitus and Hyperacusis**

    Source: in Hazell, J., ed. Proceedings of the Sixth International Tinnitus Seminar. London, England: Tinnitus and Hyperacusis Centre. 1999. p. 32-38.

    Contact: Available from Tinnitus and Hyperacusis Centre. 32 Devonshire Place, London, W1N 1PE, United Kingdom. Fax 44 + (0) 207 486 2218. E-

mail: thc@dr.com. Website: www.tinnitus.org. PRICE: Contact publisher for price. ISBN: 0953695700. Also available on CD-ROM.

Summary: This article on a neurophysiological model of tinnitus and hyperacusis (heightened sensitivity to sound) is from a lengthy document that reprints the proceedings of the Sixth International Tinnitus Seminar, held in Cambridge, United Kingdom, in September 1999 and hosted by the British Society of Audiology. The neurophysiological model of tinnitus and hyperacusis resulted from analyses of clinical and research data on tinnitus from the perspective of the basic functional properties of the central nervous system (CNS). Tinnitus induces distress in only about 25 percent of the people perceiving it, with no correlation between the distress and the psychoacoustical characterization of the tinnitus. In addition, the characterization of tinnitus in the population of people suffering from it is not related to the severity of tinnitus and to the treatment outcome. These findings support the hypothesis that the auditory system is only a secondary system, and other systems in the brain are dominant in clinically relevant tinnitus. Other evidence to support this hypothesis is the fact that essentially everyone experiences tinnitus when put in a sufficiently quiet environment (94 percent of people without tinnitus experience tinnitus when isolated for several minutes in an echo free chamber). 2 figures. 21 references.

- **Developing a Structured Interview to Assess Audiological, Aetiological and Psychological Variables of Tinnitus**

  Source: in Hazell, J., ed. Proceedings of the Sixth International Tinnitus Seminar. London, England: Tinnitus and Hyperacusis Centre. 1999. p. 277-282.

  Contact: Available from Tinnitus and Hyperacusis Centre. 32 Devonshire Place, London, W1N 1PE, United Kingdom. Fax 44 + (0) 207 486 2218. E-mail: thc@dr.com. Website: www.tinnitus.org. PRICE: Contact publisher for price. ISBN: 0953695700. Also available on CD-ROM.

  Summary: This article on a new diagnostic instrument for tinnitus is from a lengthy document that reprints the proceedings of the Sixth International Tinnitus Seminar, held in Cambridge, United Kingdom, in September 1999 and hosted by the British Society of Audiology. In this article, the authors introduce and describe the Structured Tinnitus Interview (STI). The STI represents a multidisciplinary diagnostic approach whereby major biomedical, audiological, and psychological characteristics of tinnitus are assessed in a systematic and standardized form. Separate sections of the instrument cover the patient's tinnitus history, etiological factors, and psychosocial tinnitus related complaints. Good to excellent test-retest reliability is demonstrated on both item and scale level. The dimensional scales of the STI refer to different areas of psychosocial functioning. They were found to be valid and sensitive to changes induced during cognitive behavioral treatment. The interview is very well accepted by both clinicians and patients. 1 figure. 4 tables. 14 references.

- **Children's Experience of Tinnitus**

    Source: in Hazell, J., ed. Proceedings of the Sixth International Tinnitus Seminar. London, England: Tinnitus and Hyperacusis Centre. 1999. p. 220-223.

    Contact: Available from Tinnitus and Hyperacusis Centre. 32 Devonshire Place, London, W1N 1PE, United Kingdom. Fax 44 + (0) 207 486 2218. E-mail: thc@dr.com. Website: www.tinnitus.org. PRICE: Contact publisher for price. ISBN: 0953695700. Also available on CD-ROM.

    Summary: This article on children's experience of tinnitus is from a lengthy document that reprints the proceedings of the Sixth International Tinnitus Seminar, held in Cambridge, United Kingdom, in September 1999 and hosted by the British Society of Audiology. In this article, the authors report a small scale study of 24 children (half with normal hearing and half with a hearing loss) who presented to the Psychology Department of the authors with troublesome tinnitus. Similar to findings in adult studies, results suggest that tinnitus can have as marked an impact on children's lives as it is reported to have on adults. Insomnia, emotional distress, listening and attention difficulties, are the main psychological factors associated with tinnitus in children. These in turn may have an effect on their school performances. Differences were found between children with normal hearing and those with some degree of hearing loss. Overall, children with normal hearing found tinnitus more troublesome, and presented with higher levels of anxiety than those with some level of hearing impairment. The authors conclude that children who complain of tinnitus should be taken seriously. In terms of management, individual intervention packages tailored to the needs of each child and family were found to be useful in alleviating anxiety and other associated factors. 7 tables. 10 references.

- **Gender Aspects Related to Tinnitus Complaints**

    Source: in Hazell, J., ed. Proceedings of the Sixth International Tinnitus Seminar. London, England: Tinnitus and Hyperacusis Centre. 1999. p. 266-267.

    Contact: Available from Tinnitus and Hyperacusis Centre. 32 Devonshire Place, London, W1N 1PE, United Kingdom. Fax 44 + (0) 207 486 2218. E-

mail: thc@dr.com. Website: www.tinnitus.org. PRICE: Contact publisher for price. ISBN: 0953695700. Also available on CD-ROM.

Summary: This article on gender aspects related to tinnitus complaints is from a lengthy document that reprints the proceedings of the Sixth International Tinnitus Seminar, held in Cambridge, United Kingdom, in September 1999 and hosted by the British Society of Audiology. In this article, the authors stress that when speaking with patients whose tinnitus gives rise to emotional distress, it is essential to focus on relevant gender related factors. Males, in general, tend to ignore psychological ill health more than females. The authors report on a study in which the Nottingham Health Profil (NHP), designed for the measurement of health related quality of life in medical conditions, was used in a tinnitus population including 57 females and 129 males. The severity rate for four out of six dimensions of the NHP was higher among the females. Younger women reported significantly more health problems compared to a normal female control group in four dimensions: lack of energy, pain, emotional reactions, and sleep disturbances. 6 references.

- **Effects of Publicity on Tinnitus**

    Source: in Hazell, J., ed. Proceedings of the Sixth International Tinnitus Seminar. London, England: Tinnitus and Hyperacusis Centre. 1999. p. 229-231.

    Contact: Available from Tinnitus and Hyperacusis Centre. 32 Devonshire Place, London, W1N 1PE, United Kingdom. Fax 44 + (0) 207 486 2218. E-mail: thc@dr.com. Website: www.tinnitus.org. PRICE: Contact publisher for price. ISBN: 0953695700. Also available on CD-ROM.

    Summary: This article on the effects of publicity regarding tinnitus is from a lengthy document that reprints the proceedings of the Sixth International Tinnitus Seminar, held in Cambridge, United Kingdom, in September 1999 and hosted by the British Society of Audiology. In this article, the authors report on their study which looked at the effects of publicity, self reported by new patients presenting at tinnitus clinics. The questionnaire study includes data from 316 patients, taken from 4 centers (two private and two of the British National Health Service). Results showed that of the 85 percent who had experienced publicity, more patients found publicity helpful than upsetting, while some found it both helpful and upsetting. The authors report that some types of publicity presents the worst case scenarios of tinnitus, perhaps to encourage more financial support for research and clinical services, and sympathy for those afflicted. However, medical advisors contend that this approach simply feeds the vicious cycle (symptoms causing distress which worsens the symptoms) and increase the distress of many people with tinnitus.

The authors summarize the explanatory comments that patients made, and discuss what styles of publicity should be avoided. The questionnaire used in the study is reprinted at the end of the article. 8 tables. 2 references.

- **Effects of Insomnia on Tinnitus Severity: A Follow-Up Study**

    Source: in Hazell, J., ed. Proceedings of the Sixth International Tinnitus Seminar. London, England: Tinnitus and Hyperacusis Centre. 1999. p. 271-276.

    Contact: Available from Tinnitus and Hyperacusis Centre. 32 Devonshire Place, London, W1N 1PE, United Kingdom. Fax 44 + (0) 207 486 2218. E-mail: thc@dr.com. Website: www.tinnitus.org. PRICE: Contact publisher for price. ISBN: 0953695700. Also available on CD-ROM.

    Summary: This article on the interplay between insomnia and tinnitus severity is from a lengthy document that reprints the proceedings of the Sixth International Tinnitus Seminar, held in Cambridge, United Kingdom, in September 1999 and hosted by the British Society of Audiology. In this article, the authors describe their study undertaken to investigate the effects of insomnia on tinnitus severity and to determine how this relationship may evolve with the passage of time. Questionnaires were mailed to patients prior to their initial appointment at the Oregon Health Sciences University Tinnitus Clinic between 1994 and 1997. These questionnaires requested information pertaining to insomnia, tinnitus severity, and loudness. During their initial appointment, patients received counseling, education, and reassurance about tinnitus; audiometric and tinnitus evaluations; and treatment recommendations. Follow up questionnaires were mailed to 350 patients one to four years (mean of 2.3 years) after their initial appointment at the Clinic. Questionnaires were returned by 174 patients (130 males, 44 females; mean age 55.9 years). Even though many of these patients improved in both sleep interference and tinnitus severity, a significant number (43 patients) reported on the follow up questionnaire that they continued to have difficulty sleeping. Reported loudness and severity of tinnitus were significantly greater for this group than for groups of patients who reported that they never or only sometimes have difficulty sleeping. The relationship between sleep disturbance and tinnitus severity became more pronounced with the passage of time. The authors conclude that their findings underscore the importance of identification and successful treatment of insomnia for patients with tinnitus. One appendix offers the follow up questionnaire used in the study. 6 tables. 18 references.

- **Pathophysiology of Severe Tinnitus and Chronic Pain**

    Source: in Hazell, J., ed. Proceedings of the Sixth International Tinnitus Seminar. London, England: Tinnitus and Hyperacusis Centre. 1999. p. 26-31.

    Contact: Available from Tinnitus and Hyperacusis Centre. 32 Devonshire Place, London, W1N 1PE, United Kingdom. Fax 44 + (0) 207 486 2218. E-mail: thc@dr.com. Website: www.tinnitus.org. PRICE: Contact publisher for price. ISBN: 0953695700. Also available on CD-ROM.

    Summary: This article on the pathophysiology of severe tinnitus and chronic pain is from a lengthy document that reprints the proceedings of the Sixth International Tinnitus Seminar, held in Cambridge, United Kingdom, in September 1999 and hosted by the British Society of Audiology. In this article, the author defines severe tinnitus as that which interferes with sleep, work, and social life. In most cases, severe tinnitus is believed to be caused by changes in the function of the central auditory nervous system. However, some forms are caused by changes in the function of the cochlea, as evidenced from the fact that severing the auditory nerve can relieve tinnitus in some individuals. Topics include a comparison of symptoms and signs of tinnitus and chronic pain, current hypotheses about the generation of pain and tinnitus, the generation of central tinnitus, and similarities with other hyperactive disorders. The author concludes that the changes in the function of the central nervous system that cause chronic pain and severe tinnitus are not associated with morphologic changes that can be detected by known imaging techniques, but the areas of the brain that are activated can be identified by functional imaging tests. Few electrophysiologic or behavioral tests are abnormal in individuals with chronic tinnitus and chronic pain, which complicates the diagnosis of tinnitus and the ability to monitor progress of treatment. The clinician mainly has to rely on the patients reported symptoms. 2 figures. 25 references.

- **Prevalence and Problems of Tinnitus in the Elderly**

    Source: in Hazell, J., ed. Proceedings of the Sixth International Tinnitus Seminar. London, England: Tinnitus and Hyperacusis Centre. 1999. p. 58-63.

    Contact: Available from Tinnitus and Hyperacusis Centre. 32 Devonshire Place, London, W1N 1PE, United Kingdom. Fax 44 + (0) 207 486 2218. E-mail: thc@dr.com. Website: www.tinnitus.org. PRICE: Contact publisher for price. ISBN: 0953695700. Also available on CD-ROM.

    Summary: This article on the prevalence and problems of tinnitus in the elderly is from a lengthy document that reprints the proceedings of the

Sixth International Tinnitus Seminar, held in Cambridge, United Kingdom, in September 1999 and hosted by the British Society of Audiology. In this article, the authors report on the Australian Longitudinal Study of Ageing (ALSA) which provides self report and performance based measures of sensory function and selected sociodemographic, physical, cognitive, and psychosocial information in a large sample of elderly urban Australians (n = 2087), aged 70 to 103 years. The authors' study examined tinnitus in 1,453 ALSO respondents, who provided data about tinnitus at baseline and at follow up 2 years later. Of the 1,453 respondents, 258 (17.6 percent) reported tinnitus on both occasions; 64.8 percent reported no tinnitus on either occasion; and the remainder reported tinnitus only at baseline (10.6 percent), or only at follow up (7 percent). Overall, respondents with tinnitus performed more poorly on tests of measured hearing, and appear to experience a lower quality of life in several domains than respondents who do not report tinnitus. 4 tables. 13 references.

- **Quality of Family Life of People Who Report Tinnitus**

    Source: in Hazell, J., ed. Proceedings of the Sixth International Tinnitus Seminar. London, England: Tinnitus and Hyperacusis Centre. 1999. p. 45-50.

    Contact: Available from Tinnitus and Hyperacusis Centre. 32 Devonshire Place, London, W1N 1PE, United Kingdom. Fax 44 + (0) 207 486 2218. E-mail: thc@dr.com. Website: www.tinnitus.org. PRICE: Contact publisher for price. ISBN: 0953695700. Also available on CD-ROM.

    Summary: This article on the quality of family life of people who report tinnitus is from a lengthy document that reprints the proceedings of the Sixth International Tinnitus Seminar, held in Cambridge, United Kingdom, in September 1999 and hosted by the British Society of Audiology. In this article, the authors report on their study which was undertaken to evaluate the effectiveness of the rehabilitation protocols used by the Nottingham Tinnitus Clinic by measuring how tinnitus affects the quality of life of the person reporting tinnitus and their family. The authors assessed the health related quality of life using the SF 36 Aspects of Health Questionnaire and the wider impact of tinnitus using a new Quality of Family Life Questionnaire in two groups of patients: the first awaiting a specialist appointment (group A) and the second a group of people who have attended for a specialist appointment and been discharged (group B). The results showed statistically significant better scores for individuals in group B, when controlling for other factors that might influence the measure of quality of life. Furthermore, there were systematic differences between those on the waiting list and those who had been discharged with respect to aspects of quality of family life, particularly in the areas of understanding tinnitus and allaying fears. 1 figure. 3 tables. 7 references.

- **Systematic Classification of Tinnitus**

Source: in Hazell, J., ed. Proceedings of the Sixth International Tinnitus Seminar. London, England: Tinnitus and Hyperacusis Centre. 1999. p. 17-25.

Contact: Available from Tinnitus and Hyperacusis Centre. 32 Devonshire Place, London, W1N 1PE, United Kingdom. Fax 44 + (0) 207 486 2218. E-mail: thc@dr.com. Website: www.tinnitus.org. PRICE: Contact publisher for price. ISBN: 0953695700. Also available on CD-ROM.

Summary: This article on the systematic classification of tinnitus is from a lengthy document that reprints the proceedings of the Sixth International Tinnitus Seminar, held in Cambridge, United Kingdom, in September 1999 and hosted by the British Society of Audiology. In this article, the authors offer a framework that divides tinnitus into three types, based on function and anatomy: conductive tinnitus, sensorineural tinnitus, and central tinnitus. Sensorineural tinnitus can be further subdivided into four subtypes: motor tinnitus (Type I), transduction tinnitus (Type II), transformation tinnitus (Type III), and extrasensory tinnitus (Type IV). One figure schematically illustrates the individual functional and anatomical steps involved in sound processing with the middle ear, inner ear, and brain. One table classifies some common tinnitus disorders into this new classification. 1 figure. 1 table. 21 references.

- **Use of Science to Find Successful Tinnitus Treatments**

Source: in Hazell, J., ed. Proceedings of the Sixth International Tinnitus Seminar. London, England: Tinnitus and Hyperacusis Centre. 1999. p. 3-9.

Contact: Available from Tinnitus and Hyperacusis Centre. 32 Devonshire Place, London, W1N 1PE, United Kingdom. Fax 44 + (0) 207 486 2218. E-mail: thc@dr.com. Website: www.tinnitus.org. PRICE: Contact publisher for price. ISBN: 0953695700. Also available on CD-ROM.

Summary: This article on the use of science to find successful tinnitus treatments is from a lengthy document that reprints the proceedings of the Sixth International Tinnitus Seminar, held in Cambridge, United Kingdom, in September 1999 and hosted by the British Society of Audiology. In this article, the author contends that discovering successful treatments will be facilitated by the scientific method. The author outlines a framework for clinical trials for tinnitus treatment. Patient expectations dramatically influence treatment outcomes, and therefore require careful consideration in selecting control conditions. The population under study requires careful definition of recruitment and exclusion practice, duration and severity of tinnitus, hyperacusis (heightened sensitivity to noise), and hearing loss. It is also desirable to document ear disease, psychological and psychoacoustical characteristics, treatment history, otoacoustic emissions, whether tactile or motor stimulation affects tinnitus, and whether the tinnitus is likely consistent with a peripheral or central mechanism. The author notes that the most challenging aspect is designing the appropriate control condition. A comprehensive description of the protocol is needed to facilitate replication. Benefit should be measured with established questionnaires and with measures of the magnitude of the tinnitus. A persuasive tinnitus treatment will be one that shows a large treatment effect, can be generalized across patients and clinicians, is specific and credible, and changes the way clinicians and patients think about tinnitus. 3 figures. 17 references.

- **Early Identification of Therapy Resistant Tinnitus**

    Source: in Hazell, J., ed. Proceedings of the Sixth International Tinnitus Seminar. London, England: Tinnitus and Hyperacusis Centre. 1999. p. 268-270.

    Contact: Available from Tinnitus and Hyperacusis Centre. 32 Devonshire Place, London, W1N 1PE, United Kingdom. Fax 44 + (0) 207 486 2218. E-mail: thc@dr.com. Website: www.tinnitus.org. PRICE: Contact publisher for price. ISBN: 0953695700. Also available on CD-ROM.

    Summary: This article on therapy resistant tinnitus is from a lengthy document that reprints the proceedings of the Sixth International Tinnitus Seminar, held in Cambridge, United Kingdom, in September 1999 and hosted by the British Society of Audiology. In this article, the authors report on their research study which investigated risk factors for therapy resistant tinnitus (as measured by absence from work, related to tinnitus, abbreviated at AWT). The study included 172 consecutive tinnitus patients consulting an audiological physician during a 6 month period at a university hospital in Goteborg, Sweden (54 women and 118 men). The patients were reassessed 18 months later in order to identify and investigate the therapy resistant patients. In the study, 18 out of the 79 patients who completed the study were absent from work due to tinnitus. There were significant correlations between the tinnitus severity questionnaire (TSQ) and AWT, including questions concerning how much tinnitus reduces the overall quality of life, how often tinnitus is noticed during the waking hours or impairs concentration, and how often tinnitus makes the patients feel anxious or worried, tense or irritable, or depressed and miserable. The main predictors influencing AWT were the questions concerning depression and reduced mobility, but also physical exercise on a regular basis and hearing thresholds over both ears for the low and mid frequencies. The authors conclude that it is of great importance to identify and treat depression and anxiety disorders initially, so the risks for the progression of tinnitus are minimized. 1 figure. 2 tables. 11 references.

- **Effects of Hearing Loss on Tinnitus**

Source: in Hazell, J., ed. Proceedings of the Sixth International Tinnitus Seminar. London, England: Tinnitus and Hyperacusis Centre. 1999. p. 407-414.

Contact: Available from Tinnitus and Hyperacusis Centre. 32 Devonshire Place, London, W1N 1PE, United Kingdom. Fax 44 + (0) 207 486 2218. E-mail: thc@dr.com. Website: www.tinnitus.org. PRICE: Contact publisher for price. ISBN: 0953695700. Also available on CD-ROM.

Summary: This article reports on a study in which tinnitus perception and reaction were measured in 182 individuals who received five sessions of tinnitus retraining therapy (TRT) in a 12 month period, and 159 individuals followed up after a further 12 months. The article is from a lengthy document that reprints the proceedings of the Sixth International Tinnitus Seminar, held in Cambridge, United Kingdom, in September 1999 and hosted by the British Society of Audiology. In this study, the participants were divided into three groups on the basis of hearing status: normal hearing (NORM), mild high frequency hearing loss (HF), and moderate to severe hearing loss (MOD SEV). The MOD SEV group reported that their tinnitus had worsened prior to the study, whereas the NORM and HF had started to habituate to their tinnitus. At the start of the study, the MOD SEV group had significantly greater loudness and percentage awareness, tinnitus pitch was significantly lower, and number of tinnitus sounds significantly higher than the NORM and HF groups. After 12 months of TRT, tinnitus annoyance, effect on life quality, loudness, and percentage awareness in each hearing status group improved by a similar amount. Psychological status was measured in a representative subgroup of 118 individuals. Phobic anxiety in both males and females, and depression in males were positively correlated with hearing threshold at 4000 Hz. The authors conclude that it is possible that hearing threshold influences tinnitus reaction, perception, and psychological status but it does not appear to influence response to TRT significantly. 4 figures. 3 tables. 18 references.

- **Role Psychological and Social Variables Play in Predicting Tinnitus Impairments**

    Source: in Hazell, J., ed. Proceedings of the Sixth International Tinnitus Seminar. London, England: Tinnitus and Hyperacusis Centre. 1999. p. 381-383.

    Contact: Available from Tinnitus and Hyperacusis Centre. 32 Devonshire Place, London, W1N 1PE, United Kingdom. Fax 44 + (0) 207 486 2218. E-mail: thc@dr.com. Website: www.tinnitus.org. PRICE: Contact publisher for price. ISBN: 0953695700. Also available on CD-ROM.

    Summary: This article reports on a study undertaken to investigate whether tinnitus impairments can be predicted by psychological and or social variables. The article is from a lengthy document that reprints the proceedings of the Sixth International Tinnitus Seminar, held in Cambridge, United Kingdom, in September 1999 and hosted by the British Society of Audiology. In this study, a sample of 153 patients with tinnitus (75 females and 78 males) were recruited from various treatment facilities in Austria and Germany. Patients were evaluated using the following instruments: Tinnitus Handicap Inventory (THI-12), Depression Scale (ADS-L), Quality of Life (WHOQOL BREEF), List of General and Somatic Complaints (BL), and Health Related Locus of Control Scale (KKG). The effects of depression, various dimensions of quality of life, somatic and general complaints, locus of control, as well as sleeping disorders, were assessed on emotional cognitive and functional communicative tinnitus impairments using a canonical correlation analysis. The results showed that severity of depression is the most significant predictor of emotional cognitive impairments due to tinnitus. Somatic and general complaints, physical and social domains on the quality of life scale, and depression predict the functional communicative impairments. The authors conclude that, of the variables studied, depression seems to be a general dimension influencing tinnitus related impairments. 1 table. 11 references.

- **Combining Elements of Tinnitus Retraining Therapy (TRT) and Cognitive-Behavioral Therapy: Does It Work?**

    Source: in Hazell, J., ed. Proceedings of the Sixth International Tinnitus Seminar. London, England: Tinnitus and Hyperacusis Centre. 1999. p. 399-402.

    Contact: Available from Tinnitus and Hyperacusis Centre. 32 Devonshire Place, London, W1N 1PE, United Kingdom. Fax 44 + (0) 207 486 2218. E-mail: thc@dr.com. Website: www.tinnitus.org. PRICE: Contact publisher for price. ISBN: 0953695700. Also available on CD-ROM.

Summary: This article reports on an ongoing controlled treatment study in which elements of cognitive behavioral therapy (CBT) and tinnitus retraining therapy (TRT) were combined to provide different group treatments for different target populations of patients depending on the degree of tinnitus distress. The article is from a lengthy document that reprints the proceedings of the Sixth International Tinnitus Seminar, held in Cambridge, United Kingdom, in September 1999 and hosted by the British Society of Audiology. In this study, half of the subjects in each treatment also received sound therapy by behind the ear (BTE) broadband noise generators to examine a possible therapeutic effect of additional auditory stimulation. Preliminary results show the effectiveness of both treatments, but no effect of sound therapy. The authors conclude that they find no basic contradictions between TRT and the already established cognitive behavioral treatments for chronic tinnitus. It seems very useful to combine elements of these two approaches in order to treat specific subgroups of patients. 1 figure. 3 tables. 11 references.

- **What is Tinnitus?**

    Source: in Saunders, J. Tinnitus: What is That Noise in My Head? Auckland, New Zealand: Sandalwood Enterprises. 1994. p. 17-22.

    Contact: Available from American Tinnitus Association (ATA). P.O. Box 5, Portland, OR 97207-0005. (800) 634-8978 or (503) 248-9985. Fax (503) 248-0024. E-mail: tinnitus@ata.org. Website: www.ata.org. PRICE: $14.50 for members; $18.00 for nonmembers. ISBN: 0473015625.

    Summary: This chapter is from a book that familiarizes readers with the common causes and symptoms of tinnitus and explains how people with tinnitus can take steps toward relieving the condition. Written in non-technical language, the chapter defines tinnitus and gives readers an overview of the condition. Topics covered include the five main stages in the auditory pathway, the history of tinnitus and its treatments, the classifications of tinnitus, and some of the more common causes of the condition.

- **How to Evaluate Treatments for Tinnitus**

    Source: in Vernon, J.A. Tinnitus: Treatment and Relief. Needham Heights, MA: Allyn and Bacon. 1998. p. 1-7.

    Contact: Available from Allyn and Bacon. 160 Gould Street, Needham Heights, MA 02194-2310. (800) 278-3525; Fax (617) 455-7024; E-mail: AandBpub@aol.com; http://www.abacon.com. PRICE: $26.95 plus shipping and handling. ISBN: 0205182690.

Summary: This chapter is from a book that offers information about treatment options for tinnitus. This chapter offers suggestions for evaluating treatments for tinnitus. The author notes that few patients with tinnitus can be completely cured; however, patients with tinnitus from many causes can definitely be improved by different measures, even if they are not completely cured. The author describes the differences between open studies and controlled studies when examining the effectiveness of different treatment options. From a statistical perspective, open studies have a tendency to report results that are too positive (because of participant or observer bias, for example); while controlled studies tend to give results that are too negative. The author recommends that tinnitus treatments continue to receive open studies and that those treatments that appear promising under subjective review should receive controlled trials. The ethical issues involved in treatments offered for tinnitus are discussed and there is a section of advice for the individual tinnitus patient. The ethical issues involved in treatment available for tinnitus is discussed and there is a section of advice for the individual tinnitus patient.

- **Psychological Profiles of Tinnitus Patients**

    Source: in Tyler, R.S., ed. Tinnitus Handbook. San Diego, CA: Singular Publishing Group. 2000. p. 25-57.

    Contact: Available from Singular-Thomson Learning. P.O. Box 6904, Florence, KY 41022. (800) 477-3692. Fax (606) 647-5963. Website: www.singpub.com. PRICE: $65.95 plus shipping and handling. ISBN: 1565939220.

    Summary: This chapter is from an audiology textbook that offers clinicians and recent graduates information on tinnitus (ringing or other sounds in the ears). In the chapter, the author describes psychological profiles of tinnitus patients. Topics include the relevance of investigating psychological factors in tinnitus patients, getting beyond the initial reaction of crisis, gender aspects of the subjective experience of tinnitus, tinnitus distress symptoms in different patient groups seeking medical consultation, dimensions of complaints that are appropriate for study, habituation to tinnitus and reasons for dishabituation, chronic tinnitus in comparison with chronic pain, personality patterns of people with tinnitus, perceived character and quality aspects of the tinnitus sound, anxiety as an underestimated factor in tinnitus annoyance, similarities between cognitive and emotional aspects of depression and tinnitus, how tinnitus can affect a patient's lifestyle and personal relationships, tinnitus and sleep disturbances, and causal explanations of tinnitus distress in relation to mental illness. The author concludes by emphasizing the impact of time on tinnitus and on the patient's psychosocial response to the condition. Instead of considering tinnitus a chronic condition, the author hypothesizes that tinnitus may be a signal of severe distress that interacts with crucial circumstances in the life of the individual. This model of multiple causes creates a need for repeated diagnostic and treatment methods as the condition fluctuates. 2 figures. 1 table. 121 references.

- **History of Tinnitus**

    Source: in Tyler, R.S., ed. Tinnitus Handbook. San Diego, CA: Singular Publishing Group. 2000. p. 437-448.

    Contact: Available from Singular-Thomson Learning. P.O. Box 6904, Florence, KY 41022. (800) 477-3692. Fax (606) 647-5963. Website: www.singpub.com. PRICE: $65.95 plus shipping and handling. ISBN: 1565939220.

    Summary: This chapter is the final chapter in an audiology textbook that offers clinicians and recent graduates information on tinnitus (ringing or other sounds in the ears). In the chapter, the author provides a history of tinnitus and its treatments. Tinnitus, being essentially a reflection of abnormal function of the ear, has presumably occurred in humans since evolution began. From the earliest written medical records, individuals have been consulting healers for help with this symptom. The author addresses the attitudes and approaches of such healers over the millennia towards the symptom and their subsequent approach adopted. The author concentrates on a number of representative writings, usually by well known authors and authorities of the period that reflect the then current attitudes towards the symptom. The author includes ancient Babylon, Celsus and Graeco Roman medicine, Islamic and medieval medicine, the seventeenth century and Duverney, Jean Marie Gaspard Itard, the late nineteenth century, and the Folwers and the beginning of the modern approach. 5 figures. 3 tables. 24 references.

- **Epidemiology of Tinnitus**

    Source: in Tyler, R.S., ed. Tinnitus Handbook. San Diego, CA: Singular Publishing Group. 2000. p. 1-23.

    Contact: Available from Singular-Thomson Learning. P.O. Box 6904, Florence, KY 41022. (800) 477-3692. Fax (606) 647-5963. Website: www.singpub.com. PRICE: $65.95 plus shipping and handling. ISBN: 1565939220.

    Summary: This chapter on the epidemiology of tinnitus is from an audiology textbook that offers clinicians and recent graduates information on tinnitus (ringing or other sounds in the ears). In the chapter, the authors review the prevalence of tinnitus in different populations, together with those demographic, systemic, and environmental factors that influence the prevalence. Hearing impairment and age were found to be strongly related to the prevalence of tinnitus. The effect of gender was not that clear, although some studies showed a slight increase in the proportion of females complaining of tinnitus. The effect of socioeconomic and occupational group on the prevalence of tinnitus was found to be positive. The effect of noise on the auditory system is clearly related to the prevalence of tinnitus. The authors discuss the public health and clinical implications of these data, which show that tinnitus is a widespread problem that causes considerable disability or handicap for which systematic intervention should have a high priority. Noise must have a big role in determining priorities for public health. The integration of epidemiological data into patient counseling is very important. The authors stress that patients need to be told about the causes, possible progression of the condition, and a realistic picture of the future. 67 references.

- **Psychological Management of Tinnitus**

  Source: in Tyler, R.S., ed. Tinnitus Handbook. San Diego, CA: Singular Publishing Group. 2000. p. 263-279.

  Contact: Available from Singular-Thomson Learning. P.O. Box 6904, Florence, KY 41022. (800) 477-3692. Fax (606) 647-5963. Website: www.singpub.com. PRICE: $65.95 plus shipping and handling. ISBN: 1565939220.

  Summary: This chapter on the psychological management of tinnitus is from an audiology textbook that offers clinicians and recent graduates information on tinnitus (ringing or other sounds in the ears). In the chapter, the authors provide an overview of the contributions that psychological approaches can offer in the assessment and management of tinnitus. Tinnitus is both a medical and a psychological phenomenon, in some ways similar to the experience of chronic pain. The consequences of chronic pain and tinnitus are similar: emotional effects, reduced involvement in work related activities, interpersonal problems, and decreased opportunities to engage in previously enjoyable activities. The aim of psychological treatment is to improve the ability of the individual to reduce the impact of tinnitus on their well being and lifestyle. The authors present a format of a comprehensive patient interview, including the range of available self report measures. The authors then discuss psychological treatment options, including relaxation methods, cognitive therapy, and attention control techniques. A final section discusses what can be expected as outcome of therapy. The authors conclude that multiple treatment components, such as combined cognitive therapy, attention control and relaxation training, appear to produce the most consistent positive results. Relaxation training may be useful as a vehicle for teaching some of the cognitive attention control methods, for helping people with sleep problems, or for reducing general reactivity to stress. 3 tables. 59 references.

- **Electrical Stimulation for Tinnitus Suppression**

   Source: in Tyler, R.S., ed. Tinnitus Handbook. San Diego, CA: Singular Publishing Group. 2000. p. 377-398.

   Contact: Available from Singular-Thomson Learning. P.O. Box 6904, Florence, KY 41022. (800) 477-3692. Fax (606) 647-5963. Website: www.singpub.com. PRICE: $65.95 plus shipping and handling. ISBN: 1565939220.

   Summary: This chapter on the use of electrical stimulation for tinnitus suppression is from an audiology textbook that offers clinicians and recent graduates information on tinnitus (ringing or other sounds in the ears). In the chapter, the author discusses the two forms of external electricity, the electrical potentials in the auditory system, some characteristics of biological electricity, AC potentials in the cochlea, brain electrical potentials, first attempts to alleviate tinnitus with flow of electric charges, unexpected tinnitus suppression with electricity used for other purposes, tinnitus suppression according to the site of electrical stimulation, extracochlear stimulation with transcutaneous electrodes, extracochlear implants, and intracochlear stimulation (single and multichannel cochlear implants). The author concludes by reviewing the areas where additional research is needed. 1 figure. 4 tables. 72 references.

- **Tinnitus Masking**

   Source: in Tyler, R.S., ed. Tinnitus Handbook. San Diego, CA: Singular Publishing Group. 2000. p. 313-356.

   Contact: Available from Singular-Thomson Learning. P.O. Box 6904, Florence, KY 41022. (800) 477-3692. Fax (606) 647-5963. Website: www.singpub.com. PRICE: $65.95 plus shipping and handling. ISBN: 1565939220.

   Summary: This chapter on the use of masking in the treatment of tinnitus is from an audiology textbook that offers clinicians and recent graduates information on tinnitus (ringing or other sounds in the ears). In the chapter, the authors provide a summary of the methods needed to perform tinnitus masking effectively, as well as an overview of the experience upon which those methods are based. Topics include a background and history of tinnitus masking, development of wearable masking devices, tinnitus relief from a hearing aid, bedside maskers and other nonwearable devices, initial studies of tinnitus masking, the development of the clinical procedures for masking, importance of tinnitus pitch and loudness measures, the importance of residual inhibition tests, how tinnitus masking differs from conventional masking, the effective clinical use of tinnitus masking, multiple tinnitus sounds, the efficacy of tinnitus masking, specific masking programs in the United States and in England, tinnitus and hyperacusis (over sensitivity to sound), and future directions for tinnitus research and development. One appendix offers sources of masking devices and some ideas for tapes and CDS that can be used for masking. 12 figures. 1 table. 103 references.

- **Tinnitus Habituation Therapy (THT) and Tinnitus Retraining Therapy (TRT)**

Source: in Tyler, R.S., ed. Tinnitus Handbook. San Diego, CA: Singular Publishing Group. 2000. p. 357-376.

Contact: Available from Singular-Thomson Learning. P.O. Box 6904, Florence, KY 41022. (800) 477-3692. Fax (606) 647-5963. Website: www.singpub.com. PRICE: $65.95 plus shipping and handling. ISBN: 1565939220.

Summary: This chapter on the use of Tinnitus Habituation Therapy (THT) and Tinnitus Retraining Therapy (TRT) in the treatment of tinnitus is from an audiology textbook that offers clinicians and recent graduates information on tinnitus (ringing or other sounds in the ears). In the chapter, the authors first provide an outline of the neurophysiological model of tinnitus, a prerequisite for understanding how THT and TRT work. Topics include the functions of the limbic and autonomic nervous systems, the theory of discordant damage (dysfunction), hypersensitivity of the auditory pathways, and hypersensitivity to sound (hyperacusis and phonophobia). The next section explains how the habituation approach works. The author stresses that THT is not a cure for tinnitus; when perceived, the tinnitus will have the same loudness and pitch as before the treatment. However, the habituation of tinnitus is achieved by filtering out and blocking tinnitus related neuronal activity from the conscious brain area responsible for perceiving this activity. The remainder of the chapter describes TRT, including the role of counseling, sound therapy, masking, managing sleep problems, categories of the patients, and the effectiveness of TRT. The author concludes that TRT, the simplest form of THT, seems to be effective for about 80 percent of the general tinnitus population. While it requires about 18 months to achieve a stable level of control of tinnitus, positive results are typically observed within the first six months. 2 figures. 1 table. 41 references.

- **Tinnitus: For Whom the Bell Tolls-and Tolls, and Tolls**

Source: in Rosenfeld, I. Live Now, Age Later: Proven Ways to Slow Down the Clock. New York, NY: Warner Books. 1999. p. 311-321.

Contact: Available from Warner Books. 1271 Avenue of the Americas, New York, NY 10020. (800) 759-0190. E-mail: cust.service@littlebrown.com. Website: www.twbookmark.com. PRICE: $7.99 plus shipping and handling.

Summary: This chapter on tinnitus is from a book that offers practical strategies and healthy living advice for people who want to slow down their own aging process. The book is written in casual language with an emphasis on explaining medical and health issues for the general public. The chapter first defines tinnitus (ringing or other sounds in the ears) and describes how it can occur. The author describes two types of tinnitus, objective tinnitus (someone else can hear the sounds) and subjective tinnitus (only the patient can hear the sounds). Causes of tinnitus can include wax in the ear canal, high blood pressure, prolonged bouts of high blood glucose (sugar), arthritis, neurological processes, emotional stress, drug therapy, food allergies, alcohol use, marijuana, caffeine, nicotine, Meniere's disease, otosclerosis (a bone disease), repeated exposure to loud noise, hypothyroidism (underfunction of the thyroid gland), infections, tooth grinder, and high cholesterol. The author also reviews the treatment options for the tinnitus of aging. The chapter concludes with a brief summary of the points covered, focusing on the ways to reduce the negative impact of tinnitus.

- **Chronic Tinnitus Following Electroconvulsive Therapy**

Source: in Hazell, J., ed. Proceedings of the Sixth International Tinnitus Seminar. London, England: Tinnitus and Hyperacusis Centre. 1999. p. 243-245.

Contact: Available from Tinnitus and Hyperacusis Centre. 32 Devonshire Place, London, W1N 1PE, United Kingdom. Fax 44 + (0) 207 486 2218. E-mail: thc@dr.com. Website: www.tinnitus.org. PRICE: Contact publisher for price. ISBN: 0953695700. Also available on CD-ROM.

Summary: Tinnitus can be caused by almost any pathology involving the auditory system and can also result from head trauma, a variety of medications, and electrical shock, including lightning strikes. This article is from a lengthy document that reprints the proceedings of the Sixth

International Tinnitus Seminar, held in Cambridge, United Kingdom, in September 1999 and hosted by the British Society of Audiology. In this article, the authors report a case study of chronic tinnitus that began immediately following electroconvulsive therapy (ECT). A 43 year old female with a 27 year history of obsessive compulsive disorder and major depression had previously been treated with psychotherapy, antidepressant and antipsychotic medications. Because these treatments were minimally effective and because the frequency and duration of her depressive episodes continued to increase, the patient was scheduled to undergo a series of ECT procedures. The patient received four ECT treatments during one week. Stimulating current was delivered through a unilateral electrode to the right frontotemporal region of the head. EEG seizures occurred during each of the ECT procedures. After the patient recovered from anesthesia, she complained of headaches, muscle pain, amnesia, and, after the fourth ECT, she reported a ringing sound in her right ear. Audiometric testing the day after the fourth ECT revealed a slight increase in threshold for 8000 Hz tones in her right ear. The authors conclude that it is likely that current delivered during the fourth ECT treatment triggered the perception of tinnitus for this patient. The unique organization of this patient's central nervous and auditory systems combined with her particular pharmacological history might have predisposed her to developing this symptom.

- **Approach to the Patient with Tinnitus**

    Source: in Baloh, R.W. Dizziness, Hearing Loss, and Tinnitus. Philadelphia, PA: F.A. Davis Company. 1998. p. 127-136.

    Contact: Available from Oxford University Press, Inc. Business Office, 2001 Evans Road, Cary, NC 27513. (800) 451-7556 or (919) 677-0977. Fax (919) 677-1303. PRICE: $65.00 plus shipping and handling.

    Summary: Tinnitus is a noise in the ear that is usually audible only to the patient, although occasionally the sound can be heard by the examining physician (objective tinnitus). The pathophysiology of tinnitus is largely unknown. This chapter on tinnitus is from a textbook that presents a concise approach to evaluating patients with dizziness, hearing loss, and tinnitus. The author emphasizes that key features in the patient's history can help with an accurate diagnosis of tinnitus. Particularly important is whether the tinnitus is localized to one ear or both ears or is nonlocalizable. The author outlines the causes of tinnitus, including those for objective, subjective, and drug-induced tinnitus; and reviews the workup of common presentations of tinnitus, including unilateral pulsatile tinnitus, chronic unilateral subjective tinnitus, and chronic bilateral subjective tinnitus. Numerous tables and flowcharts guide the reader through the diagnostic workup. Important points are highlighted and presented in the margins of the text. 3 figures. 1 table. 20 references.

Directories

In addition to the references and resources discussed earlier in this chapter, a number of directories relating to tinnitus have been published that consolidate information across various sources. These too might be useful in gaining access to additional guidance on tinnitus. The Combined Health Information Database lists the following, which you may wish to consult in your local medical library:[25]

- **Brain Connections: Your Source Guide to Information on Brain Diseases and Disorders. 5th ed**

    Source: New York, NY: Dana Alliance for Brain Initiatives. 2000. 49 p.

    Contact: Available from Dana Press. Charles A. Dana Foundation, 745 Fifth Avenue, Suite 700, New York, NY 10151. Fax (212) 593-7623. Website: www.dana.org. PRICE: Single copy free.

    Summary: This guide lists organizations that assist people with a brain-related disorder or disease as well as those organizations that assist caregivers and health care providers in these areas. The guide lists more than 275 organizations alphabetically by disease or disorder. Listings of particular relevance to communication disorders include: acoustic neuroma, aphasia, ataxia, attention deficit hyperactivity disorder, autism, deafness and hearing loss, disability and rehabilitation, dizziness, dyslexia, dystonia, head injury, learning disabilities, neurofibromatosis, smell and taste (chemosensory) disorders, spasmodic dysphonia, stuttering, **tinnitus,** Tourette syndrome, and vestibular disorders. Emphasis is placed on organizations that have a national focus, however, many of these groups sponsor local chapters or affiliates and make referrals to local medical professionals and organizations. For each organization listed, the guide notes mailing address, telephone numbers, e-mail and web sites; also provided are symbols which indicate that the organization offers support groups, referrals to doctors, referrals to other

---

[25] You will need to limit your search to "Directories" and tinnitus using the "Detailed Search" option. Go directly to the following hyperlink: **http://chid.nih.gov/detail/detail.html**. To find directories, use the drop boxes at the bottom of the search page where "You may refine your search by". For publication date, select "All Years", select language and the format option "Directory". By making these selections and typing in "tinnitus" (or synonyms) into the "For these words:" box, you will only receive results on directories dealing with tinnitus. You should check back periodically with this database as it is updated every three months.

sources of information, regional chapters, availability of literature, availability of speakers, and volunteer opportunities. The guide also describes the publishing body, the Dana Alliance for Brain Initiatives, and provides a list of ways in which readers can support and further brain research.

- **Self-Help Sourcebook: Finding and Forming Mutual Aid Self-Help Groups. 4th ed**

    Source: Denville, NJ: American Self-Help Clearinghouse. 1992. 226 p.

    Contact: Available from American Self-Help Clearinghouse. Attn: Sourcebook, St. Clares-Riverside Medical Center, 25 Pocono Road, Denville, NJ 07834. Voice (201) 625-7101; TTY (201) 625-9053. PRICE: $9.00 book rate; $10.00 first class mail. ISBN: 0963432206.

    Summary: This sourcebook lists self-help groups in a wide variety of topic areas, including addictions and dependencies, bereavement, disabilities, health, mental health, parenting and family, physical and/or emotional abuse, and miscellaneous categories. Topics relevant to deafness and communication disorders include acoustic neuroma, alternative/augmentative communication, autism, cleft palate and cleft lip, cochlear implants, developmental disabilities, developmentally delayed children, Down syndrome, dystonia, ear anomalies, elective mutism, hearing impairment, inner ear problems, laryngectomy, late-deafened adults, learning disabilities, Meniere's disease, neck-head-oral cancer, parents of children with hearing impairment, speech dysfunction, speech impairments, stuttering, **tinnitus,** Tourette syndrome, and Usher's syndrome. In addition to basic information about the self-help groups, the sourcebook lists self-help clearinghouses, toll-free helplines, resources for rare disorders, resources for genetic disorders, housing and neighborhood resources and resources for the homeless, how-to ideas for developing self-help groups, and using a home computer for mutual help. The book includes a bibliography and key word index.

General Home References

In addition to references for tinnitus, you may want a general home medical guide that spans all aspects of home healthcare. The following list is a recent sample of such guides (sorted alphabetically by title; hyperlinks provide rankings, information, and reviews at Amazon.com):

- **The Encyclopedia of Deafness and Hearing Disorders (Facts on File Library of Health and Living)** by Carol Turkington, Allen E. Sussman;

(Library Binding - December 2000), Facts on File, Inc.; ISBN: 081604046X; http://www.amazon.com/exec/obidos/ASIN/081604046X/icongroupinterna

- **An Introduction to Ear Disease** by Bruce Black, M.D.; Paperback - 90 pages, 1st edition (October 1, 1998), Singular Publishing Group; ISBN: 076930012X; http://www.amazon.com/exec/obidos/ASIN/076930012X/icongroupinterna

- **Living With Hearing Loss: The Sourcebook for Deafness and Hearing Disorders (The Facts for Life Series)** by Carol Turkington, Allen E. Sussman; (Paperback - December 2000), Checkmark Books; ISBN: 0816041407; http://www.amazon.com/exec/obidos/ASIN/0816041407/icongroupinterna

- **When the Brain Can't Hear: Unraveling the Mystery of Auditory Processing Disorder** by Teri James Bellis; Hardcover - 288 pages (February 2002), Pocket Books; ISBN: 0743428633; http://www.amazon.com/exec/obidos/ASIN/0743428633/icongroupinterna

Vocabulary Builder

Aging: A physiological or morphological change in the life of an organism or its parts, generally irreversible and typically associated with a decline in growth and reproductive vigor. [NIH]

Aphasia: An inability, caused by cerebral dysfunction, to communicate in reading, writing or speaking or to receive meaning from spoken or written words. [NIH]

Attenuated: Strain with weakened or reduced virulence. [NIH]

Bruit: An abnormal sound heard over an artery, related to the cardiac cycle but unrelated to the respiratory cycle or to muscle, joint, or swallowing activity. [NIH]

Canonical: A particular nucleotide sequence in which each position represents the base more often found when many actual sequences of a given class of genetic elements are compared. [NIH]

Dysphonia: Difficulty or pain in speaking; impairment of the voice. [NIH]

Gould: Turning of the head downward in walking to bring the image of the ground on the functioning position of the retina, in destructive disease of the peripheral retina. [NIH]

Habituate: Eventual cessation of response to a repeated sound. [NIH]

Neurosyphilis: A late form of syphilis that affects the brain and may lead to dementia and death. [NIH]

Niche: The ultimate unit of the habitat, i. e. the specific spot occupied by an individual organism; by extension, the more or less specialized relationships existing between an organism, individual or synusia(e), and its environment. [NIH]

CHAPTER 7. MULTIMEDIA ON TINNITUS

Overview

Information on tinnitus can come in a variety of formats. Among multimedia sources, video productions, slides, audiotapes, and computer databases are often available. In this chapter, we show you how to keep current on multimedia sources of information on tinnitus. We start with sources that have been summarized by federal agencies, and then show you how to find bibliographic information catalogued by the National Library of Medicine. If you see an interesting item, visit your local medical library to check on the availability of the title.

Video Recordings

Most diseases do not have a video dedicated to them. If they do, they are often rather technical in nature. An excellent source of multimedia information on tinnitus is the Combined Health Information Database. You will need to limit your search to "video recording" and "tinnitus" using the "Detailed Search" option. Go directly to the following hyperlink: **http://chid.nih.gov/detail/detail.html**. To find video productions, use the drop boxes at the bottom of the search page where "You may refine your search by." Select the dates and language you prefer, and the format option "Videorecording (videotape, videocassette, etc.)." By making these selections and typing "tinnitus" (or synonyms) into the "For these words:" box, you will only receive results on video productions. The following is a typical result when searching for video recordings on tinnitus:

- **Living With Tinnitus**

    Source: Timonium, MD: Milner-Fenwick, Inc. 1992. (videocassette).

Contact: Available from Milner-Fenwick, Inc. 2125 Greenspring Drive, Timonium, MD 21093. (800) 432-8433. PRICE: $250.00; discounts available. Order Number OT-15.

Summary: Designed for use in patient education, this videotape provides guidelines for living with tinnitus. The author reassures patients that tinnitus is a common problem shared by millions. Treatable causes are covered, and the association of tinnitus with sensorineural hearing loss is discussed. The author details measures that help reduce the impact of tinnitus, including hearing aids, types of masking, and changes in diet. The beneficial role of support groups and counseling is also addressed. The importance of using hearing protection to prevent the condition from worsening is also emphasized. (AA-M).

- **1996-1997 Marquam Hill Lectures. Tinnitus: Ringing in the Ears**

    Source: Portland, OR: Oregon Health Sciences University. 1996. (videocassette).

    Contact: Available from American Tinnitus Association (ATA). P.O. Box 5, Portland, OR 97207-0005. (800) 634-8978 or (503) 248-9985. Fax (503) 248-0024. E-mail: tinnitus@ata.org. Website: www.ata.org. PRICE: $20.00 for members; $25.00 for nonmembers.

    Summary: This videotape captures a lecture presented by Dr. Jack A. Vernon, an otorhinolaryngologist who specializes in researching and treating tinnitus. Dr. Vernon emphasizes that the information provided to him by patients has been the key to understanding and treating tinnitus. Dr. Vernon begins his talk with a brief description of masking and where the idea for masking came from; he also encourages listeners and patients to join the American Tinnitus Association. He then shows a series of slides, mostly audiograms, from specific patients. He presents their case studies, describes how each case was treated, and how each case furthered his understanding of tinnitus. Topics covered include the role of the patient in controlling when the tinnitus is treated (self-control of masking, for example), residual inhibition, noise-induced tinnitus (the need to be wary of noise exposure in a tinnitus affected ear), hearing loss and tinnitus experienced by dentists exposed to high-pitched noise from dental equipment, the interrelationship of tinnitus and hearing loss, and how to read an audiogram. Dr. Vernon's presentation is one in a series of Marquam Hill Lectures at the Oregon Health Sciences University (OHSU).

CHAPTER 8. PERIODICALS AND NEWS ON TINNITUS

Overview

Keeping up on the news relating to tinnitus can be challenging. Subscribing to targeted periodicals can be an effective way to stay abreast of recent developments on tinnitus. Periodicals include newsletters, magazines, and academic journals.

In this chapter, we suggest a number of news sources and present various periodicals that cover tinnitus beyond and including those which are published by patient associations mentioned earlier. We will first focus on news services, and then on periodicals. News services, press releases, and newsletters generally use more accessible language, so if you do chose to subscribe to one of the more technical periodicals, make sure that it uses language you can easily follow.

News Services and Press Releases

Well before articles show up in newsletters or the popular press, they may appear in the form of a press release or a public relations announcement. One of the simplest ways of tracking press releases on tinnitus is to search the news wires. News wires are used by professional journalists, and have existed since the invention of the telegraph. Today, there are several major "wires" that are used by companies, universities, and other organizations to announce new medical breakthroughs. In the following sample of sources, we will briefly describe how to access each service. These services only post recent news intended for public viewing.

PR Newswire

Perhaps the broadest of the wires is PR Newswire Association, Inc. To access this archive, simply go to **http://www.prnewswire.com**. Below the search box, select the option "The last 30 days." In the search box, type "tinnitus" or synonyms. The search results are shown by order of relevance. When reading these press releases, do not forget that the sponsor of the release may be a company or organization that is trying to sell a particular product or therapy. Their views, therefore, may be biased.

- **Retraining therapy shows promise as treatment for tinnitus**
  Source: Reuters Medical News
  Date: October 18, 2002

- **Pilot study suggests most chronic pain patients have tinnitus**
  Source: Reuters Medical News
  Date: September 26, 2002

- **Hearing Innovations gets FDA nod for tinnitus treatment system**
  Source: Reuters Industry Breifing
  Date: April 16, 2002

- **Patients with tinnitus as a sequela of head and neck injury need special care**
  Source: Reuters Medical News
  Date: May 08, 2001

- **Tinnitus not improved with Ginkgo biloba treatment**
  Source: Reuters Industry Breifing
  Date: January 11, 2001

- **Valproate-induced tinnitus may be mistaken for psychotic symptoms**
  Source: Reuters Medical News
  Date: November 22, 2000

- **Tinnitus relieved by lidocaine perfusion to inner ear plus IV lidocaine**
  Source: Reuters Medical News
  Date: May 19, 2000

- **Acupuncture apparently not an effective treatment for tinnitus**
  Source: Reuters Medical News
  Date: April 26, 2000

- **Studies do not back acupuncture for tinnitus**
  Source: Reuters Health eLine
  Date: April 18, 2000

- **Neuroanatomy Of Tinnitus Discovered**
  Source: Reuters Medical News
  Date: January 22, 1998

- **Brain May Play Role In Tinnitus**
  Source: Reuters Health eLine
  Date: January 22, 1998

The NIH

Within MEDLINEplus, the NIH has made an agreement with the New York Times Syndicate, the AP News Service, and Reuters to deliver news that can be browsed by the public. Search news releases at **http://www.nlm.nih.gov/medlineplus/alphanews_a.html.** MEDLINEplus allows you to browse across an alphabetical index. Or you can search by date at **http://www.nlm.nih.gov/medlineplus/newsbydate.html**. Often, news items are indexed by MEDLINEplus within their search engine.

Business Wire

Business Wire is similar to PR Newswire. To access this archive, simply go to **http://www.businesswire.com**. You can scan the news by industry category or company name.

Market Wire

Market Wire is more focused on technology than the other wires. To browse the latest press releases by topic, such as alternative medicine, biotechnology, fitness, healthcare, legal, nutrition, and pharmaceuticals, log on to Market Wire's Medical/Health channel at the following hyperlink **http://www.marketwire.com/mw/release_index?channel=MedicalHealth**. Market Wire's home page is **http://www.marketwire.com/mw/home**. From here, type "tinnitus" (or synonyms) into the search box, and click on "Search News." As this service is technology oriented, you may wish to use it when searching for press releases covering diagnostic procedures or tests.

Search Engines

Free-to-view news can also be found in the news section of your favorite search engines (see the health news page at Yahoo:

http://dir.yahoo.com/Health/News_and_Media/, or use this Web site's general news search page **http://news.yahoo.com/.** Type in "tinnitus" (or synonyms). If you know the name of a company that is relevant to tinnitus, you can go to any stock trading Web site (such as **www.etrade.com**) and search for the company name there. News items across various news sources are reported on indicated hyperlinks.

BBC

Covering news from a more European perspective, the British Broadcasting Corporation (BBC) allows the public free access to their news archive located at **http://www.bbc.co.uk/**. Search by "tinnitus" (or synonyms).

Newsletters on Tinnitus

Given their focus on current and relevant developments, newsletters are often more useful to patients than academic articles. You can find newsletters using the Combined Health Information Database (CHID). You will need to use the "Detailed Search" option. To access CHID, go directly to the following hyperlink: **http://chid.nih.gov/detail/detail.html**. Your investigation must limit the search to "Newsletter" and "tinnitus." Go to the bottom of the search page where "You may refine your search by." Select the dates and language that you prefer. For the format option, select "Newsletter." By making these selections and typing in "tinnitus" or synonyms into the "For these words:" box, you will only receive results on newsletters. The following list was generated using the options described above:

- **Steady**

    Source: Steady. 6(2): 1-8. Spring 1994.

    Contact: Available from Ear Foundation. 2000 Church Street, Box 111, Nashville, TN 37236. (800) 545-HEAR; (615) 329-7809; TTY (615) 329-7849.

    Summary: The newsletter, STEADY, is a quarterly publication of the Meniere's Network designed to provide patients with Meniere's disease with information and resources. This issue is devoted to diet, particularly sodium intake. This issue has an article on limiting sodium intake while dining out, including at fast food restaurants; nutrient exchange lists for dining out; and an article on smart low-sodium food shopping and cooking. The newsletter also includes letters to the editor; an update on the Meniere's Network members and chapters; and a brief article describing Meniere's disease. A membership form with which readers can also order reprints of earlier issues is included. Earlier issues focused on topics such as vestibular suppressants; a spouse's perspective to living with Meniere's; current research studies; allergies and Meniere's; stress; Meniere's disease in childhood; **tinnitus;** vestibular compensation; and diagnosing Meniere's disease.

- **TMJ News 'n Views: Offering Education, Support and Hope**

    Source: TMJ News 'n Views. Number 9: 1-4. November-December 1993.

    Contact: Available from MyoData-TMJ and Stress Center. P.O. Box 803394, Dallas, TX 75380. (972) 416-7676 (information). PRICE: $20.00 for one-year subscription (6 issues); $35.00 for two-year subscription; back issues $4.00 each.

    Summary: 'TMJ News 'N Views' is a bi-monthly newsletter written specifically for people who suffer from temporomandibular joint disorders (TMD). The 2-color newsletter is written by a person with TMD and is edited by a medical professional. Sections in each issue include: an article by a health professional; an article by Sharon Carr, the founder of the TMJ and Stress Center; a Question and Answer section for patients to write in and receive printed answers; Pain Pointers; and a Recipe Corner with recipes for soft, easy-to-chew food. Specific topics have included surgery for TMD; the use of acupressure for pain; the role of posture; biofeedback; caffeine; **tinnitus** and TMD; whiplash and TMD; new treatment; swallowing disorders; and stress reduction. (AA-M).

Newsletter Articles

If you choose not to subscribe to a newsletter, you can nevertheless find references to newsletter articles. We recommend that you use the Combined Health Information Database, while limiting your search criteria to "newsletter articles." Again, you will need to use the "Detailed Search" option at **http://chid.nih.gov/detail/detail.html**. Go to the bottom of the search page where "You may refine your search by." Select the dates and language that you prefer. For the format option, select "Newsletter Article."

By making these selections, and typing in "tinnitus" (or synonyms) into the "For these words:" box, you will only receive results on newsletter articles. You should check back periodically with this database as it is updated every 3 months. The following is a typical result when searching for newsletter articles on tinnitus:

- **Tinnitus and Vestibular Schwannoma (Acoustic Neuroma)**

Source: Online: RNID Tinnitus Helpline Newsletter. Number 21: 2-6. November 1999.

Contact: Available from Royal National Institute for Deaf People (RNID). RNID Helpline, P.O. Box 16464, London EC1Y8TT, United Kingdom. Fax 0171 296 8199. E-mail: helpline@rnid.org.uk. Website: www.rnid.org.uk.

Summary: This newsletter article discusses tinnitus and vestibular schwannoma (VS, also called an acoustic neuroma), which is a benign tumor arising from the Schwann cells of the nerve sheath of the vestibular nerve. The author discusses the prevalence and natural history of VS; the symptoms, including tinnitus (ringing, buzzing, or other sounds in the ears); the mechanisms by which VS may generate tinnitus; the diagnostic significance of VS; tinnitus that appears after surgery for VS; gaze evoked tinnitus; and the management of tinnitus in vestibular schwannoma. The authors note that while it is important to eliminate VS when seeking the cause of tinnitus, some patients may have problems with the noise of the MRI scanner. The authors conclude that individuals with a VS and in whom tinnitus is distressing can be identified with the Tinnitus Handicap Inventory or similar instrument at both pre and postoperative stages. If such distress is present, then tinnitus management should be considered using modern techniques for reducing tinnitus distress. 1 figure.

CHAPTER 9. PHYSICIAN GUIDELINES AND DATABASES

Overview

Doctors and medical researchers rely on a number of information sources to help patients with their conditions. Many will subscribe to journals or newsletters published by their professional associations or refer to specialized textbooks or clinical guides published for the medical profession. In this chapter, we focus on databases and Internet-based guidelines created or written for this professional audience.

NIH Guidelines

For the more common diseases, The National Institutes of Health publish guidelines that are frequently consulted by physicians. Publications are typically written by one or more of the various NIH Institutes. For physician guidelines, commonly referred to as "clinical" or "professional" guidelines, you can visit the following Institutes:

- Office of the Director (OD); guidelines consolidated across agencies available at **http://www.nih.gov/health/consumer/conkey.htm**

- National Institute of General Medical Sciences (NIGMS); fact sheets available at **http://www.nigms.nih.gov/news/facts/**

- National Library of Medicine (NLM); extensive encyclopedia (A.D.A.M., Inc.) with guidelines:
  http://www.nlm.nih.gov/medlineplus/healthtopics.html

- National Institute on Deafness and Other Communication Disorders (NIDCD); fact sheets and guidelines at
  http://www.nidcd.nih.gov/health/

NIH Databases

In addition to the various Institutes of Health that publish professional guidelines, the NIH has designed a number of databases for professionals.[26] Physician-oriented resources provide a wide variety of information related to the biomedical and health sciences, both past and present. The format of these resources varies. Searchable databases, bibliographic citations, full text articles (when available), archival collections, and images are all available. The following are referenced by the National Library of Medicine:[27]

- **Bioethics:** Access to published literature on the ethical, legal and public policy issues surrounding healthcare and biomedical research. This information is provided in conjunction with the Kennedy Institute of Ethics located at Georgetown University, Washington, D.C.: http://www.nlm.nih.gov/databases/databases_bioethics.html

- **HIV/AIDS Resources:** Describes various links and databases dedicated to HIV/AIDS research: http://www.nlm.nih.gov/pubs/factsheets/aidsinfs.html

- **NLM Online Exhibitions:** Describes "Exhibitions in the History of Medicine": http://www.nlm.nih.gov/exhibition/exhibition.html. Additional resources for historical scholarship in medicine: http://www.nlm.nih.gov/hmd/hmd.html

- **Biotechnology Information:** Access to public databases. The National Center for Biotechnology Information conducts research in computational biology, develops software tools for analyzing genome data, and disseminates biomedical information for the better understanding of molecular processes affecting human health and disease: http://www.ncbi.nlm.nih.gov/

- **Population Information:** The National Library of Medicine provides access to worldwide coverage of population, family planning, and related health issues, including family planning technology and programs, fertility, and population law and policy: http://www.nlm.nih.gov/databases/databases_population.html

- **Cancer Information:** Access to caner-oriented databases: http://www.nlm.nih.gov/databases/databases_cancer.html

---

[26] Remember, for the general public, the National Library of Medicine recommends the databases referenced in MEDLINE*plus* (http://medlineplus.gov/ or http://www.nlm.nih.gov/medlineplus/databases.html).

[27] See http://www.nlm.nih.gov/databases/databases.html.

- **Profiles in Science:** Offering the archival collections of prominent twentieth-century biomedical scientists to the public through modern digital technology: **http://www.profiles.nlm.nih.gov/**

- **Chemical Information:** Provides links to various chemical databases and references: **http://sis.nlm.nih.gov/Chem/ChemMain.html**

- **Clinical Alerts:** Reports the release of findings from the NIH-funded clinical trials where such release could significantly affect morbidity and mortality: **http://www.nlm.nih.gov/databases/alerts/clinical_alerts.html**

- **Space Life Sciences:** Provides links and information to space-based research (including NASA):
http://www.nlm.nih.gov/databases/databases_space.html

- **MEDLINE:** Bibliographic database covering the fields of medicine, nursing, dentistry, veterinary medicine, the healthcare system, and the pre-clinical sciences:
http://www.nlm.nih.gov/databases/databases_medline.html

- **Toxicology and Environmental Health Information (TOXNET):** Databases covering toxicology and environmental health:
http://sis.nlm.nih.gov/Tox/ToxMain.html

- **Visible Human Interface:** Anatomically detailed, three-dimensional representations of normal male and female human bodies:
http://www.nlm.nih.gov/research/visible/visible_human.html

While all of the above references may be of interest to physicians who study and treat tinnitus, the following are particularly noteworthy.

The Combined Health Information Database

A comprehensive source of information on clinical guidelines written for professionals is the Combined Health Information Database. You will need to limit your search to "Brochure/Pamphlet," "Fact Sheet," or "Information Package" and tinnitus using the "Detailed Search" option. Go directly to the following hyperlink: **http://chid.nih.gov/detail/detail.html**. To find associations, use the drop boxes at the bottom of the search page where "You may refine your search by." For the publication date, select "All Years," select your preferred language, and the format option "Fact Sheet." By making these selections and typing "tinnitus" (or synonyms) into the "For these words:" box above, you will only receive results on fact sheets dealing with tinnitus. The following is a sample result:

- **Facts About Concussion and Brain Injury**

    Source: Atlanta, GA: National Center for Injury Prevention and Control. 199x. 18 p.

    Contact: Available from National Center for Injury Prevention and Control. Mailstop F-41, 4770 Buford Highway, Atlanta, GA 30341. (770) 488-4642. Also available from www.cdc.gov/ncipc.tbi. PRICE: Single copy free.

    Summary: A blow or jolt to the head can disrupt the normal function of the brain. Doctors often call this type of brain injury a concussion or closed head injury. This brochure explains what can happen after a concussion, how to get better, and where to go for more information and help when needed. The brochure was written to help people who are treated for less severe brain injuries, either in hospital emergency departments or with brief hospital admission. The brochure reviews the health care provided to people with concussion, the danger signs of concussion in adults and in children, the symptoms of brain injury in adults, children, and in older adults, tips for healing (for adults and for children), and where to get help, including help for families and caregivers. Symptoms of brain injury related to communication disorders can include having trouble remembering things, experiencing slowness in thinking, acting, speaking or reading, having trouble with balance or feeling dizzy, or experiencing a ringing in the ears (tinnitus). The brochure concludes with a list of resources for additional information, including the help line and web site of the Brain Injury Association (BIA).

- **Acoustic Neuroma**

    Source: Atlanta, GA: Acoustic Neuroma Association (ANA). 1997. 20 p.

    Contact: Available from Acoustic Neuroma Association (ANA). 600 Peachtree Parkway, Suite 108, Cumming, GA 30041-8211. (770) 205-8211. Fax (770 www.ANAUSA.org. PRICE: $1.50 plus shipping and handling.

    Summary: Acoustic neuroma is a benign (non-cancerous) tissue growth that arises on the eighth cranial nerve. An acoustic neuroma can be treated by microsurgical removal or radiosurgery, or managed by observation. This booklet was written to provide patients, family members, physicians, and other health care personnel with comprehensive, nontechnical information about acoustic neuroma. The author answers questions about acoustic neuromas, covering the causes of the tumor and its growth pattern, the incidence of acoustic neuroma, symptoms, diagnostic tests used to confirm the tumor, treatment options, postoperative care and complications, and psychological factors. Postoperative complications and issues discussed include surgical recovery, hearing loss, **tinnitus,** facial weakness or paralysis, eye problems, taste disturbance and mouth dryness (or excessive salivation), swallowing and voice problems, balance problems, fatigue, headache, dental care, and protecting the other ear. The booklet includes a glossary of related terms. The booklet concludes with a brief description of the Acoustic Neuroma Association, a patient-organized support and information organization for those who face or have undergone treatment for acoustic neuroma. 4 figures. 11 references.

- **Sound and Music Therapies**

    Source: London, England: Royal National Institute for Deaf People. 1999. 2 p.

    Contact: Available from RNID Helpline. P.O. Box 16464, London EC1Y 8TT, United Kingdom. 0870 60 50 123. Fax 0171 296 8199. E-mail: helpline@rnid.org.uk. Website: www.rnid.org.uk. PRICE: Single copy free.

    Summary: It is claimed that sound and music therapies can help certain ear disorders, including **tinnitus,** by using sound or music stimulation. This fact sheet from the Royal National Institute for Deaf People (RNID, London, England) explores three types of sound and music therapies: audio psycho phonology (APP), auditory integration therapy (AIT), and Samonas sound therapy. APP uses enhanced Mozart and Gregorian chant music played through an Electronic Ear device to help people who have a variety of learning and communication disorders. AIT uses an auditory training device that plays specially selected and filtered music, and was developed to help reduce sound sensitivity in autistic children. Samonas sound therapy uses CDS of specially filtered classical music and the sounds of nature to 'work out' middle ear muscles and to stimulate the auditory system. For each type of therapy, the fact sheet includes the contact information for organizations that offer the therapy or training in that particular method.

- **What You Need to Know About TMJ Disorder**

    Source: Phoenix, AZ: SmartPractice. 199x. [4 p.].

    Contact: Available from SmartPractice. 3400 East McDowell, Phoenix, AZ 85008. (800) 522-0800. Fax (800) 522-8329. Website: www.smartpractice.com. PRICE: $34.00 for 100 brochures, plus shipping and handling.

    Summary: The temporomandibular joints connect the jaw bone to the skull and are located just in front of each ear. Temporomandibular joint (TMJ) disorder is a term used to describe dysfunction of the jaw muscles and joints. This patient education brochure outlines the signs and causes of TMJ disorders, and discusses some of the treatment options available. TMJ disorders can be characterized by pronounced noises associated with movement in the TM joints, pain when the jaw is opened fully, limited range of opening, clenching or grinding of the teeth, facial pain and a sense of facial muscle fatigue, ear pain not related to ear infection, occasional 'locking' when the jaw seems to stick open temporarily, ringing in the ears (tinnitus), and frequent headaches. TMJ disorders can develop from lost or crooked teeth, overbite, teeth that fit together poorly (malocclusion), degenerative arthritis, various head or neck injuries (such as whiplash), and stress causing clenched teeth (bruxism) and muscle spasms. Because other types of pain have been shown to mimic TMJ disorder, a careful and thorough dental and medical evaluation is essential to arrive at an accurate diagnosis. Treatment options can include correction of a malocclusion, a splint to help prevent bruxism, pain management strategies (including medication), relaxation techniques (including counseling), and physical therapy; only in rare cases is surgery required to correct a TMJ disorder. The brochure includes space for personalization by the dental office. The brochure is illustrated with full color graphics and photographs of smiling patients. 5 figures.

- **Neurofibromatosis Type 2: Information for Patients and Families**

Source: New York, NY: National Neurofibromatosis Foundation, Inc. 1994. 17 p.

Contact: Available from National Neurofibromatosis Foundation, Inc. 95 Pine Street, 16th Floor, New York, NY 10005. (800) 323-7938. (212) 344-6633. Fax (212) 747-0004. E-mail: NNFF@nf.org. Website: www.nf.org. PRICE: $1.00 plus shipping and handling.

Summary: This booklet describes neurofibromatosis (NF), a genetically determined disorder that causes tumors (mostly benign) to grow on all types of nerves in the body. The booklet defines NF and its two types (NF1 and NF2), then focuses on NF2, which includes a high risk for developing brain tumors; almost all affected individuals develop tumors on both nerves to the ears (also called the eighth cranial nerve). This nerve has two portions: the acoustic (hearing) nerve and the vestibular (balance) nerve which carries information on balance to the brain. The early symptoms of NF2 include hearing loss, ringing in the ears (tinnitus), and problems with balance. Topics include the epidemiology of NF2, the progress of the disease, complications, diagnostic tests (also used to stage the level of disease), and treatment options. The booklet concludes with some frequently asked questions about neurofibromatosis and a glossary of related terms. The contact information for the National

Neurofibromatosis Foundation (NNFF) is provided (800-323-7938 or www.nf.org).

- **Your Ears and Your Hearing**

    Source: New York, NY: League for the Hard of Hearing. 1996. 32 p.

    Contact: Available from League for the Hard of Hearing. 71 West 23rd Street, New York, NY 10010. Voice (212) 741-7650; TTY (212) 255-1932; Fax (212) 255-4413; E-mail: Postmaster@lhh.org; http://www.lhh.org. PRICE: $5.00 each. Item Number B002.

    Summary: This booklet provides basic information on ear and hearing health care. The first section describes how the ear works, the anatomy of the ear, the middle and inner ear, how hearing begins, three types of hearing loss, testing the organ of hearing, the physiology of balance, testing the organ of balance, and posturography. Three sections then cover diseases of the outer ear (ear wax, cleaning ear wax from the ears, swimmer's ear, and bony growths), the middle ear (fluid in the ear, middle ear infection, and otosclerosis), and the inner ear (acoustic neuroma, Meniere's disease, and tinnitus). Additional topics include airplane travel and the ear, motion sickness, hearing aids, cochlear implants, and noise and noise-induced hearing loss. The booklet is illustrated with full-color graphics of the ear's anatomy and physiology.

- **Altered World: Living with New Deafness**

    Source: Washington, DC: National Deaf Education Network and Clearinghouse, Laurent Clerc National Deaf Education Center. 1998. 52 p.

    Contact: National Deaf Education Network and Clearinghouse. KDES PAS-6, 800 Florida Avenue, NE, Washington, DC 20002-3695. Voice/TTY (800) 526-9105 or (202) 651-5340. Fax (202) 651-5708. E-mail: products.clerccenter@gallaudet.edu. Website: clerccenter.gallaudet.edu. PRICE: $3.00 plus shipping and handling.

    Summary: This booklet provides information for late-deafened people, focusing on the adaptations required for previously hearing people to learn to cope with their hearing loss. The booklet first identifies two crucial aspects to defining this group of people. First, late-deafened people have an acquired hearing loss; for many years they have had normal or nearly normal hearing; and their language, identities, and cultural and educational experiences are those of hearing people. Second, late-deafened people are, in the audiological sense, deaf. That is, even with the best amplification, they cannot continue to use hearing to understand speech. The authors note that this line separating hard of hearing people from deafened people is not clear or objective. People define themselves based on their experience with communication, their comfort with particular coping strategies, and on social and support groups that match their experience and preferences. After this introductory section on definitions, the booklet covers six main areas: crisis, or the diagnostic stage, including the problem of **tinnitus;** communication adaptations; work, including vocational rehabilitation, and laws that protect people with disabilities; accommodations for home and recreation; getting support; and moving on. The booklet concludes with a resources section. 19 references.

- **Discussion of Acoustic Neuromas**

    Source: Los Angeles, CA: House Ear Institute. 1995. 19 p.

    Contact: Available from House Ear Institute. 2100 West Third Street, Fifth Floor, Los Angeles, CA 90057. Voice (800) 552-HEAR; (213) 483-4431; TTY (213) 484-2642; Fax (213) 483-8789. PRICE: $1.00 per booklet. Order Number BR-14.

    Summary: This brochure describes acoustic neuromas, non-malignant fibrous growths originating from the balance or hearing nerve. Written for the person newly diagnosed with an acoustic neuroma, the booklet begins with a description of the anatomy and function of the normal ear, then discusses tumor sizes, surgical approaches (translabyrinthine, middle fossa, and retrosigmoid), partial versus total removal of an acoustic tumor, radiation therapy, and hearing impairment following surgery. A final section outlines the risks and complications of acoustic tumor surgery, including hearing loss, **tinnitus,** taste disturbance and mouth dryness, dizziness and balance disturbance, facial paralysis, eye complications, other nerve weaknesses, postoperative headache, brain complications, postoperative spinal fluid leak, postoperative bleeding and brain swelling, postoperative infection, and transfusion reactions. The booklet provides checklists and boxes to individualize the information provided to a specific patient. The address of the Acoustic Neuroma Association is given. 1 figure.

- **Communication Disorders and HIV: A Guide for Audiologists and Speech-Language Pathologists**

    Source: Rockville, MD: American Speech-Language-Hearing Association (ASHA). 199x. [4 p.].

    Contact: Available from American Speech-Language-Hearing Association (ASHA). Product Sales, 10801 Rockville Pike, Rockville, MD 20852. (888) 498-6699. TTY (301) 897-0157. Website: www.asha.org. PRICE: Single copy free.

Summary: This brochure for audiologists and speech language pathologists summarizes the interplay of HIV infection and communication disorders. The author notes that speech, language, and hearing problems frequently result as HIV attacks the central nervous system, with its manifestations occurring in the head and neck. Communication disorders may also occur as a result of treatment options. In many cases, treatments for people with HIV and AIDS and related opportunistic infections rely heavily on drug combinations that are potentially ototoxic. The brochure lists audiologic disorders, including hearing loss, **tinnitus,** and vertigo; speech language disorders, including aphasia, apraxia, confabulations, dysarthria, dysphagia, confused language, stuttering, and voice disorders; and communication disorders in pediatric AIDS, including elective mutism, hysterical aphonia, and pragmatic language disorder or delay. The brochure concludes with a brief discussion of strategies for treating people with HIV and AIDS, focusing on the professional relationship between client and practitioner, including avoiding prejudice (against lifestyle) and avoiding AIDS-phobia. The author encourages readers to call the ASHA for more information (800-638-8255).

- **Audiology: Position Statements, Practice Guidelines, Definitions, Technical Reports, Relevant Papers, Index**

  Source: Rockville, MD: American Speech-Language-Hearing Association (ASHA). 1995. 426 p.

  Contact: Available from American Speech-Language-Hearing Association (ASHA). Product Sales, 10801 Rockville Pike, Rockville, MD 20852. (888) 498-6699. TTY (301) 897-0157. Website: www.asha.org. PRICE: $75.00 plus shipping and handling. Item Number 0111974.

  Summary: This Desk Reference (Volume 2 of 4) is published by the American Speech-Language-Hearing Association to advance high quality standards and practice for the professions of audiology and speech-language pathology. Volume 2 focuses on audiology. Position Statements are included on acoustics in educational settings, the audiologist's role in occupational hearing conservation, balance system assessment, cochlear implant selection and rehabilitation, infant hearing, cerumen management, and the use of FM-amplification instruments for infants and children. Guidelines are presented on topics including audiologic assessment, management and screening, audiology services in the schools, audiometric symbols, determining threshold level for speech, audiology practice management, fitting and monitoring FM systems, graduate education in amplification, and audiometry. The Reference also includes Technical Reports and Relevant Papers on topics such as acoustic-immittance measures, central auditory processing, aural rehabilitation, cochlear implants, sound measurement, tympanometry, **tinnitus** maskers, and professionalism in audiology. This Volume includes an index to the 4-volume set.

- **Multicenter Comparative Study of Cochlear Implants: Final Reports of the Department of Veterans Affairs Cooperative Studies Program**

    Source: Annals of Otology, Rhinology and Laryngology. 104(4): 1-48. April 1995. Supplement 165, part 2.

    Contact: Available from Annals Publishing Company. 4507 Laclede Avenue, St. Louis, MO 63108.

    Summary: This document presents additional and final reports of the Department of Veterans Affairs Cooperative Studies Program 304: A Prospective Randomized Cooperative Study of Advanced Cochlear Implants. Initiated in January 1987, the study compared the efficacy and safety of the 3M-Vienna single-channel and two multichannel cochlear implants: Ineraid and Nucleus, all of which were chosen for inclusion because published data showed them to be capable of producing open-set speech understanding without lipreading. Criteria for the study were that the patient be age 18 years or older, have bilateral profound sensorineural hearing loss with no benefit from amplification (no open-set speech discrimination), have been postlingually deafened, and be English speaking. This publication includes six reports: surgical results, the influence of processing strategies on cochlear implant performance, predictors of postoperative performance with cochlear implants, performance as a function of time, **tinnitus** in the profoundly hearing impaired and the effects of cochlear implants, and change in the quality of life of adult patients with cochlear implants. The last report includes a copy of the quality of life measurement instruments used. All reports include charts and graphs, as well as relevant references.

- **Meniere Disease**

    Source: New Fairfield, CT: National Organization for Rare Disorders, Inc. (NORD). 1995. 4 p.

    Contact: Available from National Organization for Rare Disorders (NORD). P.O. Box 8923, New Fairfield, CT 6812-8923. (800) 999-6673 or (203) 746-6518. Fax (203) 746-6481. E-mail: orphan@rarediseases.org. Website: www.rarediseases.org. PRICE: $3.75 per copy; add $1.00 for delivery outside of U.S. Item Number 272.

    Summary: This fact sheet from the National Organization for Rare Disorders (NORD) summarizes information on Meniere disease, a disorder characterized by recurrent prostating dizziness (vertigo), possible hearing loss, and ringing sounds (tinnitus). The fact sheet presents a list of synonyms, a general discussion, the symptoms, causes, affected population, related disorders, standard therapies, and investigational therapies for Meniere disease. The fact sheet concludes with a list of resources for more information on Meniere disease. 1 reference.

- **Lipreading: Practical Information**

    Source: London, England: Royal National Institute for Deaf People. 1999. 3 p.

    Contact: Available from RNID Helpline. P.O. Box 16464, London EC1Y 8TT, United Kingdom. 0870 60 50 123. Fax 0171-296 8199. E-mail: helpline@rnid.org.uk. Website: www.rnid.org.uk. PRICE: Single copy free.

    Summary: This fact sheet, from the British Royal National Institute for Deaf People (RNID), gives basic information on speechreading (lipreading) for deaf, deafened, or hard of hearing people. Topics include the indications for speechreading, the use of speechreading in conjunction with a hearing aid, the use of lipspeakers (oral interpreters), how people speechread, and speechreading classes. Going to speechreading classes can boost one's confidence and offer the opportunity to talk to other people with hearing loss. Students can also find out about communication tactics, hearing aids, other equipment that can help, how the ear works and how damage may have occurred, **tinnitus,** and resources for finding more information. One section lists strategies for better speechreading.

- **How to Cope with Meniere's Disease**

    Source: American Family Physician. 55(4): 1193-1194. March 1997.

    Summary: This patient education handout provides information on Meniere's disease, a problem of the inner ear that can result in dizziness, a feeling of fullness in the ear, **tinnitus,** and hearing loss. The handout explains these symptoms, describes a typical Meniere's attack, outlines the diagnostic steps taken to confirm suspicion of Meniere's disease, lists treatment options, and provides recommendations for how to handle a Meniere's attack. The handout concludes with a few suggestions for coping with Meniere's disease, including making lifestyle changes (i.e., limiting or eliminating alcohol, caffeine, and nicotine) and handling the stress related to the disease.

- **Hearing Loss: A Guide to Prevention and Treatment**

    Source: Boston, MA: Harvard Health Publications. 2000. 41 p.

    Contact: Available from Harvard Health Publications. P.O. Box 421073, Palm Coast, FL 32142-1073. Website: www.health.harvard.edu. PRICE: $16.00 plus shipping and handling.

    Summary: This report from the Harvard Medical School offers an overview of the prevention and treatment of hearing loss. The report begins with a review of the anatomy and physiology of hearing, then describes the diagnostic tests that may be used to evaluate hearing. The next section discusses the use of hearing aids, including the new technology, hearing aid dispensing, choosing hearing aid circuitry, deciding between one hearing aid (monaural) or two (binaural), fitting a hearing aid, and adjusting to a hearing aid. Surgical options for hearing loss, including cochlear implants and other surgeries, are also considered. Additional sections cover current research and technology directions, coping with hearing loss, and preventing hearing loss. The booklet concludes with a list of resources (organizations and publications) and a glossary of related terms. Various sidebars include a do it yourself five minute hearing test, a definition of the roles of hearing professionals, a description of **tinnitus** (ringing in the ears), assistive listening devices (besides hearing aids), hearing loss and the law, and noise induced hearing loss. The report is illustrated with black and white photographs. 6 figures. Hearing.

The NLM Gateway[28]

The NLM (National Library of Medicine) Gateway is a Web-based system that lets users search simultaneously in multiple retrieval systems at the U.S. National Library of Medicine (NLM). It allows users of NLM services to initiate searches from one Web interface, providing "one-stop searching" for many of NLM's information resources or databases.[29] One target audience for the Gateway is the Internet user who is new to NLM's online resources and does not know what information is available or how best to search for it. This audience may include physicians and other healthcare providers, researchers, librarians, students, and, increasingly, patients, their families,

---

[28] Adapted from NLM: **http://gateway.nlm.nih.gov/gw/Cmd?Overview.x**.
[29] The NLM Gateway is currently being developed by the Lister Hill National Center for Biomedical Communications (LHNCBC) at the National Library of Medicine (NLM) of the National Institutes of Health (NIH).

and the public.[30] To use the NLM Gateway, simply go to the search site at **http://gateway.nlm.nih.gov/gw/Cmd**. Type "tinnitus" (or synonyms) into the search box and click "Search." The results will be presented in a tabular form, indicating the number of references in each database category.

Results Summary

Category	Items Found
Journal Articles	4708
Books / Periodicals / Audio Visual	101
Consumer Health	25
Meeting Abstracts	3
Other Collections	278
Total	5115

HSTAT[31]

HSTAT is a free, Web-based resource that provides access to full-text documents used in healthcare decision-making.[32] HSTAT's audience includes healthcare providers, health service researchers, policy makers, insurance companies, consumers, and the information professionals who serve these groups. HSTAT provides access to a wide variety of publications, including clinical practice guidelines, quick-reference guides for clinicians, consumer health brochures, evidence reports and technology assessments from the Agency for Healthcare Research and Quality (AHRQ), as well as AHRQ's Put Prevention Into Practice.[33] Simply search by "tinnitus" (or synonyms) at the following Web site: **http://text.nlm.nih.gov**.

---

[30] Other users may find the Gateway useful for an overall search of NLM's information resources. Some searchers may locate what they need immediately, while others will utilize the Gateway as an adjunct tool to other NLM search services such as PubMed® and MEDLINEplus®. The Gateway connects users with multiple NLM retrieval systems while also providing a search interface for its own collections. These collections include various types of information that do not logically belong in PubMed, LOCATORplus, or other established NLM retrieval systems (e.g., meeting announcements and pre-1966 journal citations). The Gateway will provide access to the information found in an increasing number of NLM retrieval systems in several phases.

[31] Adapted from HSTAT: **http://www.nlm.nih.gov/pubs/factsheets/hstat.html**.

[32] The HSTAT URL is **http://hstat.nlm.nih.gov/**.

[33] Other important documents in HSTAT include: the National Institutes of Health (NIH) Consensus Conference Reports and Technology Assessment Reports; the HIV/AIDS Treatment Information Service (ATIS) resource documents; the Substance Abuse and Mental Health Services Administration's Center for Substance Abuse Treatment (SAMHSA/CSAT) Treatment Improvement Protocols (TIP) and Center for Substance Abuse Prevention (SAMHSA/CSAP) Prevention Enhancement Protocols System (PEPS); the Public Health

Coffee Break: Tutorials for Biologists[34]

Some patients may wish to have access to a general healthcare site that takes a scientific view of the news and covers recent breakthroughs in biology that may one day assist physicians in developing treatments. To this end, we recommend "Coffee Break," a collection of short reports on recent biological discoveries. Each report incorporates interactive tutorials that demonstrate how bioinformatics tools are used as a part of the research process. Currently, all Coffee Breaks are written by NCBI staff.[35] Each report is about 400 words and is usually based on a discovery reported in one or more articles from recently published, peer-reviewed literature.[36] This site has new articles every few weeks, so it can be considered an online magazine of sorts, and intended for general background information. You can access Coffee Break at **http://www.ncbi.nlm.nih.gov/Coffeebreak/**.

Service (PHS) Preventive Services Task Force's *Guide to Clinical Preventive Services*; the independent, nonfederal Task Force on Community Services *Guide to Community Preventive Services*; and the Health Technology Advisory Committee (HTAC) of the Minnesota Health Care Commission (MHCC) health technology evaluations.

[34] Adapted from **http://www.ncbi.nlm.nih.gov/Coffeebreak/Archive/FAQ.html**

[35] The figure that accompanies each article is frequently supplied by an expert external to NCBI, in which case the source of the figure is cited. The result is an interactive tutorial that tells a biological story.

[36] After a brief introduction that sets the work described into a broader context, the report focuses on how a molecular understanding can provide explanations of observed biology and lead to therapies for diseases. Each vignette is accompanied by a figure and hypertext links that lead to a series of pages that interactively show how NCBI tools and resources are used in the research process.

Other Commercial Databases

In addition to resources maintained by official agencies, other databases exist that are commercial ventures addressing medical professionals. Here are some examples that may interest you:

- **CliniWeb International:** Index and table of contents to selected clinical information on the Internet; see **http://www.ohsu.edu/cliniweb/**.
- **Medical World Search:** Searches full text from thousands of selected medical sites on the Internet; see **http://www.mwsearch.com/**.

CHAPTER 10. DISSERTATIONS ON TINNITUS

Overview

University researchers are active in studying almost all known diseases. The result of research is often published in the form of Doctoral or Master's dissertations. You should understand, therefore, that applied diagnostic procedures and/or therapies can take many years to develop after the thesis that proposed the new technique or approach was written.

In this chapter, we will give you a bibliography on recent dissertations relating to tinnitus. You can read about these in more detail using the Internet or your local medical library. We will also provide you with information on how to use the Internet to stay current on dissertations.

Dissertations on Tinnitus

ProQuest Digital Dissertations is the largest archive of academic dissertations available. From this archive, we have compiled the following list covering dissertations devoted to tinnitus. You will see that the information provided includes the dissertation's title, its author, and the author's institution. To read more about the following, simply use the Internet address indicated. The following covers recent dissertations dealing with tinnitus:

- **An Investigation of the Prevalence of Tinnitus in College Music Majors and Nonmusic Majors** by Zeigler, Mark Calvin, Phd from The Florida State University, 1997, 244 pages
  http://wwwlib.umi.com/dissertations/fullcit/9735829

- **Psychological Aspects of Tinnitus the Effects of Attentional Focus, Anxiety and Fatigue** by Leader, Leslie G; Phd from The University of British Columbia (canada), 1986
  http://wwwlib.umi.com/dissertations/fullcit/NL36676

Keeping Current

As previously mentioned, an effective way to stay current on dissertations dedicated to tinnitus is to use the database called *ProQuest Digital Dissertations* via the Internet, located at the following Web address: **http://wwwlib.umi.com/dissertations**. The site allows you to freely access the last two years of citations and abstracts. Ask your medical librarian if the library has full and unlimited access to this database. From the library, you should be able to do more complete searches than with the limited 2-year access available to the general public.

Vocabulary Builder

Apraxia: Loss of ability to perform purposeful movements, in the absence of paralysis or sensory disturbance, caused by lesions in the cortex. [NIH]

Discrimination: The act of qualitative and/or quantitative differentiation between two or more stimuli. [NIH]

Splint: A rigid appliance used for the immobilization of a part or for the correction of deformity. [NIH]

PART III. APPENDICES

ABOUT PART III

Part III is a collection of appendices on general medical topics which may be of interest to patients with tinnitus and related conditions.

APPENDIX A. RESEARCHING ALTERNATIVE MEDICINE

Overview

Complementary and alternative medicine (CAM) is one of the most contentious aspects of modern medical practice. You may have heard of these treatments on the radio or on television. Maybe you have seen articles written about these treatments in magazines, newspapers, or books. Perhaps your friends or doctor have mentioned alternatives.

In this chapter, we will begin by giving you a broad perspective on complementary and alternative therapies. Next, we will introduce you to official information sources on CAM relating to tinnitus. Finally, at the conclusion of this chapter, we will provide a list of readings on tinnitus from various authors. We will begin, however, with the National Center for Complementary and Alternative Medicine's (NCCAM) overview of complementary and alternative medicine.

What Is CAM?[37]

Complementary and alternative medicine (CAM) covers a broad range of healing philosophies, approaches, and therapies. Generally, it is defined as those treatments and healthcare practices which are not taught in medical schools, used in hospitals, or reimbursed by medical insurance companies. Many CAM therapies are termed "holistic," which generally means that the healthcare practitioner considers the whole person, including physical, mental, emotional, and spiritual health. Some of these therapies are also known as "preventive," which means that the practitioner educates and

---

[37] Adapted from the NCCAM: **http://nccam.nih.gov/health/whatiscam/#4**.

treats the person to prevent health problems from arising, rather than treating symptoms after problems have occurred.

People use CAM treatments and therapies in a variety of ways. Therapies are used alone (often referred to as alternative), in combination with other alternative therapies, or in addition to conventional treatment (sometimes referred to as complementary). Complementary and alternative medicine, or "integrative medicine," includes a broad range of healing philosophies, approaches, and therapies. Some approaches are consistent with physiological principles of Western medicine, while others constitute healing systems with non-Western origins. While some therapies are far outside the realm of accepted Western medical theory and practice, others are becoming established in mainstream medicine.

Complementary and alternative therapies are used in an effort to prevent illness, reduce stress, prevent or reduce side effects and symptoms, or control or cure disease. Some commonly used methods of complementary or alternative therapy include mind/body control interventions such as visualization and relaxation, manual healing including acupressure and massage, homeopathy, vitamins or herbal products, and acupuncture.

What Are the Domains of Alternative Medicine?[38]

The list of CAM practices changes continually. The reason being is that these new practices and therapies are often proved to be safe and effective, and therefore become generally accepted as "mainstream" healthcare practices. Today, CAM practices may be grouped within five major domains: (1) alternative medical systems, (2) mind-body interventions, (3) biologically-based treatments, (4) manipulative and body-based methods, and (5) energy therapies. The individual systems and treatments comprising these categories are too numerous to list in this sourcebook. Thus, only limited examples are provided within each.

Alternative Medical Systems

Alternative medical systems involve complete systems of theory and practice that have evolved independent of, and often prior to, conventional biomedical approaches. Many are traditional systems of medicine that are

---

[38] Adapted from the NCCAM: **http://nccam.nih.gov/health/whatiscam/#4**.

practiced by individual cultures throughout the world, including a number of venerable Asian approaches.

Traditional oriental medicine emphasizes the balance or disturbances of qi (pronounced chi) or vital energy in health and disease, respectively. Traditional oriental medicine consists of a group of techniques and methods including acupuncture, herbal medicine, oriental massage, and qi gong (a form of energy therapy). Acupuncture involves stimulating specific anatomic points in the body for therapeutic purposes, usually by puncturing the skin with a thin needle.

Ayurveda is India's traditional system of medicine. Ayurvedic medicine (meaning "science of life") is a comprehensive system of medicine that places equal emphasis on body, mind, and spirit. Ayurveda strives to restore the innate harmony of the individual. Some of the primary Ayurvedic treatments include diet, exercise, meditation, herbs, massage, exposure to sunlight, and controlled breathing.

Other traditional healing systems have been developed by the world's indigenous populations. These populations include Native American, Aboriginal, African, Middle Eastern, Tibetan, and Central and South American cultures. Homeopathy and naturopathy are also examples of complete alternative medicine systems.

Homeopathic medicine is an unconventional Western system that is based on the principle that "like cures like," i.e., that the same substance that in large doses produces the symptoms of an illness, in very minute doses cures it. Homeopathic health practitioners believe that the more dilute the remedy, the greater its potency. Therefore, they use small doses of specially prepared plant extracts and minerals to stimulate the body's defense mechanisms and healing processes in order to treat illness.

Naturopathic medicine is based on the theory that disease is a manifestation of alterations in the processes by which the body naturally heals itself and emphasizes health restoration rather than disease treatment. Naturopathic physicians employ an array of healing practices, including the following: diet and clinical nutrition, homeopathy, acupuncture, herbal medicine, hydrotherapy (the use of water in a range of temperatures and methods of applications), spinal and soft-tissue manipulation, physical therapies (such as those involving electrical currents, ultrasound, and light), therapeutic counseling, and pharmacology.

Mind-Body Interventions

Mind-body interventions employ a variety of techniques designed to facilitate the mind's capacity to affect bodily function and symptoms. Only a select group of mind-body interventions having well-documented theoretical foundations are considered CAM. For example, patient education and cognitive-behavioral approaches are now considered "mainstream." On the other hand, complementary and alternative medicine includes meditation, certain uses of hypnosis, dance, music, and art therapy, as well as prayer and mental healing.

Biological-Based Therapies

This category of CAM includes natural and biological-based practices, interventions, and products, many of which overlap with conventional medicine's use of dietary supplements. This category includes herbal, special dietary, orthomolecular, and individual biological therapies.

Herbal therapy employs an individual herb or a mixture of herbs for healing purposes. An herb is a plant or plant part that produces and contains chemical substances that act upon the body. Special diet therapies, such as those proposed by Drs. Atkins, Ornish, Pritikin, and Weil, are believed to prevent and/or control illness as well as promote health. Orthomolecular therapies aim to treat disease with varying concentrations of chemicals such as magnesium, melatonin, and mega-doses of vitamins. Biological therapies include, for example, the use of laetrile and shark cartilage to treat cancer and the use of bee pollen to treat autoimmune and inflammatory diseases.

Manipulative and Body-Based Methods

This category includes methods that are based on manipulation and/or movement of the body. For example, chiropractors focus on the relationship between structure and function, primarily pertaining to the spine, and how that relationship affects the preservation and restoration of health. Chiropractors use manipulative therapy as an integral treatment tool.

In contrast, osteopaths place particular emphasis on the musculoskeletal system and practice osteopathic manipulation. Osteopaths believe that all of the body's systems work together and that disturbances in one system may have an impact upon function elsewhere in the body. Massage therapists manipulate the soft tissues of the body to normalize those tissues.

Energy Therapies

Energy therapies focus on energy fields originating within the body (biofields) or those from other sources (electromagnetic fields). Biofield therapies are intended to affect energy fields (the existence of which is not yet experimentally proven) that surround and penetrate the human body. Some forms of energy therapy manipulate biofields by applying pressure and/or manipulating the body by placing the hands in or through these fields. Examples include Qi gong, Reiki and Therapeutic Touch.

Qi gong is a component of traditional oriental medicine that combines movement, meditation, and regulation of breathing to enhance the flow of vital energy (qi) in the body, improve blood circulation, and enhance immune function. Reiki, the Japanese word representing Universal Life Energy, is based on the belief that, by channeling spiritual energy through the practitioner, the spirit is healed and, in turn, heals the physical body. Therapeutic Touch is derived from the ancient technique of "laying-on of hands." It is based on the premises that the therapist's healing force affects the patient's recovery and that healing is promoted when the body's energies are in balance. By passing their hands over the patient, these healers identify energy imbalances.

Bioelectromagnetic-based therapies involve the unconventional use of electromagnetic fields to treat illnesses or manage pain. These therapies are often used to treat asthma, cancer, and migraine headaches. Types of electromagnetic fields which are manipulated in these therapies include pulsed fields, magnetic fields, and alternating current or direct current fields.

Can Alternatives Affect My Treatment?

A critical issue in pursuing complementary alternatives mentioned thus far is the risk that these might have undesirable interactions with your medical treatment. It becomes all the more important to speak with your doctor who can offer advice on the use of alternatives. Official sources confirm this view. Though written for women, we find that the National Women's Health Information Center's advice on pursuing alternative medicine is appropriate for patients of both genders and all ages.[39]

---

[39] Adapted from **http://www.4woman.gov/faq/alternative.htm**.

Is It Okay to Want Both Traditional and Alternative or Complementary Medicine?

Should you wish to explore non-traditional types of treatment, be sure to discuss all issues concerning treatments and therapies with your healthcare provider, whether a physician or practitioner of complementary and alternative medicine. Competent healthcare management requires knowledge of both conventional and alternative therapies you are taking for the practitioner to have a complete picture of your treatment plan.

The decision to use complementary and alternative treatments is an important one. Consider before selecting an alternative therapy, the safety and effectiveness of the therapy or treatment, the expertise and qualifications of the healthcare practitioner, and the quality of delivery. These topics should be considered when selecting any practitioner or therapy.

National Center for Complementary and Alternative Medicine

The National Center for Complementary and Alternative Medicine (NCCAM) of the National Institutes of Health (http://nccam.nih.gov) has created a link to the National Library of Medicine's databases to allow patients to search for articles that specifically relate to tinnitus and complementary medicine. To search the database, go to **www.nlm.nih.gov/nccam/camonpubmed.html**. Select "CAM on PubMed." Enter "tinnitus" (or synonyms) into the search box. Click "Go." The following references provide information on particular aspects of complementary and alternative medicine (CAM) that are related to tinnitus:

- **A behavioral paradigm to judge acute sodium salicylate-induced sound experience in rats: a new approach for an animal model on tinnitus.**
  Author(s): Ruttiger L, Ciuffani J, Zenner HP, Knipper M.
  Source: Hearing Research. 2003 June; 180(1-2): 39-50.
  http://www.ncbi.nlm.nih.gov:80/entrez/query.fcgi?cmd=Retrieve&db=PubMed&list_uids=12782351&dopt=Abstract

- **A comparison of reaction times to tinnitus and nontinnitus frequencies.**
  Author(s): Goodwin PE, Johnson RM.
  Source: Ear and Hearing. 1980 May-June; 1(3): 148-55.
  http://www.ncbi.nlm.nih.gov:80/entrez/query.fcgi?cmd=Retrieve&db=PubMed&list_uids=7390072&dopt=Abstract

- **A consideration of the effect of ear canal resonance and hearing loss upon white noise generators for tinnitus retraining therapy.**
  Author(s): Baguley DM, Beynon GJ, Thornton F.
  Source: The Journal of Laryngology and Otology. 1997 September; 111(9): 810-3.
  http://www.ncbi.nlm.nih.gov:80/entrez/query.fcgi?cmd=Retrieve&db=PubMed&list_uids=9373544&dopt=Abstract

- **A controlled trial of acupuncture in tinnitus.**
  Author(s): Marks NJ, Emery P, Onisiphorou C.
  Source: The Journal of Laryngology and Otology. 1984 November; 98(11): 1103-9.
  http://www.ncbi.nlm.nih.gov:80/entrez/query.fcgi?cmd=Retrieve&db=PubMed&list_uids=6387018&dopt=Abstract

- **A controlled trial of hypnotherapy in tinnitus.**
  Author(s): Marks NJ, Karl H, Onisiphorou C.
  Source: Clinical Otolaryngology and Allied Sciences. 1985 February; 10(1): 43-6.
  http://www.ncbi.nlm.nih.gov:80/entrez/query.fcgi?cmd=Retrieve&db=PubMed&list_uids=3891159&dopt=Abstract

- **A meta-analytic review of psychological treatments for tinnitus.**
  Author(s): Andersson G, Lyttkens L.
  Source: British Journal of Audiology. 1999 August; 33(4): 201-10.
  http://www.ncbi.nlm.nih.gov:80/entrez/query.fcgi?cmd=Retrieve&db=PubMed&list_uids=10509855&dopt=Abstract

- **A multiple-baseline evaluation of the treatment of subjective tinnitus with relaxation training and biofeedback.**
  Author(s): Kirsch CA, Blanchard EB, Parnes SM.
  Source: Biofeedback Self Regul. 1987 December; 12(4): 295-312.
  http://www.ncbi.nlm.nih.gov:80/entrez/query.fcgi?cmd=Retrieve&db=PubMed&list_uids=3331298&dopt=Abstract

- **A new method of managing subjective tinnitus.**
  Author(s): Pang LQ, Pang MK, Takumi MM.
  Source: Hawaii Med J. 1979 August; 38(8): 235-9. No Abstract Available.
  http://www.ncbi.nlm.nih.gov:80/entrez/query.fcgi?cmd=Retrieve&db=PubMed&list_uids=511527&dopt=Abstract

- **A practical approach to the treatment of subjective tinnitus.**
  Author(s): Michel RG, Drawbaugh EJ, Pope TH.
  Source: Eye Ear Nose Throat Mon. 1976 March; 55(3): 96-8. No Abstract Available.
  http://www.ncbi.nlm.nih.gov:80/entrez/query.fcgi?cmd=Retrieve&db=PubMed&list_uids=1248612&dopt=Abstract

- **A review of evidence in support of a role for 5-HT in the perception of tinnitus.**
  Author(s): Simpson JJ, Davies WE.
  Source: Hearing Research. 2000 July; 145(1-2): 1-7. Review.
  http://www.ncbi.nlm.nih.gov:80/entrez/query.fcgi?cmd=Retrieve&db=PubMed&list_uids=10867271&dopt=Abstract

- **A review of randomized clinical trials in tinnitus.**
  Author(s): Dobie RA.
  Source: The Laryngoscope. 1999 August; 109(8): 1202-11. Review.
  http://www.ncbi.nlm.nih.gov:80/entrez/query.fcgi?cmd=Retrieve&db=PubMed&list_uids=10443820&dopt=Abstract

- **A tinnitus synthesizer physiological considerations.**
  Author(s): Hazell JW.
  Source: J Laryngol Otol Suppl. 1981; (4): 187-95. No Abstract Available.
  http://www.ncbi.nlm.nih.gov:80/entrez/query.fcgi?cmd=Retrieve&db=PubMed&list_uids=6946166&dopt=Abstract

- **A trial of tinnitus therapy with ear-canal magnets.**
  Author(s): Coles R, Bradley P, Donaldson I, Dingle A.
  Source: Clinical Otolaryngology and Allied Sciences. 1991 August; 16(4): 371-2.
  http://www.ncbi.nlm.nih.gov:80/entrez/query.fcgi?cmd=Retrieve&db=PubMed&list_uids=1934552&dopt=Abstract

- **Acoustic correlates of tonal tinnitus.**
  Author(s): Wilson JP, Sutton GJ.
  Source: Ciba Found Symp. 1981; 85: 82-107. Review.
  http://www.ncbi.nlm.nih.gov:80/entrez/query.fcgi?cmd=Retrieve&db=PubMed&list_uids=7035101&dopt=Abstract

- **Acupuncture for the alleviation of tinnitus.**
  Author(s): Thomas M, Laurell G, Lundeberg T.

Source: The Laryngoscope. 1988 June; 98(6 Pt 1): 664-7.
http://www.ncbi.nlm.nih.gov:80/entrez/query.fcgi?cmd=Retrieve&db=PubMed&list_uids=3374243&dopt=Abstract

- **Acupuncture for tinnitus management.**
  Author(s): Nilsson S, Axelsson A, Li De G.
  Source: Scandinavian Audiology. 1992; 21(4): 245-51.
  http://www.ncbi.nlm.nih.gov:80/entrez/query.fcgi?cmd=Retrieve&db=PubMed&list_uids=1488611&dopt=Abstract

- **Acupuncture for tinnitus: time to stop?**
  Author(s): Andersson G, Lyttkens L.
  Source: Scandinavian Audiology. 1996; 25(4): 273-5. Review.
  http://www.ncbi.nlm.nih.gov:80/entrez/query.fcgi?cmd=Retrieve&db=PubMed&list_uids=8976001&dopt=Abstract

- **Acupuncture in the management of tinnitus: a placebo-controlled study.**
  Author(s): Axelsson A, Andersson S, Gu LD.
  Source: Audiology : Official Organ of the International Society of Audiology. 1994 November-December; 33(6): 351-60.
  http://www.ncbi.nlm.nih.gov:80/entrez/query.fcgi?cmd=Retrieve&db=PubMed&list_uids=7741667&dopt=Abstract

- **Acupuncture treatment of chronic unilateral tinnitus--a double-blind cross-over trial.**
  Author(s): Hansen PE, Hansen JH, Bentzen O.
  Source: Clinical Otolaryngology and Allied Sciences. 1982 October; 7(5): 325-9.
  http://www.ncbi.nlm.nih.gov:80/entrez/query.fcgi?cmd=Retrieve&db=PubMed&list_uids=6756709&dopt=Abstract

- **Alterations in average spectrum of cochleoneural activity by long-term salicylate treatment in the guinea pig: a plausible index of tinnitus.**
  Author(s): Cazals Y, Horner KC, Huang ZW.
  Source: Journal of Neurophysiology. 1998 October; 80(4): 2113-20.
  http://www.ncbi.nlm.nih.gov:80/entrez/query.fcgi?cmd=Retrieve&db=PubMed&list_uids=9772265&dopt=Abstract

- **Alternative medications and other treatments for tinnitus: facts from fiction.**
  Author(s): Seidman MD, Babu S.

Source: Otolaryngologic Clinics of North America. 2003 April; 36(2): 359-81. Review.
http://www.ncbi.nlm.nih.gov:80/entrez/query.fcgi?cmd=Retrieve&db=PubMed&list_uids=12856304&dopt=Abstract

- **An alternative method of treating tinnitus: relaxation-hypnotherapy primarily through the home use of a recorded audio cassette.**
  Author(s): Brattberg G.
  Source: Int J Clin Exp Hypn. 1983 April; 31(2): 90-7. No Abstract Available.
  http://www.ncbi.nlm.nih.gov:80/entrez/query.fcgi?cmd=Retrieve&db=PubMed&list_uids=6339424&dopt=Abstract

- **An approach to the audit of tinnitus management.**
  Author(s): Sadlier M, Stephens SD.
  Source: The Journal of Laryngology and Otology. 1995 September; 109(9): 826-9.
  http://www.ncbi.nlm.nih.gov:80/entrez/query.fcgi?cmd=Retrieve&db=PubMed&list_uids=7494113&dopt=Abstract

- **An auditory negative after-image as a human model of tinnitus.**
  Author(s): Norena A, Micheyl C, Chery-Croze S.
  Source: Hearing Research. 2000 November; 149(1-2): 24-32.
  http://www.ncbi.nlm.nih.gov:80/entrez/query.fcgi?cmd=Retrieve&db=PubMed&list_uids=11033244&dopt=Abstract

- **An evaluation of relaxation training in the treatment of tinnitus.**
  Author(s): Ireland CE, Wilson PH, Tonkin JP, Platt-Hepworth S.
  Source: Behaviour Research and Therapy. 1985; 23(4): 423-30.
  http://www.ncbi.nlm.nih.gov:80/entrez/query.fcgi?cmd=Retrieve&db=PubMed&list_uids=3896227&dopt=Abstract

- **An experimental evaluation of the effects of transcutaneous nerve stimulation (TNS) and applied relaxation (AR) on hearing ability, tinnitus and dizziness in patients with Meniere's disease.**
  Author(s): Scott B, Larsen HC, Lyttkens L, Melin L.
  Source: British Journal of Audiology. 1994 June; 28(3): 131-40.
  http://www.ncbi.nlm.nih.gov:80/entrez/query.fcgi?cmd=Retrieve&db=PubMed&list_uids=7841897&dopt=Abstract

- **An investigation of the effect of structured teaching on a group of tinnitus patients after vestibular schwannoma removal.**
  Author(s): Baguley DM, Beynon GJ, Moffat DA.
  Source: The American Journal of Otology. 1998 November; 19(6): 828-33.
  http://www.ncbi.nlm.nih.gov:80/entrez/query.fcgi?cmd=Retrieve&db=PubMed&list_uids=9831163&dopt=Abstract

- **Animal models of tinnitus.**
  Author(s): Evans EF, Wilson JP, Borerwe TA.
  Source: Ciba Found Symp. 1981; 85: 108-38. Review.
  http://www.ncbi.nlm.nih.gov:80/entrez/query.fcgi?cmd=Retrieve&db=PubMed&list_uids=7035097&dopt=Abstract

- **Are there any studies showing whether ginkgo biloba is effective for tinnitus (ringing in the ears)?**
  Author(s): Feinberg AW.
  Source: Health News. 2003 January; 9(1): 12. No Abstract Available.
  http://www.ncbi.nlm.nih.gov:80/entrez/query.fcgi?cmd=Retrieve&db=PubMed&list_uids=12545957&dopt=Abstract

- **Assessment and treatment of tinnitus patients using a "masking approach.".**
  Author(s): Schechter MA, Henry JA.
  Source: Journal of the American Academy of Audiology. 2002 November-December; 13(10): 545-58.
  http://www.ncbi.nlm.nih.gov:80/entrez/query.fcgi?cmd=Retrieve&db=PubMed&list_uids=12503923&dopt=Abstract

- **Attempts to suppress tinnitus with transcutaneous electrical stimulation.**
  Author(s): Vernon JA, Fenwick JA.
  Source: Otolaryngology and Head and Neck Surgery. 1985 June; 93(3): 385-9.
  http://www.ncbi.nlm.nih.gov:80/entrez/query.fcgi?cmd=Retrieve&db=PubMed&list_uids=3927235&dopt=Abstract

- **Attenuation of salicylate-induced tinnitus by Ginkgo biloba extract in rats.**
  Author(s): Jastreboff PJ, Zhou S, Jastreboff MM, Kwapisz U, Gryczynska U.

Source: Audiology & Neuro-Otology. 1997 July-August; 2(4): 197-212.
http://www.ncbi.nlm.nih.gov:80/entrez/query.fcgi?cmd=Retrieve&db=PubMed&list_uids=9390833&dopt=Abstract

- **Audiological and psychological characteristics of a group of tinnitus sufferers, prior to tinnitus management training.**
  Author(s): Dineen R, Doyle J, Bench J.
  Source: British Journal of Audiology. 1997 February; 31(1): 27-38.
  http://www.ncbi.nlm.nih.gov:80/entrez/query.fcgi?cmd=Retrieve&db=PubMed&list_uids=9056041&dopt=Abstract

- **Auditory cortical basis of tinnitus.**
  Author(s): Hoke M, Pantev C, Lutkenhoner B, Lehnertz K.
  Source: Acta Otolaryngol Suppl. 1991; 491: 176-81; Discussion 182.
  http://www.ncbi.nlm.nih.gov:80/entrez/query.fcgi?cmd=Retrieve&db=PubMed&list_uids=1814151&dopt=Abstract

- **Auditory event related potentials in chronic tinnitus patients with noise induced hearing loss.**
  Author(s): Attias J, Urbach D, Gold S, Shemesh Z.
  Source: Hearing Research. 1993 December; 71(1-2): 106-13.
  http://www.ncbi.nlm.nih.gov:80/entrez/query.fcgi?cmd=Retrieve&db=PubMed&list_uids=8113129&dopt=Abstract

- **Auditory event related potentials in simulated tinnitus.**
  Author(s): Attias J, Bresloff I, Furman V, Urbach D.
  Source: J Basic Clin Physiol Pharmacol. 1995; 6(2): 173-83.
  http://www.ncbi.nlm.nih.gov:80/entrez/query.fcgi?cmd=Retrieve&db=PubMed&list_uids=8573561&dopt=Abstract

- **Auditory evoked responses in control subjects and in patients with problem-tinnitus.**
  Author(s): Gerken GM, Hesse PS, Wiorkowski JJ.
  Source: Hearing Research. 2001 July; 157(1-2): 52-64.
  http://www.ncbi.nlm.nih.gov:80/entrez/query.fcgi?cmd=Retrieve&db=PubMed&list_uids=11470185&dopt=Abstract

- **Behavioral model of chronic tinnitus in rats.**
  Author(s): Bauer CA, Brozoski TJ, Rojas R, Boley J, Wyder M.

Source: Otolaryngology and Head and Neck Surgery. 1999 October; 121(4): 457-62.
http://www.ncbi.nlm.nih.gov:80/entrez/query.fcgi?cmd=Retrieve&db=PubMed&list_uids=10504604&dopt=Abstract

- **Biofeedback therapy in the treatment of tinnitus.**
  Author(s): Ogata Y, Sekitani T, Moriya K, Watanabe K.
  Source: Auris, Nasus, Larynx. 1993; 20(2): 95-101.
  http://www.ncbi.nlm.nih.gov:80/entrez/query.fcgi?cmd=Retrieve&db=PubMed&list_uids=8216052&dopt=Abstract

- **Brain imaging of the effects of lidocaine on tinnitus.**
  Author(s): Reyes SA, Salvi RJ, Burkard RF, Coad ML, Wack DS, Galantowicz PJ, Lockwood AH.
  Source: Hearing Research. 2002 September; 171(1-2): 43-50.
  http://www.ncbi.nlm.nih.gov:80/entrez/query.fcgi?cmd=Retrieve&db=PubMed&list_uids=12204348&dopt=Abstract

- **Celebrating a decade of evaluation and treatment: the University of Maryland Tinnitus & Hyperacusis Center.**
  Author(s): Gold SL, Formby C, Gray WC.
  Source: American Journal of Audiology. 2000 December; 9(2): 69-74.
  http://www.ncbi.nlm.nih.gov:80/entrez/query.fcgi?cmd=Retrieve&db=PubMed&list_uids=11200194&dopt=Abstract

- **Central tinnitus and lateral inhibition: an auditory brainstem model.**
  Author(s): Gerken GM.
  Source: Hearing Research. 1996 August; 97(1-2): 75-83. Review.
  http://www.ncbi.nlm.nih.gov:80/entrez/query.fcgi?cmd=Retrieve&db=PubMed&list_uids=8844188&dopt=Abstract

- **Characteristics of patients with gaze-evoked tinnitus.**
  Author(s): Coad ML, Lockwood A, Salvi R, Burkard R.
  Source: Otology & Neurotology : Official Publication of the American Otological Society, American Neurotology Society [and] European Academy of Otology and Neurotology. 2001 September; 22(5): 650-4.
  http://www.ncbi.nlm.nih.gov:80/entrez/query.fcgi?cmd=Retrieve&db=PubMed&list_uids=11568674&dopt=Abstract

- **Children's experience of tinnitus: a preliminary survey of children presenting to a psychology department.**
  Author(s): Kentish RC, Crocker SR, McKenna L.

Source: British Journal of Audiology. 2000 December; 34(6): 335-40.
http://www.ncbi.nlm.nih.gov:80/entrez/query.fcgi?cmd=Retrieve&db=PubMed&list_uids=11201320&dopt=Abstract

- **Client centred hypnotherapy in the management of tinnitus--is it better than counselling?**
  Author(s): Mason JD, Rogerson DR, Butler JD.
  Source: The Journal of Laryngology and Otology. 1996 February; 110(2): 117-20.
  http://www.ncbi.nlm.nih.gov:80/entrez/query.fcgi?cmd=Retrieve&db=PubMed&list_uids=8729491&dopt=Abstract

- **Client-centered hypnotherapy for tinnitus: who is likely to benefit?**
  Author(s): Mason J, Rogerson D.
  Source: Am J Clin Hypn. 1995 April; 37(4): 294-9.
  http://www.ncbi.nlm.nih.gov:80/entrez/query.fcgi?cmd=Retrieve&db=PubMed&list_uids=7741085&dopt=Abstract

- **Comparison between self-hypnosis, masking and attentiveness for alleviation of chronic tinnitus.**
  Author(s): Attias J, Shemesh Z, Sohmer H, Gold S, Shoham C, Faraggi D.
  Source: Audiology : Official Organ of the International Society of Audiology. 1993 May-June; 32(3): 205-12.
  http://www.ncbi.nlm.nih.gov:80/entrez/query.fcgi?cmd=Retrieve&db=PubMed&list_uids=8489481&dopt=Abstract

- **Comparison of pulsed and continuous tone thresholds in patients with tinnitus.**
  Author(s): Hochberg I, Waltzman S.
  Source: Audiology : Official Organ of the International Society of Audiology. 1972 September-December; 11(5): 337-42.
  http://www.ncbi.nlm.nih.gov:80/entrez/query.fcgi?cmd=Retrieve&db=PubMed&list_uids=4671203&dopt=Abstract

- **Comparison of tinnitus masking and tinnitus retraining therapy.**
  Author(s): Henry JA, Schechter MA, Nagler SM, Fausti SA.
  Source: Journal of the American Academy of Audiology. 2002 November-December; 13(10): 559-81.
  http://www.ncbi.nlm.nih.gov:80/entrez/query.fcgi?cmd=Retrieve&db=PubMed&list_uids=12503924&dopt=Abstract

- **Comprehensive behavioral management of complex tinnitus: a case illustration.**
  Author(s): Duckro PN, Pollard CA, Bray HD, Scheiter L.
  Source: Biofeedback Self Regul. 1984 December; 9(4): 459-69.
  http://www.ncbi.nlm.nih.gov:80/entrez/query.fcgi?cmd=Retrieve&db=PubMed&list_uids=6399462&dopt=Abstract

- **Contralateral suppression of transient evoked otoacoustic emissions: intra-individual variability in tinnitus and normal subjects.**
  Author(s): Graham RL, Hazell JW.
  Source: British Journal of Audiology. 1994 August-October; 28(4-5): 235-45.
  http://www.ncbi.nlm.nih.gov:80/entrez/query.fcgi?cmd=Retrieve&db=PubMed&list_uids=7735152&dopt=Abstract

- **Contralateral suppression of transiently evoked otoacoustic emissions and tinnitus.**
  Author(s): Chery-Croze S, Truy E, Morgon A.
  Source: British Journal of Audiology. 1994 August-October; 28(4-5): 255-66.
  http://www.ncbi.nlm.nih.gov:80/entrez/query.fcgi?cmd=Retrieve&db=PubMed&list_uids=7735154&dopt=Abstract

- **Covariation of tinnitus pitch and the associated emission: a case study.**
  Author(s): Penner MJ, Glotzbach L.
  Source: Otolaryngology and Head and Neck Surgery. 1994 March; 110(3): 304-9.
  http://www.ncbi.nlm.nih.gov:80/entrez/query.fcgi?cmd=Retrieve&db=PubMed&list_uids=8134142&dopt=Abstract

- **Current concepts in the clinical management of patients with tinnitus.**
  Author(s): Parnes SM.
  Source: European Archives of Oto-Rhino-Laryngology : Official Journal of the European Federation of Oto-Rhino-Laryngological Societies (Eufos) : Affiliated with the German Society for Oto-Rhino-Laryngology - Head and Neck Surgery. 1997; 254(9-10): 406-9. Review.
  http://www.ncbi.nlm.nih.gov:80/entrez/query.fcgi?cmd=Retrieve&db=PubMed&list_uids=9438106&dopt=Abstract

- **Descending auditory system/cerebellum/tinnitus.**
  Author(s): Shulman A, Strashun A.

Source: Int Tinnitus J. 1999; 5(2): 92-106. Review.
http://www.ncbi.nlm.nih.gov:80/entrez/query.fcgi?cmd=Retrieve&db=PubMed&list_uids=10753427&dopt=Abstract

- **Diagnostic approach to tinnitus.**
  Author(s): Crummer RW, Hassan GA.
  Source: American Family Physician. 2004 January 1; 69(1): 120-6. Review.
  http://www.ncbi.nlm.nih.gov:80/entrez/query.fcgi?cmd=Retrieve&db=PubMed&list_uids=14727828&dopt=Abstract

- **Different treatment modalities of tinnitus at the EuromedClinic.**
  Author(s): Gul H, Nowak R, Buchner FA, Nagel D, Haid CT.
  Source: Int Tinnitus J. 2000; 6(1): 50-3.
  http://www.ncbi.nlm.nih.gov:80/entrez/query.fcgi?cmd=Retrieve&db=PubMed&list_uids=14689618&dopt=Abstract

- **Double-blind study on the effectiveness of a bioflavonoid in the control of tinnitus in otosclerosis.**
  Author(s): Sziklai I, Komora V, Ribari O.
  Source: Acta Chir Hung. 1992-93; 33(1-2): 101-7.
  http://www.ncbi.nlm.nih.gov:80/entrez/query.fcgi?cmd=Retrieve&db=PubMed&list_uids=1343452&dopt=Abstract

- **Effect of hyperbaric oxygen therapy in comparison to conventional or placebo therapy or no treatment in idiopathic sudden hearing loss, acoustic trauma, noise-induced hearing loss and tinnitus. A literature survey.**
  Author(s): Lamm K, Lamm H, Arnold W.
  Source: Advances in Oto-Rhino-Laryngology. 1998; 54: 86-99. Review.
  http://www.ncbi.nlm.nih.gov:80/entrez/query.fcgi?cmd=Retrieve&db=PubMed&list_uids=9547879&dopt=Abstract

- **Effect of lidocaine injection of EOAE in patients with tinnitus.**
  Author(s): Haginomori S, Makimoto K, Araki M, Kawakami M, Takahashi H.
  Source: Acta Oto-Laryngologica. 1995 July; 115(4): 488-92.
  http://www.ncbi.nlm.nih.gov:80/entrez/query.fcgi?cmd=Retrieve&db=PubMed&list_uids=7572122&dopt=Abstract

- **Effect of traditional Chinese acupuncture on severe tinnitus: a double-blind, placebo-controlled, clinical investigation with open therapeutic

control.
Author(s): Vilholm OJ, Moller K, Jorgensen K.
Source: British Journal of Audiology. 1998 June; 32(3): 197-204.
http://www.ncbi.nlm.nih.gov:80/entrez/query.fcgi?cmd=Retrieve&db=PubMed&list_uids=9710337&dopt=Abstract

- **Effective treatment of tinnitus through hypnotherapy.**
  Author(s): Marlowe FI.
  Source: Am J Clin Hypn. 1973 January; 15(3): 162-5. No Abstract Available.
  http://www.ncbi.nlm.nih.gov:80/entrez/query.fcgi?cmd=Retrieve&db=PubMed&list_uids=4780115&dopt=Abstract

- **Effectiveness of Ginkgo biloba in treating tinnitus: double blind, placebo controlled trial.**
  Author(s): Drew S, Davies E.
  Source: Bmj (Clinical Research Ed.). 2001 January 13; 322(7278): 73.
  http://www.ncbi.nlm.nih.gov:80/entrez/query.fcgi?cmd=Retrieve&db=PubMed&list_uids=11154618&dopt=Abstract

- **Effects of (-)-baclofen, clonazepam, and diazepam on tone exposure-induced hyperexcitability of the inferior colliculus in the rat: possible therapeutic implications for pharmacological management of tinnitus and hyperacusis.**
  Author(s): Szczepaniak WS, Moller AR.
  Source: Hearing Research. 1996 August; 97(1-2): 46-53.
  http://www.ncbi.nlm.nih.gov:80/entrez/query.fcgi?cmd=Retrieve&db=PubMed&list_uids=8844185&dopt=Abstract

- **Effects of EMG and thermal feedback training on tinnitus: a case study.**
  Author(s): Elfner LF, May JG, Moore JD, Mendelson JM.
  Source: Biofeedback Self Regul. 1981 December; 6(4): 517-21.
  http://www.ncbi.nlm.nih.gov:80/entrez/query.fcgi?cmd=Retrieve&db=PubMed&list_uids=7326274&dopt=Abstract

- **Efficacy of acupuncture as a treatment for tinnitus: a systematic review.**
  Author(s): Park J, White AR, Ernst E.
  Source: Archives of Otolaryngology--Head & Neck Surgery. 2000 April; 126(4): 489-92. Review.
  http://www.ncbi.nlm.nih.gov:80/entrez/query.fcgi?cmd=Retrieve&db=PubMed&list_uids=10772302&dopt=Abstract

- **Efficacy of biofeedback in the treatment of tinnitus: some considerations.**
  Author(s): Galanos AN.
  Source: Southern Medical Journal. 1982 November; 75(11): 1433.
  http://www.ncbi.nlm.nih.gov:80/entrez/query.fcgi?cmd=Retrieve&db=PubMed&list_uids=6755731&dopt=Abstract

- **Efficacy of self-hypnosis for tinnitus relief.**
  Author(s): Attias J, Shemesh Z, Shoham C, Shahar A, Sohmer H.
  Source: Scandinavian Audiology. 1990; 19(4): 245-9.
  http://www.ncbi.nlm.nih.gov:80/entrez/query.fcgi?cmd=Retrieve&db=PubMed&list_uids=2075417&dopt=Abstract

- **Electrical suppression of tinnitus.**
  Author(s): Aran JM, Cazals Y.
  Source: Ciba Found Symp. 1981; 85: 217-31.
  http://www.ncbi.nlm.nih.gov:80/entrez/query.fcgi?cmd=Retrieve&db=PubMed&list_uids=6976888&dopt=Abstract

- **Electrical tinnitus suppression (ETS) with a single channel cochlear implant.**
  Author(s): Hazell JW, Meerton LJ, Conway MJ.
  Source: J Laryngol Otol Suppl. 1989; 18: 39-44.
  http://www.ncbi.nlm.nih.gov:80/entrez/query.fcgi?cmd=Retrieve&db=PubMed&list_uids=2607193&dopt=Abstract

- **Electrical tinnitus suppression: a double-blind crossover study.**
  Author(s): Dobie RA, Hoberg KE, Rees TS.
  Source: Otolaryngology and Head and Neck Surgery. 1986 October; 95(3 Pt 1): 319-23.
  http://www.ncbi.nlm.nih.gov:80/entrez/query.fcgi?cmd=Retrieve&db=PubMed&list_uids=3108780&dopt=Abstract

- **Electrical tinnitus suppression: frequency dependence of effects.**
  Author(s): Hazell JW, Jastreboff PJ, Meerton LE, Conway MJ.
  Source: Audiology : Official Organ of the International Society of Audiology. 1993; 32(1): 68-77.
  http://www.ncbi.nlm.nih.gov:80/entrez/query.fcgi?cmd=Retrieve&db=PubMed&list_uids=8447763&dopt=Abstract

- **Electromyographic biofeedback for treatment of tinnitus.**
  Author(s): Borton TE, Clark SR.

Source: The American Journal of Otology. 1988 January; 9(1): 23-30.
http://www.ncbi.nlm.nih.gov:80/entrez/query.fcgi?cmd=Retrieve&db=PubMed&list_uids=3364533&dopt=Abstract

- **Electromyographic feedback treatment for tinnitus aurium.**
  Author(s): Borton TE, Moore WH Jr, Clark SR.
  Source: J Speech Hear Disord. 1981 February; 46(1): 39-45.
  http://www.ncbi.nlm.nih.gov:80/entrez/query.fcgi?cmd=Retrieve&db=PubMed&list_uids=7206677&dopt=Abstract

- **Electrophysiological indices of selective auditory attention in subjects with and without tinnitus.**
  Author(s): Jacobson GP, Calder JA, Newman CW, Peterson EL, Wharton JA, Ahmad BK.
  Source: Hearing Research. 1996 August; 97(1-2): 66-74.
  http://www.ncbi.nlm.nih.gov:80/entrez/query.fcgi?cmd=Retrieve&db=PubMed&list_uids=8844187&dopt=Abstract

- **Elevated fusiform cell activity in the dorsal cochlear nucleus of chinchillas with psychophysical evidence of tinnitus.**
  Author(s): Brozoski TJ, Bauer CA, Caspary DM.
  Source: The Journal of Neuroscience : the Official Journal of the Society for Neuroscience. 2002 March 15; 22(6): 2383-90.
  http://www.ncbi.nlm.nih.gov:80/entrez/query.fcgi?cmd=Retrieve&db=PubMed&list_uids=11896177&dopt=Abstract

- **EMG biofeedback in the treatment of tinnitus: an experimental evaluation.**
  Author(s): Haralambous G, Wilson PH, Platt-Hepworth S, Tonkin JP, Hensley VR, Kavanagh D.
  Source: Behaviour Research and Therapy. 1987; 25(1): 49-55.
  http://www.ncbi.nlm.nih.gov:80/entrez/query.fcgi?cmd=Retrieve&db=PubMed&list_uids=3593161&dopt=Abstract

- **Evidence for a cochlear origin for acoustic re-emissions, threshold fine-structure and tonal tinnitus.**
  Author(s): Wilson JP.
  Source: Hearing Research. 1980 June; 2(3-4): 233-52.
  http://www.ncbi.nlm.nih.gov:80/entrez/query.fcgi?cmd=Retrieve&db=PubMed&list_uids=7410230&dopt=Abstract

- **External electrical tinnitus suppression: a review.**
  Author(s): Shulman A.
  Source: The American Journal of Otology. 1987 November; 8(6): 479-84. Review.
  http://www.ncbi.nlm.nih.gov:80/entrez/query.fcgi?cmd=Retrieve&db=PubMed&list_uids=3324768&dopt=Abstract

- **Focal metabolic activation in the predominant left auditory cortex in patients suffering from tinnitus: a PET study with [18F]deoxyglucose.**
  Author(s): Arnold W, Bartenstein P, Oestreicher E, Romer W, Schwaiger M.
  Source: Orl; Journal for Oto-Rhino-Laryngology and Its Related Specialties. 1996 July-August; 58(4): 195-9.
  http://www.ncbi.nlm.nih.gov:80/entrez/query.fcgi?cmd=Retrieve&db=PubMed&list_uids=8883104&dopt=Abstract

- **Functional brain imaging of tinnitus-like perception induced by aversive auditory stimuli.**
  Author(s): Mirz F, Gjedde A, Sodkilde-Jrgensen H, Pedersen CB.
  Source: Neuroreport. 2000 February 28; 11(3): 633-7.
  http://www.ncbi.nlm.nih.gov:80/entrez/query.fcgi?cmd=Retrieve&db=PubMed&list_uids=10718327&dopt=Abstract

- **Gingko biloba (Rokan) therapy in tinnitus patients and measurable interactions between tinnitus and vestibular disturbances.**
  Author(s): Schneider D, Schneider L, Shulman A, Claussen CF, Just E, Koltchev C, Kersebaum M, Dehler R, Goldstein B, Claussen E.
  Source: Int Tinnitus J. 2000; 6(1): 56-62.
  http://www.ncbi.nlm.nih.gov:80/entrez/query.fcgi?cmd=Retrieve&db=PubMed&list_uids=14689620&dopt=Abstract

- **Ginkgo biloba extract for the treatment of tinnitus.**
  Author(s): Holgers KM, Axelsson A, Pringle I.
  Source: Audiology : Official Organ of the International Society of Audiology. 1994 March-April; 33(2): 85-92.
  http://www.ncbi.nlm.nih.gov:80/entrez/query.fcgi?cmd=Retrieve&db=PubMed&list_uids=8179518&dopt=Abstract

- **Ginkgo biloba for tinnitus: a review.**
  Author(s): Ernst E, Stevinson C.

Source: Clinical Otolaryngology and Allied Sciences. 1999 June; 24(3): 164-7. Review.
http://www.ncbi.nlm.nih.gov:80/entrez/query.fcgi?cmd=Retrieve&db=PubMed&list_uids=10384838&dopt=Abstract

- **Ginkgo ineffective for tinnitus.**
  Author(s): DeBisschop M.
  Source: The Journal of Family Practice. 2003 October; 52(10): 766, 769.
  http://www.ncbi.nlm.nih.gov:80/entrez/query.fcgi?cmd=Retrieve&db=PubMed&list_uids=14529599&dopt=Abstract

- **Health and Nutrition Examination Survey of 1971-75: Part II. Tinnitus, subjective hearing loss, and well-being.**
  Author(s): Cooper JC Jr.
  Source: Journal of the American Academy of Audiology. 1994 January; 5(1): 37-43.
  http://www.ncbi.nlm.nih.gov:80/entrez/query.fcgi?cmd=Retrieve&db=PubMed&list_uids=8155893&dopt=Abstract

- **Homolateral and contralateral masking of tinnitus by noise-bands and by pure tones.**
  Author(s): Feldmann H.
  Source: Audiology : Official Organ of the International Society of Audiology. 1971 May-June; 10(3): 138-44.
  http://www.ncbi.nlm.nih.gov:80/entrez/query.fcgi?cmd=Retrieve&db=PubMed&list_uids=5163656&dopt=Abstract

- **Hyperactivity in the dorsal cochlear nucleus after intense sound exposure and its resemblance to tone-evoked activity: a physiological model for tinnitus.**
  Author(s): Kaltenbach JA, Afman CE.
  Source: Hearing Research. 2000 February; 140(1-2): 165-72.
  http://www.ncbi.nlm.nih.gov:80/entrez/query.fcgi?cmd=Retrieve&db=PubMed&list_uids=10675644&dopt=Abstract

- **Hypnosis as an aid for tinnitus patients.**
  Author(s): Kaye JM, Marlowe FI, Ramchandani D, Berman S, Schindler B, Loscalzo G.
  Source: Ear, Nose, & Throat Journal. 1994 May; 73(5): 309-12, 315.
  http://www.ncbi.nlm.nih.gov:80/entrez/query.fcgi?cmd=Retrieve&db=PubMed&list_uids=8045234&dopt=Abstract

- **Hypnosis for tinnitus.**
  Author(s): GUILD J.
  Source: Can Med Assoc J. 1958 March 15; 78(6): 426-7. No Abstract Available.
  http://www.ncbi.nlm.nih.gov:80/entrez/query.fcgi?cmd=Retrieve&db=PubMed&list_uids=13511321&dopt=Abstract

- **Idiopathic Subjective Tinnitus Treated by Amitriptyline Hydrochloride/Biofeedback.**
  Author(s): Podoshin L, Ben-David Y, Fradis M, Malatskey S, Hafner H.
  Source: Int Tinnitus J. 1995; 1(1): 54-60.
  http://www.ncbi.nlm.nih.gov:80/entrez/query.fcgi?cmd=Retrieve&db=PubMed&list_uids=10753321&dopt=Abstract

- **Idiopathic subjective tinnitus treated by biofeedback, acupuncture and drug therapy.**
  Author(s): Podoshin L, Ben-David Y, Fradis M, Gerstel R, Felner H.
  Source: Ear, Nose, & Throat Journal. 1991 May; 70(5): 284-9.
  http://www.ncbi.nlm.nih.gov:80/entrez/query.fcgi?cmd=Retrieve&db=PubMed&list_uids=1914952&dopt=Abstract

- **Impact of a relaxation training on psychometric and immunologic parameters in tinnitus sufferers.**
  Author(s): Weber C, Arck P, Mazurek B, Klapp BF.
  Source: Journal of Psychosomatic Research. 2002 January; 52(1): 29-33.
  http://www.ncbi.nlm.nih.gov:80/entrez/query.fcgi?cmd=Retrieve&db=PubMed&list_uids=11801262&dopt=Abstract

- **Incurrence and alterations in contralateral tinnitus following monaural exposure to a pure tone.**
  Author(s): Young IM, Lowry LD.
  Source: The Journal of the Acoustical Society of America. 1983 June; 73(6): 2219-21.
  http://www.ncbi.nlm.nih.gov:80/entrez/query.fcgi?cmd=Retrieve&db=PubMed&list_uids=6875103&dopt=Abstract

- **Interrupted noise as a tinnitus masker: an annoyance study.**
  Author(s): Letowski TR, Thompson MV.
  Source: Ear and Hearing. 1985 March-April; 6(2): 65-70.
  http://www.ncbi.nlm.nih.gov:80/entrez/query.fcgi?cmd=Retrieve&db=PubMed&list_uids=3996786&dopt=Abstract

- **Intracochlear electrical tinnitus reduction.**
  Author(s): Dauman R, Tyler RS, Aran JM.
  Source: Acta Oto-Laryngologica. 1993 May; 113(3): 291-5.
  http://www.ncbi.nlm.nih.gov:80/entrez/query.fcgi?cmd=Retrieve&db=PubMed&list_uids=8517130&dopt=Abstract

- **Intratympanic steroid treatment of inner ear disease and tinnitus (preliminary report).**
  Author(s): Silverstein H, Choo D, Rosenberg SI, Kuhn J, Seidman M, Stein I.
  Source: Ear, Nose, & Throat Journal. 1996 August; 75(8): 468-71, 474, 476 Passim.
  http://www.ncbi.nlm.nih.gov:80/entrez/query.fcgi?cmd=Retrieve&db=PubMed&list_uids=8828271&dopt=Abstract

- **Is biofeedback effective for chronic tinnitus? An intensive study with seven subjects.**
  Author(s): Landis B, Landis E.
  Source: American Journal of Otolaryngology. 1992 November-December; 13(6): 349-56.
  http://www.ncbi.nlm.nih.gov:80/entrez/query.fcgi?cmd=Retrieve&db=PubMed&list_uids=1443390&dopt=Abstract

- **Judgments and measurements of the loudness of tinnitus before and after masking.**
  Author(s): Penner MJ.
  Source: Journal of Speech and Hearing Research. 1988 December; 31(4): 582-7.
  http://www.ncbi.nlm.nih.gov:80/entrez/query.fcgi?cmd=Retrieve&db=PubMed&list_uids=3230887&dopt=Abstract

- **Lateral inhibition in the auditory cortex: an EEG index of tinnitus?**
  Author(s): Kadner A, Viirre E, Wester DC, Walsh SF, Hestenes J, Vankov A, Pineda JA.
  Source: Neuroreport. 2002 March 25; 13(4): 443-6.
  http://www.ncbi.nlm.nih.gov:80/entrez/query.fcgi?cmd=Retrieve&db=PubMed&list_uids=11930157&dopt=Abstract

- **Lateralized tinnitus studied with functional magnetic resonance imaging: abnormal inferior colliculus activation.**
  Author(s): Melcher JR, Sigalovsky IS, Guinan JJ Jr, Levine RA.

Source: Journal of Neurophysiology. 2000 February; 83(2): 1058-72.
http://www.ncbi.nlm.nih.gov:80/entrez/query.fcgi?cmd=Retrieve&db=PubMed&list_uids=10669517&dopt=Abstract

- **Learned self-control of tinnitus through a matching-to-sample feedback technique: a clinical investigation.**
  Author(s): Ince LP, Greene RY, Alba A, Zaretsky HH.
  Source: Journal of Behavioral Medicine. 1984 December; 7(4): 355-65.
  http://www.ncbi.nlm.nih.gov:80/entrez/query.fcgi?cmd=Retrieve&db=PubMed&list_uids=6520867&dopt=Abstract

- **Long-term effect of hyperbaric oxygenation treatment on chronic distressing tinnitus.**
  Author(s): Tan J, Tange RA, Dreschler WA, vd Kleij A, Tromp EC.
  Source: Scandinavian Audiology. 1999; 28(2): 91-6.
  http://www.ncbi.nlm.nih.gov:80/entrez/query.fcgi?cmd=Retrieve&db=PubMed&list_uids=10384896&dopt=Abstract

- **Management of the patient with tinnitus.**
  Author(s): Schleuning AJ 2nd.
  Source: The Medical Clinics of North America. 1991 November; 75(6): 1225-37. Review.
  http://www.ncbi.nlm.nih.gov:80/entrez/query.fcgi?cmd=Retrieve&db=PubMed&list_uids=1943314&dopt=Abstract

- **Management of the tinnitus patient.**
  Author(s): House JW.
  Source: The Annals of Otology, Rhinology, and Laryngology. 1981 November-December; 90(6 Pt 1): 597-601.
  http://www.ncbi.nlm.nih.gov:80/entrez/query.fcgi?cmd=Retrieve&db=PubMed&list_uids=7316384&dopt=Abstract

- **Management of tinnitus aurium with lidocaine and carbamazepine.**
  Author(s): Shea JJ, Harell M.
  Source: The Laryngoscope. 1978 September; 88(9 Pt 1): 1477-84.
  http://www.ncbi.nlm.nih.gov:80/entrez/query.fcgi?cmd=Retrieve&db=PubMed&list_uids=682804&dopt=Abstract

- **Managing tinnitus: a comparison of different approaches to tinnitus management training.**
  Author(s): Dineen R, Doyle J, Bench J.

Source: British Journal of Audiology. 1997 October; 31(5): 331-44.
http://www.ncbi.nlm.nih.gov:80/entrez/query.fcgi?cmd=Retrieve&db=PubMed&list_uids=9373742&dopt=Abstract

- **Masking of tinnitus and central masking.**
  Author(s): Penner MJ.
  Source: Journal of Speech and Hearing Research. 1987 June; 30(2): 147-52.
  http://www.ncbi.nlm.nih.gov:80/entrez/query.fcgi?cmd=Retrieve&db=PubMed&list_uids=3599946&dopt=Abstract

- **Masking of tinnitus and mental activity.**
  Author(s): Andersson G, Khakpoor A, Lyttkens L.
  Source: Clinical Otolaryngology and Allied Sciences. 2002 August; 27(4): 270-4.
  http://www.ncbi.nlm.nih.gov:80/entrez/query.fcgi?cmd=Retrieve&db=PubMed&list_uids=12169130&dopt=Abstract

- **Masking of tinnitus through a cochlear implant.**
  Author(s): Vernon JA.
  Source: Journal of the American Academy of Audiology. 2000 June; 11(6): 293-4.
  http://www.ncbi.nlm.nih.gov:80/entrez/query.fcgi?cmd=Retrieve&db=PubMed&list_uids=10857999&dopt=Abstract

- **Measurement of tinnitus in humans.**
  Author(s): Hazell JW.
  Source: Ciba Found Symp. 1981; 85: 35-53.
  http://www.ncbi.nlm.nih.gov:80/entrez/query.fcgi?cmd=Retrieve&db=PubMed&list_uids=6915837&dopt=Abstract

- **Measures of tinnitus: step size, matches to imagined tones, and masking patterns.**
  Author(s): Penner MJ, Klafter EJ.
  Source: Ear and Hearing. 1992 December; 13(6): 410-6.
  http://www.ncbi.nlm.nih.gov:80/entrez/query.fcgi?cmd=Retrieve&db=PubMed&list_uids=1487103&dopt=Abstract

- **Measuring tinnitus parameters: loudness, pitch, and maskability.**
  Author(s): Mitchell CR, Vernon JA, Creedon TA.

Source: Journal of the American Academy of Audiology. 1993 May; 4(3): 139-51.

http://www.ncbi.nlm.nih.gov:80/entrez/query.fcgi?cmd=Retrieve&db=PubMed&list_uids=8318704&dopt=Abstract

- **Myths in neurotology, revisited: smoke and mirrors in tinnitus therapy.**
  Author(s): Howard ML.
  Source: Otology & Neurotology : Official Publication of the American Otological Society, American Neurotology Society [and] European Academy of Otology and Neurotology. 2001 November; 22(6): 711-4.
  http://www.ncbi.nlm.nih.gov:80/entrez/query.fcgi?cmd=Retrieve&db=PubMed&list_uids=11698785&dopt=Abstract

- **Neuronavigated repetitive transcranial magnetic stimulation in patients with tinnitus: a short case series.**
  Author(s): Eichhammer P, Langguth B, Marienhagen J, Kleinjung T, Hajak G.
  Source: Biological Psychiatry. 2003 October 15; 54(8): 862-5.
  http://www.ncbi.nlm.nih.gov:80/entrez/query.fcgi?cmd=Retrieve&db=PubMed&list_uids=14550687&dopt=Abstract

- **Neuronavigated rTMS in a patient with chronic tinnitus. Effects of 4 weeks treatment.**
  Author(s): Langguth B, Eichhammer P, Wiegand R, Marienhegen J, Maenner P, Jacob P, Hajak G.
  Source: Neuroreport. 2003 May 23; 14(7): 977-80.
  http://www.ncbi.nlm.nih.gov:80/entrez/query.fcgi?cmd=Retrieve&db=PubMed&list_uids=12802186&dopt=Abstract

- **Neurophysiological model of tinnitus: dependence of the minimal masking level on treatment outcome.**
  Author(s): Jastreboff PJ, Hazell JW, Graham RL.
  Source: Hearing Research. 1994 November; 80(2): 216-32.
  http://www.ncbi.nlm.nih.gov:80/entrez/query.fcgi?cmd=Retrieve&db=PubMed&list_uids=7896580&dopt=Abstract

- **Neuropsychiatric aspects of tinnitus.**
  Author(s): Ambrosino SV.
  Source: J Laryngol Otol Suppl. 1981; (4): 169-72. No Abstract Available.
  http://www.ncbi.nlm.nih.gov:80/entrez/query.fcgi?cmd=Retrieve&db=PubMed&list_uids=6946165&dopt=Abstract

- **Objective evidence for tinnitus in auditory-evoked magnetic fields.**
  Author(s): Hoke M.
  Source: Acta Otolaryngol Suppl. 1990; 476: 189-94.
  http://www.ncbi.nlm.nih.gov:80/entrez/query.fcgi?cmd=Retrieve&db=PubMed&list_uids=2087962&dopt=Abstract

- **Objective evidence of tinnitus in auditory evoked magnetic fields.**
  Author(s): Hoke M, Feldmann H, Pantev C, Lutkenhoner B, Lehnertz K.
  Source: Hearing Research. 1989 February; 37(3): 281-6.
  http://www.ncbi.nlm.nih.gov:80/entrez/query.fcgi?cmd=Retrieve&db=PubMed&list_uids=2708150&dopt=Abstract

- **On helping people with tinnitus to help themselves.**
  Author(s): Hayes R.
  Source: British Journal of Audiology. 1987 November; 21(4): 327-8.
  http://www.ncbi.nlm.nih.gov:80/entrez/query.fcgi?cmd=Retrieve&db=PubMed&list_uids=3690071&dopt=Abstract

- **On helping people with tinnitus to help themselves.**
  Author(s): Slater R.
  Source: British Journal of Audiology. 1987 May; 21(2): 87-90.
  http://www.ncbi.nlm.nih.gov:80/entrez/query.fcgi?cmd=Retrieve&db=PubMed&list_uids=3594018&dopt=Abstract

- **On the evidence of auditory evoked magnetic fields as an objective measure of tinnitus.**
  Author(s): Colding-Jorgensen E, Lauritzen M, Johnsen NJ, Mikkelsen KB, Saermark K.
  Source: Electroencephalography and Clinical Neurophysiology. 1992 November; 83(5): 322-7.
  http://www.ncbi.nlm.nih.gov:80/entrez/query.fcgi?cmd=Retrieve&db=PubMed&list_uids=1385088&dopt=Abstract

- **On the pathophysiology of tinnitus; a review and a peripheral model.**
  Author(s): Eggermont JJ.
  Source: Hearing Research. 1990 September; 48(1-2): 111-23. Review.
  http://www.ncbi.nlm.nih.gov:80/entrez/query.fcgi?cmd=Retrieve&db=PubMed&list_uids=2249954&dopt=Abstract

- **Otoacoustic emissions and tinnitus.**
  Author(s): Wilson JP.

- **Personality of the tinnitus patient.**
  Author(s): House PR.
  Source: Ciba Found Symp. 1981; 85: 193-203.
  http://www.ncbi.nlm.nih.gov:80/entrez/query.fcgi?cmd=Retrieve&db=PubMed&list_uids=7035099&dopt=Abstract

- **Physiologically active cochlear micromechanics--one source of tinnitus.**
  Author(s): Kemp DT.
  Source: Ciba Found Symp. 1981; 85: 54-81. Review.
  http://www.ncbi.nlm.nih.gov:80/entrez/query.fcgi?cmd=Retrieve&db=PubMed&list_uids=7035100&dopt=Abstract

- **Prior treatments in a group of tinnitus sufferers seeking treatment.**
  Author(s): Andersson G.
  Source: Psychotherapy and Psychosomatics. 1997; 66(2): 107-10.
  http://www.ncbi.nlm.nih.gov:80/entrez/query.fcgi?cmd=Retrieve&db=PubMed&list_uids=9097339&dopt=Abstract

- **Psychological aspects of tinnitus and the application of cognitive-behavioral therapy.**
  Author(s): Andersson G.
  Source: Clinical Psychology Review. 2002 September; 22(7): 977-90. Review.
  http://www.ncbi.nlm.nih.gov:80/entrez/query.fcgi?cmd=Retrieve&db=PubMed&list_uids=12238249&dopt=Abstract

- **Psychological factors affecting outcome of treatment after transcutaneous electrotherapy for persistent tinnitus.**
  Author(s): Collet L, Moussu MF, Dubreuil C, Disant F, Chanal JM, Morgon A.
  Source: Arch Otorhinolaryngol. 1987; 244(1): 20-2.
  http://www.ncbi.nlm.nih.gov:80/entrez/query.fcgi?cmd=Retrieve&db=PubMed&list_uids=3497623&dopt=Abstract

- **Psychological profile of help-seeking and non-help-seeking tinnitus patients.**
  Author(s): Attias J, Shemesh Z, Bleich A, Solomon Z, Bar-Or G, Alster J, Sohmer H.

Source: Scandinavian Audiology. 1995; 24(1): 13-8.
http://www.ncbi.nlm.nih.gov:80/entrez/query.fcgi?cmd=Retrieve&db=PubMed&list_uids=7761793&dopt=Abstract

- **Psychological treatment of tinnitus. An experimental group study.**
  Author(s): Scott B, Lindberg P, Lyttkens L, Melin L.
  Source: Scandinavian Audiology. 1985; 14(4): 223-30.
  http://www.ncbi.nlm.nih.gov:80/entrez/query.fcgi?cmd=Retrieve&db=PubMed&list_uids=3912955&dopt=Abstract

- **Psychophysiological therapy for tinnitus.**
  Author(s): White TP, Hoffman SR, Gale EN.
  Source: Ear and Hearing. 1986 December; 7(6): 397-9.
  http://www.ncbi.nlm.nih.gov:80/entrez/query.fcgi?cmd=Retrieve&db=PubMed&list_uids=3539680&dopt=Abstract

- **Regional cerebral blood flow during tinnitus: a PET case study with lidocaine and auditory stimulation.**
  Author(s): Andersson G, Lyttkens L, Hirvela C, Furmark T, Tillfors M, Fredrikson M.
  Source: Acta Oto-Laryngologica. 2000 October; 120(8): 967-72.
  http://www.ncbi.nlm.nih.gov:80/entrez/query.fcgi?cmd=Retrieve&db=PubMed&list_uids=11200593&dopt=Abstract

- **Relaxation-biofeedback in the treatment of tinnitus.**
  Author(s): Carmen R, Svihovec D.
  Source: The American Journal of Otology. 1984 July; 5(5): 376-81.
  http://www.ncbi.nlm.nih.gov:80/entrez/query.fcgi?cmd=Retrieve&db=PubMed&list_uids=6383065&dopt=Abstract

- **Reliability of tinnitus loudness matches under procedural variation.**
  Author(s): Henry JA, Flick CL, Gilbert A, Ellingson RM, Fausti SA.
  Source: Journal of the American Academy of Audiology. 1999 October; 10(9): 502-20.
  http://www.ncbi.nlm.nih.gov:80/entrez/query.fcgi?cmd=Retrieve&db=PubMed&list_uids=10522624&dopt=Abstract

- **Reorganization of auditory cortex in tinnitus.**
  Author(s): Muhlnickel W, Elbert T, Taub E, Flor H.

Source: Proceedings of the National Academy of Sciences of the United States of America. 1998 August 18; 95(17): 10340-3.
http://www.ncbi.nlm.nih.gov:80/entrez/query.fcgi?cmd=Retrieve&db=PubMed&list_uids=9707649&dopt=Abstract

- **Results of combined low-power laser therapy and extracts of Ginkgo biloba in cases of sensorineural hearing loss and tinnitus.**
  Author(s): Plath P, Olivier J.
  Source: Advances in Oto-Rhino-Laryngology. 1995; 49: 101-4.
  http://www.ncbi.nlm.nih.gov:80/entrez/query.fcgi?cmd=Retrieve&db=PubMed&list_uids=7653339&dopt=Abstract

- **Results of leucotomy operations for tinnitus.**
  Author(s): Beard AW.
  Source: Journal of Psychosomatic Research. 1965 September; 9(1): 29-32.
  http://www.ncbi.nlm.nih.gov:80/entrez/query.fcgi?cmd=Retrieve&db=PubMed&list_uids=5857613&dopt=Abstract

- **Retraining therapy for chronic tinnitus. A critical analysis of its status.**
  Author(s): Kroener-Herwig B, Biesinger E, Gerhards F, Goebel G, Verena Greimel K, Hiller W.
  Source: Scandinavian Audiology. 2000; 29(2): 67-78. Review.
  http://www.ncbi.nlm.nih.gov:80/entrez/query.fcgi?cmd=Retrieve&db=PubMed&list_uids=10888343&dopt=Abstract

- **Severe tinnitus: treatment with biofeedback training (results in 41 cases).**
  Author(s): House JW, Miller L, House PR.
  Source: Trans Am Acad Ophthalmol Otolaryngol. 1977 July-August; 84(4 Pt 1): Orl-697-703. No Abstract Available.
  http://www.ncbi.nlm.nih.gov:80/entrez/query.fcgi?cmd=Retrieve&db=PubMed&list_uids=898522&dopt=Abstract

- **Simple custom-made disposable surface electrode system for non-invasive "electro-acupuncture" or TNS and its clinical applications including treatment of cephalic hypertension and hypotension syndromes as well as temporo-mandibular joint problems, tinnitus, shoulder and lower back pain, etc.**
  Author(s): Omura Y.

Source: Acupuncture & Electro-Therapeutics Research. 1981; 6(2-3): 109-34.
http://www.ncbi.nlm.nih.gov:80/entrez/query.fcgi?cmd=Retrieve&db=PubMed&list_uids=6120617&dopt=Abstract

- **Simultaneous measurement of tinnitus pitch and loudness.**
  Author(s): Penner MJ, Saran A.
  Source: Ear and Hearing. 1994 December; 15(6): 416-21.
  http://www.ncbi.nlm.nih.gov:80/entrez/query.fcgi?cmd=Retrieve&db=PubMed&list_uids=7895937&dopt=Abstract

- **Soft-laser/Ginkgo therapy in chronic tinnitus. A placebo-controlled study.**
  Author(s): von Wedel H, Calero L, Walger M, Hoenen S, Rutwalt D.
  Source: Advances in Oto-Rhino-Laryngology. 1995; 49: 105-8.
  http://www.ncbi.nlm.nih.gov:80/entrez/query.fcgi?cmd=Retrieve&db=PubMed&list_uids=7653340&dopt=Abstract

- **Some preliminary observations on the effect of galvanic current on tinnitus aurium.**
  Author(s): HATTON DS, ERULKAR SD, ROSENBERG PE.
  Source: The Laryngoscope. 1960 February; 70: 123-30.
  http://www.ncbi.nlm.nih.gov:80/entrez/query.fcgi?cmd=Retrieve&db=PubMed&list_uids=13852045&dopt=Abstract

- **Some psychological aspects of tinnitus.**
  Author(s): Reiss M, Reiss G.
  Source: Percept Mot Skills. 1999 June; 88(3 Pt 1): 790-2. Review.
  http://www.ncbi.nlm.nih.gov:80/entrez/query.fcgi?cmd=Retrieve&db=PubMed&list_uids=10407886&dopt=Abstract

- **Sound stimulation via bone conduction for tinnitus relief: a pilot study.**
  Author(s): Holgers KM, Hakansson BE.
  Source: International Journal of Audiology. 2002 July; 41(5): 293-300.
  http://www.ncbi.nlm.nih.gov:80/entrez/query.fcgi?cmd=Retrieve&db=PubMed&list_uids=12166689&dopt=Abstract

- **Study of the so-called cochlear mechanical tinnitus.**
  Author(s): O-Uchi T, Tanaka Y.

Source: Acta Otolaryngol Suppl. 1988; 447: 94-9.
http://www.ncbi.nlm.nih.gov:80/entrez/query.fcgi?cmd=Retrieve&db=PubMed&list_uids=3188900&dopt=Abstract

- **Subjective idiopathic tinnitus.**
  Author(s): Billue JS.
  Source: Clin Excell Nurse Pract. 1998 March; 2(2): 73-82. Review.
  http://www.ncbi.nlm.nih.gov:80/entrez/query.fcgi?cmd=Retrieve&db=PubMed&list_uids=10451267&dopt=Abstract

- **The effects of reassurance, relaxation training and distraction on chronic tinnitus sufferers.**
  Author(s): Jakes SC, Hallam RS, Rachman S, Hinchcliffe R.
  Source: Behaviour Research and Therapy. 1986; 24(5): 497-507.
  http://www.ncbi.nlm.nih.gov:80/entrez/query.fcgi?cmd=Retrieve&db=PubMed&list_uids=3530238&dopt=Abstract

- **The efficacy of Ginkgo special extract EGb 761 in patients with tinnitus.**
  Author(s): Morgenstern C, Biermann E.
  Source: Int J Clin Pharmacol Ther. 2002 May; 40(5): 188-97.
  http://www.ncbi.nlm.nih.gov:80/entrez/query.fcgi?cmd=Retrieve&db=PubMed&list_uids=12051570&dopt=Abstract

- **The functional neuroanatomy of tinnitus: evidence for limbic system links and neural plasticity.**
  Author(s): Lockwood AH, Salvi RJ, Coad ML, Towsley ML, Wack DS, Murphy BW.
  Source: Neurology. 1998 January; 50(1): 114-20.
  http://www.ncbi.nlm.nih.gov:80/entrez/query.fcgi?cmd=Retrieve&db=PubMed&list_uids=9443467&dopt=Abstract

- **The influence of training on tinnitus perception: an evaluation 12 months after tinnitus management training.**
  Author(s): Dineen R, Doyle J, Bench J, Perry A.
  Source: British Journal of Audiology. 1999 February; 33(1): 29-51.
  http://www.ncbi.nlm.nih.gov:80/entrez/query.fcgi?cmd=Retrieve&db=PubMed&list_uids=10219721&dopt=Abstract

- **The management of chronic tinnitus--comparison of a cognitive-behavioural group training with yoga.**

Author(s): Kroner-Herwig B, Hebing G, van Rijn-Kalkmann U, Frenzel A, Schilkowsky G, Esser G.
Source: Journal of Psychosomatic Research. 1995 February; 39(2): 153-65.
http://www.ncbi.nlm.nih.gov:80/entrez/query.fcgi?cmd=Retrieve&db=PubMed&list_uids=7595873&dopt=Abstract

- **The medical audiological evaluation of tinnitus patients.**
  Author(s): Seabra JC.
  Source: Int Tinnitus J. 1999; 5(1): 53-6.
  http://www.ncbi.nlm.nih.gov:80/entrez/query.fcgi?cmd=Retrieve&db=PubMed&list_uids=10753421&dopt=Abstract

- **The medical treatment of tinnitus.**
  Author(s): Shea JJ, Emmett JR.
  Source: J Laryngol Otol Suppl. 1981; (4): 130-8.
  http://www.ncbi.nlm.nih.gov:80/entrez/query.fcgi?cmd=Retrieve&db=PubMed&list_uids=6946161&dopt=Abstract

- **The psychological treatment of tinnitus: an experimental evaluation.**
  Author(s): Lindberg P, Scott B, Melin L, Lyttkens L.
  Source: Behaviour Research and Therapy. 1989; 27(6): 593-603.
  http://www.ncbi.nlm.nih.gov:80/entrez/query.fcgi?cmd=Retrieve&db=PubMed&list_uids=2692553&dopt=Abstract

- **The relationship of tinnitus to craniocervical mandibular disorders.**
  Author(s): Gelb H, Gelb ML, Wagner ML.
  Source: Cranio. 1997 April; 15(2): 136-43. Review.
  http://www.ncbi.nlm.nih.gov:80/entrez/query.fcgi?cmd=Retrieve&db=PubMed&list_uids=9586516&dopt=Abstract

- **The treatment of tinnitus--a historical perspective.**
  Author(s): Stephens SD.
  Source: The Journal of Laryngology and Otology. 1984 October; 98(10): 963-72.
  http://www.ncbi.nlm.nih.gov:80/entrez/query.fcgi?cmd=Retrieve&db=PubMed&list_uids=6387016&dopt=Abstract

- **The use of Walkman Mini-stereo system as a tinnitus masker.**
  Author(s): Al-Jassim AH.

Source: The Journal of Laryngology and Otology. 1988 January; 102(1): 27-8.
http://www.ncbi.nlm.nih.gov:80/entrez/query.fcgi?cmd=Retrieve&db=PubMed&list_uids=3343558&dopt=Abstract

- **Therapies for tinnitus.**
  Author(s): House JW.
  Source: The American Journal of Otology. 1989 May; 10(3): 163-5. Review.
  http://www.ncbi.nlm.nih.gov:80/entrez/query.fcgi?cmd=Retrieve&db=PubMed&list_uids=2665506&dopt=Abstract

- **Thermal biofeedback and the treatment of tinnitus.**
  Author(s): Walsh WM, Gerley PP.
  Source: The Laryngoscope. 1985 August; 95(8): 987-9.
  http://www.ncbi.nlm.nih.gov:80/entrez/query.fcgi?cmd=Retrieve&db=PubMed&list_uids=3894844&dopt=Abstract

- **Time patterns and related parameters in masking of tinnitus.**
  Author(s): Feldmann H.
  Source: Acta Oto-Laryngologica. 1983 May-June; 95(5-6): 594-8.
  http://www.ncbi.nlm.nih.gov:80/entrez/query.fcgi?cmd=Retrieve&db=PubMed&list_uids=6880672&dopt=Abstract

- **Tinnitus after head injury: evidence from otoacoustic emissions.**
  Author(s): Ceranic BJ, Prasher DK, Raglan E, Luxon LM.
  Source: Journal of Neurology, Neurosurgery, and Psychiatry. 1998 October; 65(4): 523-9.
  http://www.ncbi.nlm.nih.gov:80/entrez/query.fcgi?cmd=Retrieve&db=PubMed&list_uids=9771778&dopt=Abstract

- **Tinnitus and craniomandibular disorders--is there a link?**
  Author(s): Rubinstein B.
  Source: Swed Dent J Suppl. 1993; 95: 1-46.
  http://www.ncbi.nlm.nih.gov:80/entrez/query.fcgi?cmd=Retrieve&db=PubMed&list_uids=8503098&dopt=Abstract

- **Tinnitus and otoacoustic emissions.**
  Author(s): Ceranic BJ, Prasher DK, Luxon LM.

Source: Clinical Otolaryngology and Allied Sciences. 1995 June; 20(3): 192-200. Review.
http://www.ncbi.nlm.nih.gov:80/entrez/query.fcgi?cmd=Retrieve&db=PubMed&list_uids=7554325&dopt=Abstract

- **Tinnitus as a function of duration and etiology: counselling implications.**
Author(s): Stouffer JL, Tyler RS, Kileny PR, Dalzell LE.
Source: The American Journal of Otology. 1991 May; 12(3): 188-94.
http://www.ncbi.nlm.nih.gov:80/entrez/query.fcgi?cmd=Retrieve&db=PubMed&list_uids=1882967&dopt=Abstract

- **Tinnitus diagnosis and therapy in the aged.**
Author(s): von Wedel H, von Wedel UC, Zorowka P.
Source: Acta Otolaryngol Suppl. 1990; 476: 195-201.
http://www.ncbi.nlm.nih.gov:80/entrez/query.fcgi?cmd=Retrieve&db=PubMed&list_uids=2087963&dopt=Abstract

- **Tinnitus due to abnormal contraction of stapedial muscle. An abnormal phenomenon in the course of facial nerve paralysis and its audiological significance.**
Author(s): Watanabe I, Kumagami H, Tsuda Y.
Source: Orl; Journal for Oto-Rhino-Laryngology and Its Related Specialties. 1974; 36(4): 217-26.
http://www.ncbi.nlm.nih.gov:80/entrez/query.fcgi?cmd=Retrieve&db=PubMed&list_uids=4474647&dopt=Abstract

- **Tinnitus in hamsters following exposure to intense sound.**
Author(s): Heffner HE, Harrington IA.
Source: Hearing Research. 2002 August; 170(1-2): 83-95.
http://www.ncbi.nlm.nih.gov:80/entrez/query.fcgi?cmd=Retrieve&db=PubMed&list_uids=12208543&dopt=Abstract

- **Tinnitus induced by tones.**
Author(s): Kemp S, Plaisted ID.
Source: Journal of Speech and Hearing Research. 1986 March; 29(1): 65-70.
http://www.ncbi.nlm.nih.gov:80/entrez/query.fcgi?cmd=Retrieve&db=PubMed&list_uids=3702380&dopt=Abstract

- **Tinnitus maskers in the treatment of tinnitus. The MICROTEK 321Q.**
Author(s): Vierstraete K, Debruyne F, Vantrappen G, Feenstra L.

Source: Acta Otorhinolaryngol Belg. 1996; 50(3): 211-20.
http://www.ncbi.nlm.nih.gov:80/entrez/query.fcgi?cmd=Retrieve&db=PubMed&list_uids=8888905&dopt=Abstract

- **Tinnitus masking-a significant contribution to tinnitus management.**
  Author(s): Hazell JW, Wood S.
  Source: British Journal of Audiology. 1981 November; 15(4): 223-30.
  http://www.ncbi.nlm.nih.gov:80/entrez/query.fcgi?cmd=Retrieve&db=PubMed&list_uids=7296101&dopt=Abstract

- **Tinnitus program at Brasilia University Medical School.**
  Author(s): Oliveira CA, Venosa A, Araujo MF.
  Source: Int Tinnitus J. 1999; 5(2): 141-3.
  http://www.ncbi.nlm.nih.gov:80/entrez/query.fcgi?cmd=Retrieve&db=PubMed&list_uids=10753434&dopt=Abstract

- **Tinnitus reduction using transcutaneous electrical stimulation.**
  Author(s): Steenerson RL, Cronin GW.
  Source: Otolaryngologic Clinics of North America. 2003 April; 36(2): 337-44.
  http://www.ncbi.nlm.nih.gov:80/entrez/query.fcgi?cmd=Retrieve&db=PubMed&list_uids=12856301&dopt=Abstract

- **Tinnitus remission objectified by neuromagnetic measurements.**
  Author(s): Pantev C, Hoke M, Lutkenhoner B, Lehnertz K, Kumpf W.
  Source: Hearing Research. 1989 July; 40(3): 261-4.
  http://www.ncbi.nlm.nih.gov:80/entrez/query.fcgi?cmd=Retrieve&db=PubMed&list_uids=2793608&dopt=Abstract

- **Tinnitus retraining therapy for patients with tinnitus and decreased sound tolerance.**
  Author(s): Jastreboff PJ, Jastreboff MM.
  Source: Otolaryngologic Clinics of North America. 2003 April; 36(2): 321-36. Review.
  http://www.ncbi.nlm.nih.gov:80/entrez/query.fcgi?cmd=Retrieve&db=PubMed&list_uids=12856300&dopt=Abstract

- **Tinnitus suppression by electrical promontory stimulation (EPS) in patients with sensorineural hearing loss.**
  Author(s): Konopka W, Zalewski P, Olszewski J, Olszewska-Ziaber A, Pietkiewicz P.

Source: Auris, Nasus, Larynx. 2001 January; 28(1): 35-40.
http://www.ncbi.nlm.nih.gov:80/entrez/query.fcgi?cmd=Retrieve&db=
PubMed&list_uids=11137361&dopt=Abstract

- **Tinnitus suppression in cochlear implant users.**
  Author(s): Dauman R, Tyler RS.
  Source: Advances in Oto-Rhino-Laryngology. 1993; 48: 168-73.
  http://www.ncbi.nlm.nih.gov:80/entrez/query.fcgi?cmd=Retrieve&db=
  PubMed&list_uids=8273472&dopt=Abstract

- **Tinnitus treatment by transcutaneous nerve stimulation (TNS).**
  Author(s): Rahko T, Kotti V.
  Source: Acta Otolaryngol Suppl. 1997; 529: 88-9.
  http://www.ncbi.nlm.nih.gov:80/entrez/query.fcgi?cmd=Retrieve&db=
  PubMed&list_uids=9288279&dopt=Abstract

- **Tinnitus, quackery and folklore.**
  Author(s): Job A, Raman R.
  Source: Trop Doct. 1991 July; 21(3): 122. No Abstract Available.
  http://www.ncbi.nlm.nih.gov:80/entrez/query.fcgi?cmd=Retrieve&db=
  PubMed&list_uids=1926555&dopt=Abstract

- **Tinnitus.**
  Author(s): Marion MS, Cevette MJ.
  Source: Mayo Clinic Proceedings. 1991 June; 66(6): 614-20. Review.
  http://www.ncbi.nlm.nih.gov:80/entrez/query.fcgi?cmd=Retrieve&db=
  PubMed&list_uids=2046400&dopt=Abstract

- **Tinnitus.**
  Author(s): Alleva M, Loch WE, Paparella MM.
  Source: Primary Care. 1990 June; 17(2): 289-97. Review.
  http://www.ncbi.nlm.nih.gov:80/entrez/query.fcgi?cmd=Retrieve&db=
  PubMed&list_uids=2196610&dopt=Abstract

- **Tinnitus.**
  Author(s): Neher A.
  Source: Southern Medical Journal. 1989 December; 82(12): 1589.
  http://www.ncbi.nlm.nih.gov:80/entrez/query.fcgi?cmd=Retrieve&db=
  PubMed&list_uids=2595438&dopt=Abstract

- **Tinnitus. Diagnosis and treatment of this elusive symptom.**
  Author(s): Noell CA, Meyerhoff WL.
  Source: Geriatrics. 2003 February; 58(2): 28-34. Review.
  http://www.ncbi.nlm.nih.gov:80/entrez/query.fcgi?cmd=Retrieve&db=PubMed&list_uids=12596495&dopt=Abstract

- **Tinnitus: a stepwise workup to quiet the noise within.**
  Author(s): Ciocon JO, Amede F, Lechtenberg C, Astor F.
  Source: Geriatrics. 1995 February; 50(2): 18-25. Erratum In: Geriatrics 1995 March; 50(3): 16.
  http://www.ncbi.nlm.nih.gov:80/entrez/query.fcgi?cmd=Retrieve&db=PubMed&list_uids=7835722&dopt=Abstract

- **Tinnitus: diagnosis and treatment.**
  Author(s): Pulec JL, Hodell SF, Anthony PF.
  Source: The Annals of Otology, Rhinology, and Laryngology. 1978 November-December; 87(6 Pt 1): 821-33.
  http://www.ncbi.nlm.nih.gov:80/entrez/query.fcgi?cmd=Retrieve&db=PubMed&list_uids=310651&dopt=Abstract

- **Tinnitus: differential effects of therapy in a single case.**
  Author(s): Hallam RS, Jakes SC.
  Source: Behaviour Research and Therapy. 1985; 23(6): 691-4.
  http://www.ncbi.nlm.nih.gov:80/entrez/query.fcgi?cmd=Retrieve&db=PubMed&list_uids=3907616&dopt=Abstract

- **Tinnitus: evaluation and treatment.**
  Author(s): House JW.
  Source: The American Journal of Otology. 1984 October; 5(6): 472-5.
  http://www.ncbi.nlm.nih.gov:80/entrez/query.fcgi?cmd=Retrieve&db=PubMed&list_uids=6334995&dopt=Abstract

- **Tinnitus: evaluation of biofeedback and stomatognathic treatment.**
  Author(s): Erlandsson SI, Rubinstein B, Carlsson SG.
  Source: British Journal of Audiology. 1991 June; 25(3): 151-61.
  http://www.ncbi.nlm.nih.gov:80/entrez/query.fcgi?cmd=Retrieve&db=PubMed&list_uids=1873582&dopt=Abstract

- **Towards an objectification by classification of tinnitus.**
  Author(s): Norena A, Cransac H, Chery-Croze S.

Source: Clinical Neurophysiology : Official Journal of the International Federation of Clinical Neurophysiology. 1999 April; 110(4): 666-75.
http://www.ncbi.nlm.nih.gov:80/entrez/query.fcgi?cmd=Retrieve&db=PubMed&list_uids=10378736&dopt=Abstract

- **Transcutaneous electrical stimulation for tinnitus.**
  Author(s): Engelberg M, Bauer W.
  Source: The Laryngoscope. 1985 October; 95(10): 1167-73.
  http://www.ncbi.nlm.nih.gov:80/entrez/query.fcgi?cmd=Retrieve&db=PubMed&list_uids=3900611&dopt=Abstract

- **Transcutaneous electrotherapy for severe tinnitus.**
  Author(s): Chouard CH, Meyer B, Maridat D.
  Source: Acta Oto-Laryngologica. 1981 May-June; 91(5-6): 415-22.
  http://www.ncbi.nlm.nih.gov:80/entrez/query.fcgi?cmd=Retrieve&db=PubMed&list_uids=6973909&dopt=Abstract

- **Transcutaneous nerve stimulation (TNS) in tinnitus.**
  Author(s): Kaada B, Hognestad S, Havstad J.
  Source: Scandinavian Audiology. 1989; 18(4): 211-7.
  http://www.ncbi.nlm.nih.gov:80/entrez/query.fcgi?cmd=Retrieve&db=PubMed&list_uids=2609098&dopt=Abstract

- **Transient suppression of tinnitus by transcranial magnetic stimulation.**
  Author(s): Plewnia C, Bartels M, Gerloff C.
  Source: Annals of Neurology. 2003 February; 53(2): 263-6.
  http://www.ncbi.nlm.nih.gov:80/entrez/query.fcgi?cmd=Retrieve&db=PubMed&list_uids=12557296&dopt=Abstract

- **Transient-evoked otoacoustic emissions and contralateral suppression in patients with unilateral tinnitus.**
  Author(s): Lind O.
  Source: Scandinavian Audiology. 1996; 25(3): 167-72.
  http://www.ncbi.nlm.nih.gov:80/entrez/query.fcgi?cmd=Retrieve&db=PubMed&list_uids=8881004&dopt=Abstract

- **Treatment of severe tinnitus with biofeedback training.**
  Author(s): House JW.
  Source: The Laryngoscope. 1978 March; 88(3): 406-12.
  http://www.ncbi.nlm.nih.gov:80/entrez/query.fcgi?cmd=Retrieve&db=PubMed&list_uids=628294&dopt=Abstract

- **Treatment of severe tinnitus.**
  Author(s): Laurikainen E, Johansson R, Akaan-Penttila E, Haapaniemi J.
  Source: Acta Otolaryngol Suppl. 2000; 543: 77-8.
  http://www.ncbi.nlm.nih.gov:80/entrez/query.fcgi?cmd=Retrieve&db=PubMed&list_uids=10908984&dopt=Abstract

- **Treatment of subjective tinnitus with biofeedback.**
  Author(s): Grossan M.
  Source: Ear, Nose, & Throat Journal. 1976 October; 55(10): 314-8.
  http://www.ncbi.nlm.nih.gov:80/entrez/query.fcgi?cmd=Retrieve&db=PubMed&list_uids=991780&dopt=Abstract

- **Treatment of tinnitus by intratympanic instillation of lignocaine (lidocaine) 2 per cent through ventilation tubes.**
  Author(s): Podoshin L, Fradis M, David YB.
  Source: The Journal of Laryngology and Otology. 1992 July; 106(7): 603-6.
  http://www.ncbi.nlm.nih.gov:80/entrez/query.fcgi?cmd=Retrieve&db=PubMed&list_uids=1527456&dopt=Abstract

- **Treatment of tinnitus with alternative therapy.**
  Author(s): Bentzen O.
  Source: Acta Otorhinolaryngol Belg. 1986; 40(3): 487-91. No Abstract Available.
  http://www.ncbi.nlm.nih.gov:80/entrez/query.fcgi?cmd=Retrieve&db=PubMed&list_uids=3788551&dopt=Abstract

- **Treatment of tinnitus with electrical stimulation.**
  Author(s): Steenerson RL, Cronin GW.
  Source: Otolaryngology and Head and Neck Surgery. 1999 November; 121(5): 511-3.
  http://www.ncbi.nlm.nih.gov:80/entrez/query.fcgi?cmd=Retrieve&db=PubMed&list_uids=10547461&dopt=Abstract

- **Treatment of tinnitus.**
  Author(s): Busis SN.
  Source: Jama : the Journal of the American Medical Association. 1992 September 16; 268(11): 1467.
  http://www.ncbi.nlm.nih.gov:80/entrez/query.fcgi?cmd=Retrieve&db=PubMed&list_uids=1512918&dopt=Abstract

- **Trial of an extract of Ginkgo biloba (EGB) for tinnitus and hearing loss.**
  Author(s): Coles R.

Source: Clinical Otolaryngology and Allied Sciences. 1988 December; 13(6): 501-2.
http://www.ncbi.nlm.nih.gov:80/entrez/query.fcgi?cmd=Retrieve&db=PubMed&list_uids=3228994&dopt=Abstract

- **Use of homeopathy in the treatment of tinnitus.**
  Author(s): Simpson JJ, Donaldson I, Davies WE.
  Source: British Journal of Audiology. 1998 August; 32(4): 227-33.
  http://www.ncbi.nlm.nih.gov:80/entrez/query.fcgi?cmd=Retrieve&db=PubMed&list_uids=9923984&dopt=Abstract

- **Variability in matches to subjective tinnitus.**
  Author(s): Penner MJ.
  Source: Journal of Speech and Hearing Research. 1983 June; 26(2): 263-7.
  http://www.ncbi.nlm.nih.gov:80/entrez/query.fcgi?cmd=Retrieve&db=PubMed&list_uids=6887813&dopt=Abstract

- **Vascular decompression of the cochlear nerve in tinnitus sufferers.**
  Author(s): Meyerhoff WL, Mickey BE.
  Source: The Laryngoscope. 1988 June; 98(6 Pt 1): 602-4.
  http://www.ncbi.nlm.nih.gov:80/entrez/query.fcgi?cmd=Retrieve&db=PubMed&list_uids=3374234&dopt=Abstract

- **Vertigo, tinnitus, and hearing loss in the geriatric patient.**
  Author(s): Kessinger RC, Boneva DV.
  Source: Journal of Manipulative and Physiological Therapeutics. 2000 June; 23(5): 352-62.
  http://www.ncbi.nlm.nih.gov:80/entrez/query.fcgi?cmd=Retrieve&db=PubMed&list_uids=10863256&dopt=Abstract

Additional Web Resources

A number of additional Web sites offer encyclopedic information covering CAM and related topics. The following is a representative sample:

- Alternative Medicine Foundation, Inc.: **http://www.herbmed.org/**
- AOL: **http://search.aol.com/cat.adp?id=169&layer=&from=subcats**
- Chinese Medicine: **http://www.newcenturynutrition.com/**
- Family Village: **http://www.familyvillage.wisc.edu/med_altn.htm**
- Google: **http://directory.google.com/Top/Health/Alternative/**

- Open Directory Project: **http://dmoz.org/Health/Alternative/**
- TPN.com: **http://www.tnp.com/**
- Yahoo.com: **http://dir.yahoo.com/Health/Alternative_Medicine/**
- WebMD®Health: **http://my.webmd.com/drugs_and_herbs**
- WholeHealthMD.com:
  http://www.wholehealthmd.com/reflib/0,1529,,00.html

The following is a specific Web list relating to tinnitus; please note that any particular subject below may indicate either a therapeutic use, or a contraindication (potential danger), and does not reflect an official recommendation:

- **General Overview**

    Iron-Deficiency Anemia
    Source: Healthnotes, Inc.; www.healthnotes.com

    Ménière's Disease
    Source: Healthnotes, Inc.; www.healthnotes.com

    Tinnitus
    Source: Healthnotes, Inc.; www.healthnotes.com

    Vertigo
    Source: Healthnotes, Inc.; www.healthnotes.com

- **Alternative Therapy**

    Acupuncture
    Source: Healthnotes, Inc.; www.healthnotes.com

    Acupuncture
    Source: WholeHealthMD.com, LLC.; www.wholehealthmd.com
    Hyperlink:
    http://www.wholehealthmd.com/refshelf/substances_view/0,1525,663,00.html

    Biofeedback
    Source: WholeHealthMD.com, LLC.; www.wholehealthmd.com

Hyperlink:
http://www.wholehealthmd.com/refshelf/substances_view/0,1525,675,00.html

Craniosacral Therapy
Source: WholeHealthMD.com, LLC.; www.wholehealthmd.com
Hyperlink:
http://www.wholehealthmd.com/refshelf/substances_view/0,1525,685,00.html

Mind & Body Medicine
Source: Integrative Medicine Communications; www.drkoop.com

- **Chinese Medicine**

    ### Anshen Buxin Wan
    Alternative names: Anshen Buxin Pills
    Source: Pharmacopoeia Commission of the Ministry of Health, People's Republic of China

    ### Bushen Yinao Pian
    Alternative names: Bushen Yinao Tablets
    Source: Pharmacopoeia Commission of the Ministry of Health, People's Republic of China

    ### Cishi
    Alternative names: Magnetite; Magnetitum
    Source: Chinese Materia Medica

    ### Dabuyin Wan
    Alternative names: Dabuyin Pills
    Source: Pharmacopoeia Commission of the Ministry of Health, People's Republic of China

    ### Daige San
    Alternative names: Daige Powder
    Source: Pharmacopoeia Commission of the Ministry of Health, People's Republic of China

    ### Danggui Longhui Wan
    Alternative names: Danggui Longhui Pills
    Source: Pharmacopoeia Commission of the Ministry of Health, People's Republic of China

Dihuang
Alternative names: Digitalis Leaf; Yangdihuangye; Folium Digitalis
Source: Chinese Materia Medica

Erlong Zuoci Wan
Alternative names: Erlong Zuoci Pills; Erlong Zuoci Wan (Er Long Zuo Ci Wan)
Source: Pharmacopoeia Commission of the Ministry of Health, People's Republic of China

Erzhi Wan
Alternative names: Erzhi Pills; Erzhi Wan (Er Zhi Wan)
Source: Pharmacopoeia Commission of the Ministry of Health, People's Republic of China

Gengnian'an Pian
Alternative names: Gengnian'an Tablets
Source: Pharmacopoeia Commission of the Ministry of Health, People's Republic of China

Gouqizi
Alternative names: Barbary Wolfberry Fruit; Fructus Lycii
Source: Chinese Materia Medica

Gusuibu
Alternative names: Fortune's Drynaria Rhizome; Rhizoma Drynariae
Source: Chinese Materia Medica

Heizhima
Alternative names: Black Sesame; Semen Sesami Nigrum
Source: Chinese Materia Medica

Heizhongcaozi
Alternative names: Fennelflower Seed; Semen Nigellae
Source: Chinese Materia Medica

Heshi
Alternative names: Wild Carrot Fruit; Nanheshi; Fructus Carotae
Source: Chinese Materia Medica

Heshouwu
Alternative names: Fleeceflower Root; Radix Polygoni Multiflori
Source: Chinese Materia Medica

Longdan Xiegan Wan
Alternative names: Longdan Xiegan Pills
Source: Pharmacopoeia Commission of the Ministry of Health, People's Republic of China

Lurong
Alternative names: Hairy Deer-horn (Hairy Antler); Cornu Cervi Pantotrichum
Source: Chinese Materia Medica

Maiwei Dihuang Wan
Alternative names: Maiwei Dihuang Pills
Source: Pharmacopoeia Commission of the Ministry of Health, People's Republic of China

Mohanlian
Alternative names: Yerbadetajo Herb; Herba Ecliptae
Source: Chinese Materia Medica

Muli
Alternative names: Oyster Shell; Concha Ostreae
Source: Chinese Materia Medica

Nuzhenzi
Alternative names: Glossy Privet Fruit; Fructus Ligustri Lucidi
Source: Chinese Materia Medica

Qingning Wan
Alternative names: Qingning Pills
Source: Pharmacopoeia Commission of the Ministry of Health, People's Republic of China

Sangshen
Alternative names: Mulberry Fruit; Fructus Mori
Source: Chinese Materia Medica

Shanzhuyu
Alternative names: Asiatic Cornelian Cherry Fruit; Fructus Corni
Source: Chinese Materia Medica

Shenrong Guben Pian
Alternative names: Shenrong Guben Tablets; Shenrong Guben Pian (Shen Rong Gu Ben Pi An)
Source: Pharmacopoeia Commission of the Ministry of Health, People's Republic of China

Shouwu Wan
Alternative names: Shouwu Pills; Shouwu Wan (Shou Wu Wan)
Source: Pharmacopoeia Commission of the Ministry of Health, People's Republic of China

Shudihuang
Alternative names: Prepared Rehmannia Root; Radix Rehmanniae Preparata
Source: Chinese Materia Medica

Suoyang Gujing Wan
Alternative names: Suoyang Gujing Pills; Suoyang Gujing Wan (Suo Yang Gu Jing Wan)
Source: Pharmacopoeia Commission of the Ministry of Health, People's Republic of China

Tusizi
Alternative names: Dodder Seed; Semen Cuseutae
Source: Chinese Materia Medica

Zhiheshouwu
Alternative names: Prepared FLeeceflower Root; Radix Polygoni Multiflori Preparata
Source: Chinese Materia Medica

- Homeopathy

    ### Actaea Racemosa
    Source: Healthnotes, Inc.; www.healthnotes.com

    ### Calcarea Carbonica
    Source: Healthnotes, Inc.; www.healthnotes.com

    ### Carbo Vegetabilis
    Source: Healthnotes, Inc.; www.healthnotes.com

China (chinchona)
Source: Healthnotes, Inc.; www.healthnotes.com

Chininum Sulphuricum
Source: Healthnotes, Inc.; www.healthnotes.com

Cimicifuga
Source: Healthnotes, Inc.; www.healthnotes.com

Graphites
Source: Healthnotes, Inc.; www.healthnotes.com

Kali Carbonicum
Source: Healthnotes, Inc.; www.healthnotes.com

Lycopodium
Source: Healthnotes, Inc.; www.healthnotes.com

Natrum Salicylicum
Source: Healthnotes, Inc.; www.healthnotes.com

Salicylic Acid
Source: Healthnotes, Inc.; www.healthnotes.com

- **Herbs and Supplements**

    Black Cohosh
    Source: Prima Communications, Inc.www.personalhealthzone.com

    Feverfew
    Source: The Canadian Internet Directory for Holistic Help, WellNet, Health and Wellness Network; www.wellnet.ca

    Ginkgo
    Alternative names: Ginkgo biloba
    Source: Alternative Medicine Foundation, Inc.;
    www.amfoundation.org

    Ginkgo
    Source: Prima Communications, Inc.www.personalhealthzone.com

Ginkgo
Source: The Canadian Internet Directory for Holistic Help, WellNet, Health and Wellness Network; www.wellnet.ca

Ginkgo Biloba
Source: Healthnotes, Inc.; www.healthnotes.com

Ginkgo Biloba
Source: Integrative Medicine Communications; www.drkoop.com

Ginkgo Biloba
Source: WholeHealthMD.com, LLC.; www.wholehealthmd.com
Hyperlink:
http://www.wholehealthmd.com/refshelf/substances_view/0,1525,788,00.html

Ligustrum
Alternative names: Ligustrum lucidum
Source: Healthnotes, Inc.; www.healthnotes.com

Maidenhair Tree
Source: Integrative Medicine Communications; www.drkoop.com

Melatonin
Source: Healthnotes, Inc.; www.healthnotes.com

Melatonin
Source: WholeHealthMD.com, LLC.; www.wholehealthmd.com
Hyperlink:
http://www.wholehealthmd.com/refshelf/substances_view/0,1525,804,00.html

Plantago Psyllium
Alternative names: Psyllium, Ispaghula; Plantago psyllium/ovata
Source: Alternative Medicine Foundation, Inc.;
www.amfoundation.org

Salsalate
Source: Healthnotes, Inc.; www.healthnotes.com

Uncaria Asian
Alternative names: Asian species; Uncaria sp.
Source: Alternative Medicine Foundation, Inc.; www.amfoundation.org

White Willow Bark
Source: WholeHealthMD.com, LLC.; www.wholehealthmd.com
Hyperlink: http://www.wholehealthmd.com/refshelf/substances_view/0,1525,10069,00.html

Willow Bark
Alternative names: There are several species of willow includingSalix alba, Salix nigra, Salix fragilis, Salix purpurea, Salix babylonica, White Willow, European Willow, Black Willow, Pussy Willow, Crack Willow, Purple Willow, Weeping Willow, Liu-zhi
Source: Integrative Medicine Communications; www.drkoop.com

General References

A good place to find general background information on CAM is the National Library of Medicine. It has prepared within the MEDLINEplus system an information topic page dedicated to complementary and alternative medicine. To access this page, go to the MEDLINEplus site at: **www.nlm.nih.gov/medlineplus/alternativemedicine.html.** This Web site provides a general overview of various topics and can lead to a number of general sources. The following additional references describe, in broad terms, alternative and complementary medicine (sorted alphabetically by title; hyperlinks provide rankings, information, and reviews at Amazon.com):

- **No More Amoxicillin: Preventing and Treating Ear and Respiratory Infections Without Antibiotics** by Mary Ann Block; Paperback: 144 pages; (August 1998), Kensington Publishing Corp.; ISBN: 1575663163; **http://www.amazon.com/exec/obidos/ASIN/1575663163/icongroupinterna**

- **Alternative Medicine for Dummies** by James Dillard (Author); Audio Cassette, Abridged edition (1998), Harper Audio; ISBN: 0694520659; **http://www.amazon.com/exec/obidos/ASIN/0694520659/icongroupinterna**

- **Complementary and Alternative Medicine Secrets** by W. Kohatsu (Editor); Hardcover (2001), Hanley & Belfus; ISBN: 1560534400;

http://www.amazon.com/exec/obidos/ASIN/1560534400/icongroupinterna

- **Dictionary of Alternative Medicine** by J. C. Segen; Paperback-2nd edition (2001), Appleton & Lange; ISBN: 0838516211;
  http://www.amazon.com/exec/obidos/ASIN/0838516211/icongroupinterna

- **Eat, Drink, and Be Healthy: The Harvard Medical School Guide to Healthy Eating** by Walter C. Willett, MD, et al; Hardcover - 352 pages (2001), Simon & Schuster; ISBN: 0684863375;
  http://www.amazon.com/exec/obidos/ASIN/0684863375/icongroupinterna

- **Encyclopedia of Natural Medicine, Revised 2nd Edition** by Michael T. Murray, Joseph E. Pizzorno; Paperback - 960 pages, 2nd Rev edition (1997), Prima Publishing; ISBN: 0761511571;
  http://www.amazon.com/exec/obidos/ASIN/0761511571/icongroupinterna

- **Integrative Medicine: An Introduction to the Art & Science of Healing** by Andrew Weil (Author); Audio Cassette, Unabridged edition (2001), Sounds True; ISBN: 1564558541;
  http://www.amazon.com/exec/obidos/ASIN/1564558541/icongroupinterna

- **New Encyclopedia of Herbs & Their Uses** by Deni Bown; Hardcover - 448 pages, Revised edition (2001), DK Publishing; ISBN: 078948031X;
  http://www.amazon.com/exec/obidos/ASIN/078948031X/icongroupinterna

- **Textbook of Complementary and Alternative Medicine** by Wayne B. Jonas; Hardcover (2003), Lippincott, Williams & Wilkins; ISBN: 0683044370;
  http://www.amazon.com/exec/obidos/ASIN/0683044370/icongroupinterna

For additional information on complementary and alternative medicine, ask your doctor or write to:

National Center for Complementary and Alternative Medicine Clearinghouse
National Institutes of Health
P. O. Box 8218
Silver Spring, MD 20907-8218

Vocabulary Builder

The following vocabulary builder gives definitions of words used in this chapter that have not been defined in previous chapters:

EMG: Recording of electrical activity or currents in a muscle. [NIH]

APPENDIX B. RESEARCHING NUTRITION

Overview

Since the time of Hippocrates, doctors have understood the importance of diet and nutrition to patients' health and well-being. Since then, they have accumulated an impressive archive of studies and knowledge dedicated to this subject. Based on their experience, doctors and healthcare providers may recommend particular dietary supplements to patients with tinnitus. Any dietary recommendation is based on a patient's age, body mass, gender, lifestyle, eating habits, food preferences, and health condition. It is therefore likely that different patients with tinnitus may be given different recommendations. Some recommendations may be directly related to tinnitus, while others may be more related to the patient's general health. These recommendations, themselves, may differ from what official sources recommend for the average person.

In this chapter we will begin by briefly reviewing the essentials of diet and nutrition that will broadly frame more detailed discussions of tinnitus. We will then show you how to find studies dedicated specifically to nutrition and tinnitus.

Food and Nutrition: General Principles

What Are Essential Foods?

Food is generally viewed by official sources as consisting of six basic elements: (1) fluids, (2) carbohydrates, (3) protein, (4) fats, (5) vitamins, and (6) minerals. Consuming a combination of these elements is considered to be a healthy diet:

- **Fluids** are essential to human life as 80-percent of the body is composed of water. Water is lost via urination, sweating, diarrhea, vomiting, diuretics (drugs that increase urination), caffeine, and physical exertion.

- **Carbohydrates** are the main source for human energy (thermoregulation) and the bulk of typical diets. They are mostly classified as being either simple or complex. Simple carbohydrates include sugars which are often consumed in the form of cookies, candies, or cakes. Complex carbohydrates consist of starches and dietary fibers. Starches are consumed in the form of pastas, breads, potatoes, rice, and other foods. Soluble fibers can be eaten in the form of certain vegetables, fruits, oats, and legumes. Insoluble fibers include brown rice, whole grains, certain fruits, wheat bran and legumes.

- **Proteins** are eaten to build and repair human tissues. Some foods that are high in protein are also high in fat and calories. Food sources for protein include nuts, meat, fish, cheese, and other dairy products.

- **Fats** are consumed for both energy and the absorption of certain vitamins. There are many types of fats, with many general publications recommending the intake of unsaturated fats or those low in cholesterol.

Vitamins and minerals are fundamental to human health, growth, and, in some cases, disease prevention. Most are consumed in your diet (exceptions being vitamins K and D which are produced by intestinal bacteria and sunlight on the skin, respectively). Each vitamin and mineral plays a different role in health. The following outlines essential vitamins:

- **Vitamin A** is important to the health of your eyes, hair, bones, and skin; sources of vitamin A include foods such as eggs, carrots, and cantaloupe.

- **Vitamin B^1**, also known as thiamine, is important for your nervous system and energy production; food sources for thiamine include meat, peas, fortified cereals, bread, and whole grains.

- **Vitamin B^2**, also known as riboflavin, is important for your nervous system and muscles, but is also involved in the release of proteins from nutrients; food sources for riboflavin include dairy products, leafy vegetables, meat, and eggs.

- **Vitamin B^3**, also known as niacin, is important for healthy skin and helps the body use energy; food sources for niacin include peas, peanuts, fish, and whole grains

- **Vitamin B^6**, also known as pyridoxine, is important for the regulation of cells in the nervous system and is vital for blood formation; food sources for pyridoxine include bananas, whole grains, meat, and fish.

- **Vitamin B¹²** is vital for a healthy nervous system and for the growth of red blood cells in bone marrow; food sources for vitamin B¹² include yeast, milk, fish, eggs, and meat.
- **Vitamin C** allows the body's immune system to fight various diseases, strengthens body tissue, and improves the body's use of iron; food sources for vitamin C include a wide variety of fruits and vegetables.
- **Vitamin D** helps the body absorb calcium which strengthens bones and teeth; food sources for vitamin D include oily fish and dairy products.
- **Vitamin E** can help protect certain organs and tissues from various degenerative diseases; food sources for vitamin E include margarine, vegetables, eggs, and fish.
- **Vitamin K** is essential for bone formation and blood clotting; common food sources for vitamin K include leafy green vegetables.
- **Folic Acid** maintains healthy cells and blood and, when taken by a pregnant woman, can prevent her fetus from developing neural tube defects; food sources for folic acid include nuts, fortified breads, leafy green vegetables, and whole grains.

It should be noted that it is possible to overdose on certain vitamins which become toxic if consumed in excess (e.g. vitamin A, D, E and K).

Like vitamins, minerals are chemicals that are required by the body to remain in good health. Because the human body does not manufacture these chemicals internally, we obtain them from food and other dietary sources. The more important minerals include:

- **Calcium** is needed for healthy bones, teeth, and muscles, but also helps the nervous system function; food sources for calcium include dry beans, peas, eggs, and dairy products.
- **Chromium** is helpful in regulating sugar levels in blood; food sources for chromium include egg yolks, raw sugar, cheese, nuts, beets, whole grains, and meat.
- **Fluoride** is used by the body to help prevent tooth decay and to reinforce bone strength; sources of fluoride include drinking water and certain brands of toothpaste.
- **Iodine** helps regulate the body's use of energy by synthesizing into the hormone thyroxine; food sources include leafy green vegetables, nuts, egg yolks, and red meat.

- **Iron** helps maintain muscles and the formation of red blood cells and certain proteins; food sources for iron include meat, dairy products, eggs, and leafy green vegetables.

- **Magnesium** is important for the production of DNA, as well as for healthy teeth, bones, muscles, and nerves; food sources for magnesium include dried fruit, dark green vegetables, nuts, and seafood.

- **Phosphorous** is used by the body to work with calcium to form bones and teeth; food sources for phosphorous include eggs, meat, cereals, and dairy products.

- **Selenium** primarily helps maintain normal heart and liver functions; food sources for selenium include wholegrain cereals, fish, meat, and dairy products.

- **Zinc** helps wounds heal, the formation of sperm, and encourage rapid growth and energy; food sources include dried beans, shellfish, eggs, and nuts.

The United States government periodically publishes recommended diets and consumption levels of the various elements of food. Again, your doctor may encourage deviations from the average official recommendation based on your specific condition. To learn more about basic dietary guidelines, visit the Web site: **http://www.health.gov/dietaryguidelines/**. Based on these guidelines, many foods are required to list the nutrition levels on the food's packaging. Labeling Requirements are listed at the following site maintained by the Food and Drug Administration: **http://www.cfsan.fda.gov/~dms/lab-cons.html**. When interpreting these requirements, the government recommends that consumers become familiar with the following abbreviations before reading FDA literature:[40]

- **DVs (Daily Values):** A new dietary reference term that will appear on the food label. It is made up of two sets of references, DRVs and RDIs.

- **DRVs (Daily Reference Values):** A set of dietary references that applies to fat, saturated fat, cholesterol, carbohydrate, protein, fiber, sodium, and potassium.

- **RDIs (Reference Daily Intakes):** A set of dietary references based on the Recommended Dietary Allowances for essential vitamins and minerals and, in selected groups, protein. The name "RDI" replaces the term "U.S. RDA."

---

[40] Adapted from the FDA: **http://www.fda.gov/fdac/special/foodlabel/dvs.html**.

- **RDAs (Recommended Dietary Allowances):** A set of estimated nutrient allowances established by the National Academy of Sciences. It is updated periodically to reflect current scientific knowledge.

What Are Dietary Supplements?[41]

Dietary supplements are widely available through many commercial sources, including health food stores, grocery stores, pharmacies, and by mail. Dietary supplements are provided in many forms including tablets, capsules, powders, gel-tabs, extracts, and liquids. Historically in the United States, the most prevalent type of dietary supplement was a multivitamin/mineral tablet or capsule that was available in pharmacies, either by prescription or "over the counter." Supplements containing strictly herbal preparations were less widely available. Currently in the United States, a wide array of supplement products are available, including vitamin, mineral, other nutrients, and botanical supplements as well as ingredients and extracts of animal and plant origin.

The Office of Dietary Supplements (ODS) of the National Institutes of Health is the official agency of the United States which has the expressed goal of acquiring "new knowledge to help prevent, detect, diagnose, and treat disease and disability, from the rarest genetic disorder to the common cold."[42] According to the ODS, dietary supplements can have an important impact on the prevention and management of disease and on the maintenance of health.[43] The ODS notes that considerable research on the effects of dietary supplements has been conducted in Asia and Europe where the use of plant products, in particular, has a long tradition. However, the overwhelming majority of supplements have not been studied scientifically. To explore the role of dietary supplements in the improvement of health care, the ODS plans, organizes, and supports conferences, workshops, and symposia on scientific topics related to dietary supplements. The ODS often works in conjunction with other NIH Institutes and Centers, other

---

[41] This discussion has been adapted from the NIH: **http://ods.od.nih.gov/showpage.aspx?pageid=46**.

[42] Contact: The Office of Dietary Supplements, National Institutes of Health, Building 31, Room 1B29, 31 Center Drive, MSC 2086, Bethesda, Maryland 20892-2086, Tel: (301) 435-2920, Fax: (301) 480-1845, E-mail: ods@nih.gov.

[43] Adapted from **http://ods.od.nih.gov/showpage.aspx?pageid=2**. The Dietary Supplement Health and Education Act defines dietary supplements as "a product (other than tobacco) intended to supplement the diet that bears or contains one or more of the following dietary ingredients: a vitamin, mineral, amino acid, herb or other botanical; or a dietary substance for use to supplement the diet by increasing the total dietary intake; or a concentrate, metabolite, constituent, extract, or combination of any ingredient described above; and intended for ingestion in the form of a capsule, powder, softgel, or gelcap, and not represented as a conventional food or as a sole item of a meal or the diet."

government agencies, professional organizations, and public advocacy groups.

To learn more about official information on dietary supplements, visit the ODS site at **http://dietary-supplements.info.nih.gov/**. Or contact:

The Office of Dietary Supplements
National Institutes of Health
Building 31, Room 1B29
31 Center Drive, MSC 2086
Bethesda, Maryland 20892-2086
Tel: (301) 435-2920
Fax: (301) 480-1845
E-mail: ods@nih.gov

Finding Studies on Tinnitus

The NIH maintains an office dedicated to patient nutrition and diet. The National Institutes of Health's Office of Dietary Supplements (ODS) offers a searchable bibliographic database called the IBIDS (International Bibliographic Information on Dietary Supplements). The IBIDS contains over 460,000 scientific citations and summaries about dietary supplements and nutrition as well as references to published international, scientific literature on dietary supplements such as vitamins, minerals, and botanicals.[44] IBIDS is available to the public free of charge through the ODS Internet page: **http://ods.od.nih.gov/databases/ibids.html**.

After entering the search area, you have three choices: (1) IBIDS Consumer Database, (2) Full IBIDS Database, or (3) Peer Reviewed Citations Only. We recommend that you start with the Consumer Database. While you may not find references for the topics that are of most interest to you, check back periodically as this database is frequently updated. More studies can be found by searching the Full IBIDS Database. Healthcare professionals and researchers generally use the third option, which lists peer-reviewed citations. In all cases, we suggest that you take advantage of the "Advanced Search" option that allows you to retrieve up to 100 fully explained

---

[44] Adapted from **http://ods.od.nih.gov**. IBIDS is produced by the Office of Dietary Supplements (ODS) at the National Institutes of Health to assist the public, healthcare providers, educators, and researchers in locating credible, scientific information on dietary supplements. IBIDS was developed and will be maintained through an interagency partnership with the Food and Nutrition Information Center of the National Agricultural Library, U.S. Department of Agriculture.

references in a comprehensive format. Type "tinnitus" (or synonyms) into the search box. To narrow the search, you can also select the "Title" field.

The following information is typical of that found when using the "Full IBIDS Database" when searching using "tinnitus" (or a synonym):

- **A review of randomized clinical trials in tinnitus.**
  Author(s): Department of Otolaryngology-Head and Neck Surgery, The University of Texas Health Science Center at San Antonio, 78284-7777, USA.
  Source: Dobie, R A Laryngoscope. 1999 August; 109(8): 1202-11 0023-852X

- **Acupuncture in the management of tinnitus: a placebo-controlled study.**
  Author(s): Department of Audiology, Sahlgrenska University Hospital, Gothenburg, Sweden.
  Source: Axelsson, A Andersson, S Gu, L D Audiology. 1994 Nov-December; 33(6): 351-60 0020-6091

- **Are there any studies showing whether ginkgo biloba is effective for tinnitus (ringing in the ears)?**
  Source: Feinberg, A W Health-News. 2003 January; 9(1): 12 1081-5880

- **Assessing tinnitus and prospective tinnitus therapeutics using a psychophysical animal model.**
  Author(s): Department of Surgery, Southern Illinois University School of Medicine, Springfield 62794, USA. cbauer@siumed.edu
  Source: Bauer, C A Brozoski, T J J-Assoc-Res-Otolaryngol. 2001 March; 2(1): 54-64 1525-3961

- **Audiological and psychological characteristics of a group of tinnitus sufferers, prior to tinnitus management training.**
  Author(s): School of Communication Disorders, La Trobe University, Australia.
  Source: Dineen, R Doyle, J Bench, J Br-J-Audiol. 1997 February; 31(1): 27-38 0300-5364

- **Cerebellar arteriovenous malformation with facial paralysis, hearing loss, and tinnitus: a case report.**
  Author(s): Department of Otolaryngology, Kobe City General Hospital, Japan. Masahiro.Kikuchi@ma2.seikyou.ne.jp
  Source: Kikuchi, M Funabiki, K Hasebe, S Takahashi, H Otol-Neurotol. 2002 September; 23(5): 723-6 1531-7129

- **Detrimental effects of alcohol on tinnitus.**
  Author(s): Welsh Hearing Institute, University Hospital of Wales, Heath Park, Cardiff, UK.
  Source: Stephens, D Clin-Otolaryngol. 1999 April; 24(2): 114-6 0307-7772

- **Double-blind study on the effectiveness of a bioflavonoid in the control of tinnitus in otosclerosis.**
  Author(s): Department of Otorhinolaryngology, Semmelweis University Medical School, Budapest, Hungary.
  Source: Sziklai, I Komora, V Ribari, O Acta-Chir-Hung. 1992-93; 33(1-2): 101-7 0231-4614

- **Effect of melatonin on tinnitus.**
  Author(s): Ear Research Foundation, Sarasota, Florida 34239, USA.
  Source: Rosenberg, S I Silverstein, H Rowan, P T Olds, M J Laryngoscope. 1998 March; 108(3): 305-10 0023-852X

- **Effect of traditional Chinese acupuncture on severe tinnitus: a double-blind, placebo-controlled, clinical investigation with open therapeutic control.**
  Author(s): Department of Audiology, Vejle Hospital, Denmark.
  Source: Vilholm, O J Moller, K Jorgensen, K Br-J-Audiol. 1998 June; 32(3): 197-204 0300-5364

- **Effectiveness of Ginkgo biloba in treating tinnitus: double blind, placebo controlled trial.**
  Author(s): Pharmacology Department, Division of Neuroscience, University of Birmingham, Birmingham B15 2TT, UK. s.j.drew@bham.ac.uk
  Source: Drew, S Davies, E BMJ. 2001 January 13; 322(7278): 73 0959-8138

- **Efficacy of oral oxpentifylline in the management of idiopathic tinnitus.**
  Author(s): ENT Department, Lewisham Hospital, London, UK.
  Source: Salama, N Y Bhatia, P Robb, P J ORL-J-Otorhinolaryngol-Relat-Spec. 1989; 51(5): 300-4 0301-1569

- **Evaluation of amino-oxyacetic acid as a palliative in tinnitus.**
  Author(s): Department of Pharmacology, Tulane University School of Medicine, New Orleans, LA.
  Source: Guth, P S Risey, J Briner, W Blair, P Reed, H T Bryant, G Norris, C Housley, G Miller, R Ann-Otol-Rhinol-Laryngol. 1990 January; 99(1): 74-9 0003-4894

- **Evaluation of tinnitus patients by peroral multi-drug treatment.**
  Author(s): Division of Clinical Otology, University Hospital, University of Tokushima, School of Medicine, Japan.
  Source: Ohsaki, K Ueno, M Zheng, H X Wang, Q C Nishizaki, K Nobuto, Y Fujimura, T Auris-Nasus-Larynx. 1998 May; 25(2): 149-54 0385-8146

- **Gabapentin for the treatment of tinnitus: a case report.**
  Author(s): Pain Institute of Northeast Florida, 2021 Kingsley Ave., Suite 102, Orange Park, FL 32073, USA.

Source: Zapp, J J Ear-Nose-Throat-J. 2001 February; 80(2): 114-6 0145-5613

- **Ginkgo biloba extract for the treatment of tinnitus.**
  Author(s): Department of Audiology, Sahlgren's Hospital, Goteborg, Sweden.
  Source: Holgers, K M Axelsson, A Pringle, I Audiology. 1994 Mar-April; 33(2): 85-92 0020-6091

- **Ginkgo biloba for tinnitus: a review.**
  Author(s): Department of Complementary Medicine, School of Postgraduate Medicine and Health Sciences, University of Exeter, UK. E.Ernst@exeter.ac.uk
  Source: Ernst, E Stevinson, C Clin-Otolaryngol. 1999 June; 24(3): 164-7 0307-7772

- **Glutamic acid in the treatment of tinnitus.**
  Source: McIlwain, J C J-Laryngol-Otol. 1987 June; 101(6): 552-4 0022-2151

- **Intradermal injection vs. oral treatment of tinnitus.**
  Author(s): Dept. of Medical-Surgical Specialities, Section of Otorhinolaringology, Padua University, via D. Monegario 6/c, 35127 Padova, Italie.
  Source: Savastano, M Tomaselli, F Maggiori, S Therapie. 2001 Jul-August; 56(4): 403-7 0040-5957

- **Misoprostol for tinnitus.**
  Author(s): Pharmaceutical Services, University of California, San Francisco 94143, USA.
  Source: Crinnion, C L McCart, G M Ann-Pharmacother. 1995 Jul-August; 29(7-8): 782-4 1060-0280

- **Neurophysiologic mechanisms of tinnitus.**
  Author(s): Department of Otolaryngology--Head and Neck Surgery, Wayne State University, Detroit, Michigan 48201, USA.
  Source: Kaltenbach, J A J-Am-Acad-Audiol. 2000 March; 11(3): 125-37 1050-0545

- **Progressive sensorineural hearing loss, subjective tinnitus and vertigo caused by elevated blood lipids.**
  Author(s): Pulec Ear Clinic and Ear International, Los Angeles, California, USA.
  Source: Pulec, J L Pulec, M B Mendoza, I Ear-Nose-Throat-J. 1997 October; 76(10): 716-20, 725-6, 728 passim 0145-5613

- **Quinine-induced tinnitus in rats.**
  Author(s): Department of Surgery, Yale University School of Medicine, New Haven, Conn.

Source: Jastreboff, P J Brennan, J F Sasaki, C T Arch-Otolaryngol-Head-Neck-Surg. 1991 October; 117(10): 1162-6 0886-4470

- **Support for the central theory of tinnitus generation: a military epidemiological study.**
  Author(s): Institute for Noise Hazards Research and Evoked Potentials Laboratory, Medical Corps, Petach-Tikva, Israel. attiasj@clalit.org.il
  Source: Attias, J Reshef, I Shemesh, Z Salomon, G Int-J-Audiol. 2002 July; 41(5): 301-7 1499-2027

- **Synthetic prostaglandin E1 misoprostol as a treatment for tinnitus.**
  Author(s): House Ear Institute, Los Angeles, Calif.
  Source: Briner, W House, J O'Leary, M Arch-Otolaryngol-Head-Neck-Surg. 1993 June; 119(6): 652-4 0886-4470

- **The effect of nicotinamide on tinnitus: a double-blind controlled study.**
  Source: Hulshof, J H Vermeij, P Clin-Otolaryngol. 1987 June; 12(3): 211-4 0307-7772

- **The efficacy of Arlevert therapy for vertigo and tinnitus.**
  Author(s): Department of Otolaryngology, University Hospital, Brno-Bohunice, Czech Republic.
  Source: Novotny, M Kostrica, R Cirek, Z Int-Tinnitus-J. 1999; 5(1): 60-2 0946-5448

- **The efficacy of Ginkgo special extract EGb 761 in patients with tinnitus.**
  Author(s): Allgemeines Krankenhaus St. Georg. Hamburg, Germany.
  Source: Morgenstern, C Biermann, E Int-J-Clin-Pharmacol-Ther. 2002 May; 40(5): 188-97 0946-1965

- **The efficacy of medication on tinnitus due to acute acoustic trauma.**
  Author(s): Department of Otorhinolaryngology-Head & Neck Surgery, Aristotelian University of Thessaloniki, General District Hospital AHEPA, Greece. kdmarcos@axd.forthnet.gr
  Source: Markou, K Lalaki, P Barbetakis, N Tsalighopoulos, M G Daniilidis, I Scand-Audiol-Suppl. 2001; (52): 180-4 0107-8593

- **The role of zinc in management of tinnitus.**
  Author(s): Department of ORL and HNS, Gulhane Medical School, Etlik, 06018 Ankara, Turkey. syetiser@yahoo.com
  Source: Yetiser, S Tosun, F Satar, B Arslanhan, M Akcam, T Ozkaptan, Y Auris-Nasus-Larynx. 2002 October; 29(4): 329-33 0385-8146

- **Tinnitus-induced weight loss in rats. An animal model for tinnitus research.**
  Author(s): University ENT Department, Inselspital, Bern, Switzerland.

Source: Kellerhals, B Zogg, R ORL-J-Otorhinolaryngol-Relat-Spec. 1991; 53(6): 331-4 0301-1569

- **Transitory endolymph leakage induced hearing loss and tinnitus: depolarization, biphasic shortening and loss of electromotility of outer hair cells.**
Author(s): Department of Otolaryngology, University of Tubingen, Germany.
Source: Zenner, H P Reuter, G Zimmermann, U Gitter, A H Fermin, C LePage, E L Eur-Arch-Otorhinolaryngol. 1994; 251(3): 143-53 0937-4477

- **Valproate-induced tinnitus misinterpreted as psychotic symptoms.**
Author(s): Department of Psychiatry, Montgomery VA Medical Center, USA.
Source: Reeves, R R Mustain, D W Pendarvis, J E South-Med-J. 2000 October; 93(10): 1030-1 0038-4348

- **Vitamin B12 deficiency in patients with chronic-tinnitus and noise-induced hearing loss.**
Author(s): Institute of Noise Hazards Research and Evoked Potentials Laboratory, IDF, Chaim-Sheba Medical Center, Ramat-Gan, Israel.
Source: Shemesh, Z Attias, J Ornan, M Shapira, N Shahar, A Am-J-Otolaryngol. 1993 Mar-April; 14(2): 94-9 0196-0709

- **Zinc and diet for tinnitus.**
Source: DeBartolo, H M Am-J-Otol. 1989 May; 10(3): 256 0192-9763

- **Zinc in the management of tinnitus. Placebo-controlled trial.**
Author(s): Audiological and ENT Department, University Hospital of Aarhus, Denmark.
Source: Paaske, P B Pedersen, C B Kjems, G Sam, I L Ann-Otol-Rhinol-Laryngol. 1991 August; 100(8): 647-9 0003-4894

Federal Resources on Nutrition

In addition to the IBIDS, the United States Department of Health and Human Services (HHS) and the United States Department of Agriculture (USDA) provide many sources of information on general nutrition and health. Recommended resources include:

- healthfinder®, HHS's gateway to health information, including diet and nutrition:
http://www.healthfinder.gov/scripts/SearchContext.asp?topic=238&page=0

- The United States Department of Agriculture's Web site dedicated to nutrition information: **www.nutrition.gov**

- The Food and Drug Administration's Web site for federal food safety information: **www.foodsafety.gov**

- The National Action Plan on Overweight and Obesity sponsored by the United States Surgeon General: **http://www.surgeongeneral.gov/topics/obesity/**

- The Center for Food Safety and Applied Nutrition has an Internet site sponsored by the Food and Drug Administration and the Department of Health and Human Services: **http://vm.cfsan.fda.gov/**

- Center for Nutrition Policy and Promotion sponsored by the United States Department of Agriculture: **http://www.usda.gov/cnpp/**

- Food and Nutrition Information Center, National Agricultural Library sponsored by the United States Department of Agriculture: **http://www.nal.usda.gov/fnic/**

- Food and Nutrition Service sponsored by the United States Department of Agriculture: **http://www.fns.usda.gov/fns/**

Additional Web Resources

A number of additional Web sites offer encyclopedic information covering food and nutrition. The following is a representative sample:

- AOL: **http://search.aol.com/cat.adp?id=174&layer=&from=subcats**
- Family Village: **http://www.familyvillage.wisc.edu/med_nutrition.html**
- Google: **http://directory.google.com/Top/Health/Nutrition/**
- Open Directory Project: **http://dmoz.org/Health/Nutrition/**
- Yahoo.com: **http://dir.yahoo.com/Health/Nutrition/**
- WebMD®Health: **http://my.webmd.com/nutrition**
- WholeHealthMD.com: **http://www.wholehealthmd.com/reflib/0,1529,,00.html**

The following is a specific Web list relating to tinnitus; please note that any particular subject below may indicate either a therapeutic use, or a contraindication (potential danger), and does not reflect an official recommendation:

- **Vitamins**

    Folic Acid/Vitamin B
    Source: WholeHealthMD.com, LLC.; www.wholehealthmd.com
    Hyperlink:
    http://www.wholehealthmd.com/refshelf/substances_view/0,1525,936,00.html

    Niacin
    Source: WholeHealthMD.com, LLC.; www.wholehealthmd.com
    Hyperlink:
    http://www.wholehealthmd.com/refshelf/substances_view/0,1525,892,00.html

    Vitamin B
    Source: WholeHealthMD.com, LLC.; www.wholehealthmd.com
    Hyperlink:
    http://www.wholehealthmd.com/refshelf/substances_view/0,1525,10067,00.html

    Vitamin B12
    Source: Healthnotes, Inc.; www.healthnotes.com

    Vitamin B12
    Source: Prima Communications, Inc.www.personalhealthzone.com

- **Minerals**

    Magnesium
    Source: WholeHealthMD.com, LLC.; www.wholehealthmd.com
    Hyperlink:
    http://www.wholehealthmd.com/refshelf/substances_view/0,1525,890,00.html

    Manganese
    Source: Integrative Medicine Communications; www.drkoop.com

Vinpocetine
Source: WholeHealthMD.com, LLC.; www.wholehealthmd.com
Hyperlink:
http://www.wholehealthmd.com/refshelf/substances_view/0,1525,10065,00.html

Zinc
Source: Healthnotes, Inc.; www.healthnotes.com

Zinc
Source: Prima Communications, Inc.www.personalhealthzone.com

Zinc
Source: WholeHealthMD.com, LLC.; www.wholehealthmd.com
Hyperlink:
http://www.wholehealthmd.com/refshelf/substances_view/0,1525,10071,00.html

Zinc/Copper
Source: WholeHealthMD.com, LLC.; www.wholehealthmd.com
Hyperlink:
http://www.wholehealthmd.com/refshelf/substances_view/0,1525,938,00.html

- **Food and Diet**

  ### Wheat
  Source: Healthnotes, Inc.; www.healthnotes.com

Vocabulary Builder

The following vocabulary builder defines words used in the references in this chapter that have not been defined in previous chapters:

Consumption: Pulmonary tuberculosis. [NIH]

Sperm: The fecundating fluid of the male. [NIH]

Wound: Any interruption, by violence or by surgery, in the continuity of the external surface of the body or of the surface of any internal organ. [NIH]

APPENDIX C. FINDING MEDICAL LIBRARIES

Overview

At a medical library you can find medical texts and reference books, consumer health publications, specialty newspapers and magazines, as well as medical journals. In this Appendix, we show you how to quickly find a medical library in your area.

Preparation

Before going to the library, highlight the references mentioned in this sourcebook that you find interesting. Focus on those items that are not available via the Internet, and ask the reference librarian for help with your search. He or she may know of additional resources that could be helpful to you. Most importantly, your local public library and medical libraries have Interlibrary Loan programs with the National Library of Medicine (NLM), one of the largest medical collections in the world. According to the NLM, most of the literature in the general and historical collections of the National Library of Medicine is available on interlibrary loan to any library. NLM's interlibrary loan services are only available to libraries. If you would like to access NLM medical literature, then visit a library in your area that can request the publications for you.[45]

---

[45] Adapted from the NLM: http://www.nlm.nih.gov/psd/cas/interlibrary.html

Finding a Local Medical Library

The quickest method to locate medical libraries is to use the Internet-based directory published by the National Network of Libraries of Medicine (NN/LM). This network includes 4626 members and affiliates that provide many services to librarians, health professionals, and the public. To find a library in your area, simply visit **http://nnlm.gov/members/adv.html** or call 1-800-338-7657.

Medical Libraries in the U.S. and Canada

In addition to the NN/LM, the National Library of Medicine (NLM) lists a number of libraries with reference facilities that are open to the public. The following is the NLM's list and includes hyperlinks to each library's Web site. These Web pages can provide information on hours of operation and other restrictions. The list below is a small sample of libraries recommended by the National Library of Medicine (sorted alphabetically by name of the U.S. state or Canadian province where the library is located)[46]:

- **Alabama:** Health InfoNet of Jefferson County (Jefferson County Library Cooperative, Lister Hill Library of the Health Sciences), **http://www.uab.edu/infonet/**

- **Alabama:** Richard M. Scrushy Library (American Sports Medicine Institute)

- **Arizona:** Samaritan Regional Medical Center: The Learning Center (Samaritan Health System, Phoenix, Arizona), **http://www.samaritan.edu/library/bannerlibs.htm**

- **California:** Kris Kelly Health Information Center (St. Joseph Health System, Humboldt), **http://www.humboldt1.com/~kkhic/index.html**

- **California:** Community Health Library of Los Gatos, **http://www.healthlib.org/orgresources.html**

- **California:** Consumer Health Program and Services (CHIPS) (County of Los Angeles Public Library, Los Angeles County Harbor-UCLA Medical Center Library) - Carson, CA, **http://www.colapublib.org/services/chips.html**

- **California:** Gateway Health Library (Sutter Gould Medical Foundation)

- **California:** Health Library (Stanford University Medical Center), **http://www-med.stanford.edu/healthlibrary/**

---
[46] Abstracted from **http://www.nlm.nih.gov/medlineplus/libraries.html**.

- **California:** Patient Education Resource Center - Health Information and Resources (University of California, San Francisco), http://sfghdean.ucsf.edu/barnett/PERC/default.asp
- **California:** Redwood Health Library (Petaluma Health Care District), http://www.phcd.org/rdwdlib.html
- **California:** Los Gatos PlaneTree Health Library, http://planetreesanjose.org/
- **California:** Sutter Resource Library (Sutter Hospitals Foundation, Sacramento), http://suttermedicalcenter.org/library/
- **California:** Health Sciences Libraries (University of California, Davis), http://www.lib.ucdavis.edu/healthsci/
- **California:** ValleyCare Health Library & Ryan Comer Cancer Resource Center (ValleyCare Health System, Pleasanton), http://gaelnet.stmarys-ca.edu/other.libs/gbal/east/vchl.html
- **California:** Washington Community Health Resource Library (Fremont), http://www.healthlibrary.org/
- **Colorado:** William V. Gervasini Memorial Library (Exempla Healthcare), http://www.saintjosephdenver.org/yourhealth/libraries/
- **Connecticut:** Hartford Hospital Health Science Libraries (Hartford Hospital), http://www.harthosp.org/library/
- **Connecticut:** Healthnet: Connecticut Consumer Health Information Center (University of Connecticut Health Center, Lyman Maynard Stowe Library), http://library.uchc.edu/departm/hnet/
- **Connecticut:** Waterbury Hospital Health Center Library (Waterbury Hospital, Waterbury), http://www.waterburyhospital.com/library/consumer.shtml
- **Delaware:** Consumer Health Library (Christiana Care Health System, Eugene du Pont Preventive Medicine & Rehabilitation Institute, Wilmington), http://www.christianacare.org/health_guide/health_guide_pmri_health_info.cfm
- **Delaware:** Lewis B. Flinn Library (Delaware Academy of Medicine, Wilmington), http://www.delamed.org/chls.html
- **Georgia:** Family Resource Library (Medical College of Georgia, Augusta), http://cmc.mcg.edu/kids_families/fam_resources/fam_res_lib/frl.htm
- **Georgia:** Health Resource Center (Medical Center of Central Georgia, Macon), http://www.mccg.org/hrc/hrchome.asp

- **Hawaii:** Hawaii Medical Library: Consumer Health Information Service (Hawaii Medical Library, Honolulu), http://hml.org/CHIS/
- **Idaho:** DeArmond Consumer Health Library (Kootenai Medical Center, Coeur d'Alene), http://www.nicon.org/DeArmond/index.htm
- **Illinois:** Health Learning Center of Northwestern Memorial Hospital (Chicago), http://www.nmh.org/health_info/hlc.html
- **Illinois:** Medical Library (OSF Saint Francis Medical Center, Peoria), http://www.osfsaintfrancis.org/general/library/
- **Kentucky:** Medical Library - Services for Patients, Families, Students & the Public (Central Baptist Hospital, Lexington), http://www.centralbap.com/education/community/library.cfm
- **Kentucky:** University of Kentucky - Health Information Library (Chandler Medical Center, Lexington), http://www.mc.uky.edu/PatientEd/
- **Louisiana:** Alton Ochsner Medical Foundation Library (Alton Ochsner Medical Foundation, New Orleans), http://www.ochsner.org/library/
- **Louisiana:** Louisiana State University Health Sciences Center Medical Library-Shreveport, http://lib-sh.lsuhsc.edu/
- **Maine:** Franklin Memorial Hospital Medical Library (Franklin Memorial Hospital, Farmington), http://www.fchn.org/fmh/lib.htm
- **Maine:** Gerrish-True Health Sciences Library (Central Maine Medical Center, Lewiston), http://www.cmmc.org/library/library.html
- **Maine:** Hadley Parrot Health Science Library (Eastern Maine Healthcare, Bangor), http://www.emh.org/hll/hpl/guide.htm
- **Maine:** Maine Medical Center Library (Maine Medical Center, Portland), http://www.mmc.org/library/
- **Maine:** Parkview Hospital (Brunswick), http://www.parkviewhospital.org/
- **Maine:** Southern Maine Medical Center Health Sciences Library (Southern Maine Medical Center, Biddeford), http://www.smmc.org/services/service.php3?choice=10
- **Maine:** Stephens Memorial Hospital's Health Information Library (Western Maine Health, Norway), http://www.wmhcc.org/Library/
- **Manitoba, Canada:** Consumer & Patient Health Information Service (University of Manitoba Libraries), http://www.umanitoba.ca/libraries/units/health/reference/chis.html

- **Manitoba, Canada:** J.W. Crane Memorial Library (Deer Lodge Centre, Winnipeg), **http://www.deerlodge.mb.ca/crane_library/about.asp**
- **Maryland:** Health Information Center at the Wheaton Regional Library (Montgomery County, Dept. of Public Libraries, Wheaton Regional Library), **http://www.mont.lib.md.us/healthinfo/hic.asp**
- **Massachusetts:** Baystate Medical Center Library (Baystate Health System), **http://www.baystatehealth.com/1024/**
- **Massachusetts:** Boston University Medical Center Alumni Medical Library (Boston University Medical Center), **http://med-libwww.bu.edu/library/lib.html**
- **Massachusetts:** Lowell General Hospital Health Sciences Library (Lowell General Hospital, Lowell), **http://www.lowellgeneral.org/library/HomePageLinks/WWW.htm**
- **Massachusetts:** Paul E. Woodard Health Sciences Library (New England Baptist Hospital, Boston), **http://www.nebh.org/health_lib.asp**
- **Massachusetts:** St. Luke's Hospital Health Sciences Library (St. Luke's Hospital, Southcoast Health System, New Bedford), **http://www.southcoast.org/library/**
- **Massachusetts:** Treadwell Library Consumer Health Reference Center (Massachusetts General Hospital), **http://www.mgh.harvard.edu/library/chrcindex.html**
- **Massachusetts:** UMass HealthNet (University of Massachusetts Medical School, Worcester), **http://healthnet.umassmed.edu/**
- **Michigan:** Botsford General Hospital Library - Consumer Health (Botsford General Hospital, Library & Internet Services), **http://www.botsfordlibrary.org/consumer.htm**
- **Michigan:** Helen DeRoy Medical Library (Providence Hospital and Medical Centers), **http://www.providence-hospital.org/library/**
- **Michigan:** Marquette General Hospital - Consumer Health Library (Marquette General Hospital, Health Information Center), **http://www.mgh.org/center.html**
- **Michigan:** Patient Education Resouce Center - University of Michigan Cancer Center (University of Michigan Comprehensive Cancer Center, Ann Arbor), **http://www.cancer.med.umich.edu/learn/leares.htm**
- **Michigan:** Sladen Library & Center for Health Information Resources - Consumer Health Information (Detroit), **http://www.henryford.com/body.cfm?id=39330**

- **Montana:** Center for Health Information (St. Patrick Hospital and Health Sciences Center, Missoula)
- **National:** Consumer Health Library Directory (Medical Library Association, Consumer and Patient Health Information Section), http://caphis.mlanet.org/directory/index.html
- **National:** National Network of Libraries of Medicine (National Library of Medicine) - provides library services for health professionals in the United States who do not have access to a medical library, http://nnlm.gov/
- **National:** NN/LM List of Libraries Serving the Public (National Network of Libraries of Medicine), http://nnlm.gov/members/
- **Nevada:** Health Science Library, West Charleston Library (Las Vegas-Clark County Library District, Las Vegas), http://www.lvccld.org/special_collections/medical/index.htm
- **New Hampshire:** Dartmouth Biomedical Libraries (Dartmouth College Library, Hanover), http://www.dartmouth.edu/~biomed/resources.htmld/conshealth.htmld
- **New Jersey:** Consumer Health Library (Rahway Hospital, Rahway), http://www.rahwayhospital.com/library.htm
- **New Jersey:** Dr. Walter Phillips Health Sciences Library (Englewood Hospital and Medical Center, Englewood), http://www.englewoodhospital.com/links/index.htm
- **New Jersey:** Meland Foundation (Englewood Hospital and Medical Center, Englewood), http://www.geocities.com/ResearchTriangle/9360/
- **New York:** Choices in Health Information (New York Public Library) - NLM Consumer Pilot Project participant, http://www.nypl.org/branch/health/links.html
- **New York:** Health Information Center (Upstate Medical University, State University of New York, Syracuse), http://www.upstate.edu/library/hic/
- **New York:** Health Sciences Library (Long Island Jewish Medical Center, New Hyde Park), http://www.lij.edu/library/library.html
- **New York:** ViaHealth Medical Library (Rochester General Hospital), http://www.nyam.org/library/
- **Ohio:** Consumer Health Library (Akron General Medical Center, Medical & Consumer Health Library), http://www.akrongeneral.org/hwlibrary.htm

- **Oklahoma:** The Health Information Center at Saint Francis Hospital (Saint Francis Health System, Tulsa), **http://www.sfh-tulsa.com/services/healthinfo.asp**

- **Oregon:** Planetree Health Resource Center (Mid-Columbia Medical Center, The Dalles), **http://www.mcmc.net/phrc/**

- **Pennsylvania:** Community Health Information Library (Milton S. Hershey Medical Center, Hershey), **http://www.hmc.psu.edu/commhealth/**

- **Pennsylvania:** Community Health Resource Library (Geisinger Medical Center, Danville), **http://www.geisinger.edu/education/commlib.shtml**

- **Pennsylvania:** HealthInfo Library (Moses Taylor Hospital, Scranton), **http://www.mth.org/healthwellness.html**

- **Pennsylvania:** Hopwood Library (University of Pittsburgh, Health Sciences Library System, Pittsburgh), **http://www.hsls.pitt.edu/guides/chi/hopwood/index_html**

- **Pennsylvania:** Koop Community Health Information Center (College of Physicians of Philadelphia), **http://www.collphyphil.org/kooppg1.shtml**

- **Pennsylvania:** Learning Resources Center - Medical Library (Susquehanna Health System, Williamsport), **http://www.shscares.org/services/lrc/index.asp**

- **Pennsylvania:** Medical Library (UPMC Health System, Pittsburgh), **http://www.upmc.edu/passavant/library.htm**

- **Quebec, Canada:** Medical Library (Montreal General Hospital), **http://www.mghlib.mcgill.ca/**

- **South Dakota:** Rapid City Regional Hospital Medical Library (Rapid City Regional Hospital), **http://www.rcrh.org/Services/Library/Default.asp**

- **Texas:** Houston HealthWays (Houston Academy of Medicine-Texas Medical Center Library), **http://hhw.library.tmc.edu/**

- **Washington:** Community Health Library (Kittitas Valley Community Hospital), **http://www.kvch.com/**

- **Washington:** Southwest Washington Medical Center Library (Southwest Washington Medical Center, Vancouver), **http://www.swmedicalcenter.com/body.cfm?id=72**

APPENDIX D. NIH CONSENSUS STATEMENT ON NOISE AND HEARING LOSS

Overview

NIH Consensus Development Conferences are convened to evaluate available scientific information and resolve safety and efficacy issues related to biomedical technology. The resultant NIH Consensus Statements are intended to advance understanding of the technology or issue in question and to be useful to health professionals and the public.[47] Each NIH consensus statement is the product of an independent, non-Federal panel of experts and is based on the panel's assessment of medical knowledge available at the time the statement was written. Therefore, a consensus statement provides a "snapshot in time" of the state of knowledge of the conference topic.

The NIH makes the following caveat: "When reading or downloading NIH consensus statements, keep in mind that new knowledge is inevitably accumulating through medical research. Nevertheless, each NIH consensus statement is retained on this website in its original form as a record of the NIH Consensus Development Program."[48] The following consensus statement was posted on the NIH site and not indicated as "out of date" in March 2002. It was originally published, however, in January 1990.[49]

---

[47] This paragraph is adapted from the NIH: **http://odp.od.nih.gov/consensus/cons/cons.htm**.
[48] Adapted from the NIH: **http://odp.od.nih.gov/consensus/cons/consdate.htm**.
[49] *Noise and Hearing Loss.* NIH Consensus Statement Online 1990 Jan 22-24 [cited 2002 February 21];8(1):1-24. **http://consensus.nih.gov/cons/076/076_statement.htm**.

Abstract

The National Institutes of Health Consensus Development Conference on Noise and Hearing Loss brought together biomedical and behavioral scientists, health care providers, and the public to address the characteristics of noise-induced hearing loss, acoustic parameters of hazardous noise exposure, individual and age-specific susceptibility, and prevention strategies. Following a day and a half of presentations by experts and discussion by the audience, a consensus panel weighed the evidence and prepared a consensus statement.

Among their findings, the panel concluded that sounds of sufficient intensity and duration will damage the ear and result in temporary or permanent hearing loss at any age. Sound levels of less than 75 dB(A) are unlikely to cause permanent hearing loss, while sound levels about 85 dB(A) with exposures of 8 hours per day will produce permanent hearing loss after many years. Current scientific knowledge is inadequate to predict that any particular individual will be safe when exposed to a hazardous noise. Strategies to prevent damage from sound exposure should include the use of individual hearing protection devices, education programs beginning with school-age children, consumer guidance, increased product noise labeling, and hearing conservation programs for occupational settings.

The full text of the consensus panel's statement follows.

Introduction

Hearing loss afflicts approximately 28 million people in the United States. Approximately 10 million of these impairments are at least partially attributable to damage from exposure to loud sounds. Sounds that are sufficiently loud to damage sensitive inner ear structures can produce hearing loss that is not reversible by any presently available medical or surgical treatment. Hearing impairment associated with noise exposure can occur at any age, including early infancy, and is often characterized by difficulty in understanding speech and the potentially troublesome symptom, tinnitus (i.e., ringing in the ears). Very loud sounds of short duration, such as an explosion or gunfire, can produce immediate, severe, and permanent loss of hearing. Longer exposure to less intense but still hazardous sounds, commonly encountered in the workplace or in certain leisure time activities, exacts a gradual toll on hearing sensitivity, initially without the victim's awareness.

More than 20 million Americans are exposed on a regular basis to hazardous noise levels that could result in hearing loss. Occupational noise exposure, the most common cause of noise-induced hearing loss (NIHL), threatens the hearing of firefighters, police officers, military personnel, construction and factory workers, musicians, farmers, and truck drivers, to name a few. Live or recorded high-volume music, recreational vehicles, airplanes, lawn-care equipment, woodworking tools, some household appliances, and chain saws are examples of nonoccupational sources of potentially hazardous noise. One important feature of NIHL is that it is preventable in all but certain cases of accidental exposure. Legislation and regulations have been enacted that spell out guidelines for protecting workers from hazardous noise levels in the workplace and consumers from hazardous noise during leisure time pursuits. Inconsistent compliance and spotty enforcement of existing governmental regulations have been the underlying cause for their relative ineffectiveness in achieving prevention of NIHL. A particularly unfortunate occurrence was the elimination of the Office of Noise Abatement and Control within the Environmental Protection Agency in 1982.

On January 22-24, 1990, the National Institute on Deafness and Other Communication Disorders, together with the Office of Medical Applications of Research of the National Institutes of Health, convened a Consensus Development Conference on Noise and Hearing Loss. Cosponsors of the conference were the National Institute of Child Health and Human Development, the National Institute on Aging, and the National Institute for Occupational Safety and Health of the Centers for Disease Control. The effects of environmental sounds on human listeners may include:

- Interference with speech communication and other auditory signals.
- Annoyance and aversion.
- Noise-induced hearing loss.
- Changes in various body systems.
- Interference with sleep.

This conference was entirely centered on NIHL. The panel focused on five questions related to noise and hearing loss:

- What is noise-induced hearing loss?
- What sounds can damage hearing?
- What factors, including age, determine an individual's susceptibility to noise-induced hearing loss?

- What can be done to prevent noise-induced hearing loss?
- What are the directions for future research?

Following a day and a half of presentations by experts in the relevant fields and discussion from the audience, a consensus panel comprising specialists and generalists from the medical and other related scientific disciplines, together with public representatives, considered the evidence and formulated a consensus statement in response to the five previously stated questions.

What Is Noise-Induced Hearing Loss?

Sounds of sufficient intensity and duration will damage the ear and result in temporary or permanent hearing loss. The hearing loss may range from mild to profound and may also result in tinnitus. The effect of repeated sound overstimulation is cumulative over a lifetime and is not currently treatable. Hearing impairment has a major impact on one's communication ability and even mild impairment may adversely affect the quality of life. Unfortunately, although NIHL is preventable, our increasingly noisy environment places more and more people at risk.

Studies of NIHL

Most studies of the association between sound exposure and hearing loss in humans are retrospective measurements of the hearing sensitivities of numerous individuals correlated with their noise exposures. The variability within these studies is usually large; thus, it is difficult to predict the precise magnitude of hearing loss that will result from a specific sound exposure. Prospective studies of selected workers' hearing levels over a long time while their sound exposures are carefully monitored are costly and time-consuming and, due to attrition, require a large number of subjects. When significant hearing loss is found, for ethical reasons, exposures must be reduced, interfering with the relationships under study. Although studies of NIHL in humans are difficult, they provide valuable information not available from animal studies and should be continued.

In prospective animal studies, sound exposures can be carefully controlled, and the anatomic and physiologic correlates of NIHL can be precisely defined. Although there may be interspecies differences with respect to the absolute sound exposure that will injure the ear, the basic mechanisms that lead to damage appear to be similar in all mammalian ears.

Anatomic and Physiologic Correlates of NIHL

Two types of injury are recognized: acoustic trauma and NIHL. Short-duration sound of sufficient intensity (e.g., a gunshot or explosion) may result in an immediate, severe, and permanent hearing loss, which is termed acoustic trauma. Virtually all of the structures of the ear can be damaged, in particular the organ of Corti, the delicate sensory structure of the auditory portion of the inner ear (cochlea), which may be torn apart.

Moderate exposure may initially cause temporary hearing loss, termed temporary threshold shift (TTS). Structural changes associated with TTS have not been fully established but may include subtle intracellular changes in the sensory cells (hair cells) and swelling of the auditory nerve endings. Other potentially reversible effects include vascular changes, metabolic exhaustion, and chemical changes within the hair cells. There is also evidence of a regional decrease in the stiffness of the stereocilia (the hair bundles at the top of the hair cells), which may recover. This decrease in stereocilia stiffness may lead to a decrease in the coupling of sound energy to the hair cells, which thereby alters hearing sensitivity.

Repeated exposure to sounds that cause TTS may gradually cause permanent NIHL in experimental animals. In this type of injury, cochlear blood flow may be impaired, and a few scattered hair cells are damaged with each exposure. With continued exposure, the number of damaged hair cells increases. Although most structures in the inner ear can be harmed by excessive sound exposure, the sensory cells are the most vulnerable. Damage to the stereocilia is often the first change, specifically, alteration of the rootlet structures that normally anchor the stereocilia into the top of the hair cell. Once destroyed, the sensory cells are not replaced. During the recovery period between some sound exposures, damaged regions of the organ of Corti heal by scar formation. This process is very important because it reestablishes the barrier between the two fluids of the inner ear (perilymph and endolymph). If this barrier is not reestablished, degeneration of hair cells may continue. Further, once a sufficient number of hair cells are lost, the nerve fibers to that region also degenerate. With degeneration of the cochlear nerve fibers, there is corresponding degeneration within the central nervous system. The extent to which these neural changes contribute to NIHL is not clear.

With moderate periods of exposure to potentially hazardous high-frequency sound, the damage is usually confined to a restricted area in the high-frequency region of the cochlea. With a comparable exposure to low-frequency noise, hair cell damage is not confined to the low-frequency region but may also affect the high-frequency regions. The predominance of damage in different cochlear regions with different frequency exposures reflects factors such as the resonance of the ear canal, the middle-ear transfer characteristics, and the mechanical characteristics of the organ of Corti and basilar membrane.

Assessment of NIHL

Hearing loss is measured by determining auditory thresholds (sensitivity) at various frequencies (pure-tone audiometry). Complete assessment should also include measures of speech understanding and middle-ear status (immittance audiometry). Pure-tone audiometry is also used in industrial hearing conservation programs to determine whether adequate protection against hazardous sound levels is provided.

The first audiometric sign of NIHL resulting from broadband noise is usually a loss of sensitivity in the higher frequencies from 3,000 through 6,000 Hertz (Hz) (i.e., cycles per second), resulting in a characteristic audiometric "notch." With additional hearing loss from noise or aging, the threshold at 8,000 Hz may worsen and eliminate this characteristic audiometric pattern. Thus, the presence or absence of NIHL cannot be established on the basis of audiometric shape, per se. The hearing loss is usually bilateral, but some degree of asymmetry is not unusual, especially with lateralized noise sources such as rifles. After moderate sound exposure, TTS may occur, and, during a period of relative quiet, thresholds will return to normal levels. If the exposure continues on a regular basis, permanent threshold shifts (PTS) will result, increasing in magnitude and extending to lower and higher frequencies. If the exposures continue, NIHL increases, more rapidly in the early years. After many years of exposure, NIHL levels off in the high frequencies, but continues to worsen in the low frequencies. Although TTS and PTS are correlated, the relation is not strong enough to use TTS to predict the magnitude of permanent hearing loss.

An important consequence of the sensitivity loss associated with NIHL is difficulty in understanding speech. Whereas a large proportion of the energy in speech is contained within the low-frequency range, much of the information required to differentiate one speech sound from another is contained within the higher frequencies. With significant hearing loss in the high frequencies, important speech information is often inaudible or unusable. Other interfering sounds such as background noise, competing voices, or room reverberation may reduce even further the hearing-impaired listener's receptive communication ability. The presence of tinnitus may be an additional debilitating condition.

NIHL may interfere with daily life, especially those social activities that occur in noisy settings. Increased effort is required for understanding speech in these situations, which leads to fatigue, anxiety, and stress. Decreased participation in these activities often results, affecting not only hearing-impaired individuals but also friends and family members. Hearing loss is associated with depression in the elderly and may be related to dementia and cognitive dysfunction. Systematic study of the effects of hearing loss on the quality of life have only lately focused specifically on individuals with NIHL; therefore, continued studies of this kind are desirable.

The impairment in hearing ability resulting from NIHL may vary from mild to severe. An individual's ability to communicate and function in daily life varies with the degree of loss and the individual's communication needs although these relationships are complex. The magnitude of the effect on communication ability may be estimated by a variety of scales, which are often used in disability determinations. These scales, which vary substantially in the frequencies used, the upper and lower limits of impairment, age correction, and adjustment for asymmetric hearing loss, attempt to predict the degree of communication impairment (understanding of speech) on the basis of pure-tone thresholds. There is no consensus about the validity or utility of the scales, which scale should be used, whether measures of speech understanding should be included, or whether self-assessment ratings should be incorporated into either impairment rating scales or disability determinations.

What Sounds Can Damage Hearing?

Some sounds are so weak physically that they are not heard. Some sounds are audible but do not have any temporary or permanent after-effects. Some sounds are strong enough to produce a temporary hearing loss from which there may appear to be complete recovery. Damaging sounds are those that are sufficiently strong, sufficiently long-lasting, and involve appropriate frequencies so that permanent hearing loss will ensue.

Most of the sounds in the environment that produce such permanent effects occur over a very long time (for example, about 8 hours per workday over a period of 10 or more years). On the other hand, there are some particularly abrupt or explosive sounds that can cause damage even with a single exposure.

The line between these categories of sounds cannot be stated simply because not all persons respond to sound in the same manner. Thus, if a sound of given frequency bandwidth, level, and duration is considered hazardous, one must specify for what proportion of the population it will be hazardous and, within that proportion, by what criterion of damage (whether anatomical, audiometric, speech understanding) it is hazardous.

The most widely used measure of a sound's strength or amplitude is called "sound level," measured by a sound-level meter in units called "decibels" (dB). For example, the sound level of speech at typical conversational distances is between 65 and 70 dB. There are weaker sounds, still audible, and of course much stronger sounds. Those above 85 dB are potentially hazardous.

Sounds must also be specified in terms of frequency or bandwidth, roughly like the span of keys on a piano. The range of audible frequencies extends from about 20 Hz, below the lowest notes on a piano, to at least 16,000 or 20,000 Hz, well above the highest notes on a piccolo. Most environmental noises include a wide band of frequencies and, by convention, are measured through the "A" filter in the sound-level meter and thus are designated in dB(A) units. It is not clear what effect, if any, sound outside the frequency range covered in dB(A) measurements may have on hearing. At this time, it is not known whether ultrasonic vibration will damage hearing.

To define what sounds can damage hearing, sound level, whether across all frequency bands or taken band by band, is not enough. The duration of exposure--typical for a day and accumulated over many years--is critical. Sound levels associated with particular sources such as snowmobiles, rock music, and chain saws, are often cited, but predicting the likelihood of NIHL from such sources also requires knowledge of typical durations and the number of exposures.

There appears to be reasonable agreement that sound levels below 75 dB(A) will not engender a permanent hearing loss, even at 4000 Hz. At higher levels, the amount of hearing loss is directly related to sound level for comparable durations.

According to some existing rules and regulations, a noise level of 85 dB(A) for an 8-hour daily exposure is potentially damaging. If total sound energy were the important predictor, an equivalent exposure could be as high as 88 dB(A) if restricted to 4 hours. (A 3-dB increase is equivalent to doubling the sound intensity.) This relation, enshrined in some standards and regulations, is a theory based on a dose or exposure defined by total energy.

In spite of the physical simplicity of a total-energy concept, other principles have been invoked to define equivalent exposures of different sound levels and durations. Early research suggested that NIHL after 10 years could be predicted from temporary threshold shifts (TTS) measured 2 minutes after a comparable single-day exposure. Those results, however, were taken to indicate that a halving of duration could be offset by a 5-dB change in sound level rather than a 3-dB change. This 5-dB rule is implemented in the Walsh-Healey Act of 1969 and subsequent Occupational Safety and Health Administration regulations for the purpose of requiring preventive efforts for noise-exposed workers. The 3-dB trading rule is agreed to in International Standards Organization (ISO) Standard 1999.2 (1989) for the purpose of predicting the amount of noise-induced hearing loss resulting from different exposures. There is no consensus concerning a single rule to be used for all purposes in the United States.

Generally, for sound levels below about 140 dB, different temporal forms of sound, whether impulse (gunshot), impact (drop forge) or steady state (turbine), when specified with respect to their level and duration, produce the same hearing loss. This does not appear to follow at levels above 140 dB, where impulse noise creates more damage than would be predicted. This may imply that impulse noise above a certain critical level results in acoustic trauma from which the ear cannot recover.

Although sound exposures that are potentially hazardous to hearing are usually defined in terms of sound level, frequency bandwidths, and duration, there are several simple approximations that indicate that a sound exposure may be suspected as hazardous. These include the following: If the sound is appreciably louder than conversational level, it is potentially harmful, provided that the sound is present for a sufficient period of time. Hazardous noise may also be suspected if the listener experiences: (a) difficulty in communication while in the sound, (b) ringing in the ear (tinnitus) after exposure to the sound, and/or (c) the experience that sounds seem muffled after leaving the sound-exposure area.

In the consideration of sounds that can damage hearing, one point is clear: it is the acoustic energy of the sound reaching the ear, not its source, which is important. That is, it does not matter if the hazardous sound is generated by a machine in the workplace, by an amplifier/loudspeaker at a rock concert, or by a snowmobile ridden by the listener. Significant amounts of acoustic energy reaching the ear will create damage--at work, at school, at home, or during leisure activities. Although there has been a tendency to concentrate on the more significant occupational and transportation noise, the same rules apply to all potential noise hazards.

What Factors, Including Age, Determine an Individual's Susceptibility to Noise-Induced Hearing Loss?

One thoroughly established characteristic of NIHL is that, on the average, more intense and longer-duration noise exposures cause more severe hearing loss. A second is that there is a remarkably broad range of individual differences in sensitivity to any given noise exposure. Several factors have been proposed to explain differences in NIHL among individuals; others may be associated with differences over time within the same individual. It is important to distinguish those factors whose roles in determining susceptibility are supported by a consistent body of theory and empirical evidence from other factors whose roles have been proposed but for which theory, data, or both are less conclusive.

Differences among Individuals

Both temporary threshold shift (TTS) and permanent threshold shift (PTS) in response to a given intense noise may differ as much as 30 to 50 dB among individuals. Both animal research and retrospective studies of humans exposed to industrial noise have demonstrated this remarkable variation in susceptibility. The biological bases for these differences are unknown. A number of extrinsic factors (e.g., characteristics of the ear canal and middle ear, drugs, and prior exposure to noise) may influence an individual's susceptibility to NIHL. However, animal studies that have controlled these variables suggest that individual differences in inner ear anatomy and physiology also may be significant. Additional research is necessary to determine whether vascular, neural feedback (efferent system), or other mechanisms can account for and predict such individual variation.

One factor that may be associated with decreased susceptibility to NIHL is conductive hearing loss; the cochlear structures may be protected by any form of acoustic attenuation. For similar reasons, middle ear muscles, which normally serve a protective function by contracting in response to intense sound, when inoperative, can result in increased susceptibility. Among the other factors that are theoretically associated with differences in susceptibility are (a) unusually efficient acoustic transfer through the external and middle ear, as a determinant of the amount of energy coupled to the inner ear structures, and (b) preexisting hearing loss, which could imply that less additional loss would occur if the sensitive structures have already been damaged. Support for these hypotheses has been modest, in the case of the transfer function, because little empirical work has been done to test that hypothesis, and, in the case of reduced sensitivity, because several studies disagree. In general, when there is a difference in average loss to a given noise exposure, those ears with previous PTS or TTS have shown somewhat less additional loss than those not previously exposed.

Findings have sometimes implicated degree of pigmentation, both of the receptor structures (melanization) and of the eye and skin, as related to susceptibility. However, these results too are equivocal.

Gender

There is little difference in hearing thresholds between young male and female children. Between ages 10 and 20, males begin to show reduced high-frequency auditory sensitivity relative to females. Women continue to demonstrate better hearing than men into advanced age. These gender differences are probably due to greater exposure of males to noise rather than to their inherent susceptibility to its effects.

Differences within Individuals

Ototoxic Drugs

Among the causes of differences of susceptibility to noise exposure within individuals are ototoxic drugs and other chemicals. In animal research, certain antibiotics (aminoglycosides) appear to exacerbate the damaging effects of noise exposure. Clinical evidence of corresponding effects in human patients has not been established, but precautions should be taken with regard to noise exposures of individual patients treated with these medications. Although high doses of aspirin are widely known to cause TTS and tinnitus, aspirin has not been shown to increase susceptibility to NIHL.

Age

In certain animal models there is evidence of heightened susceptibility to noise exposure shortly after birth--a "critical period" (possibly following the time when fluids fill the middle ear but before complete development of the cochlear structures). However, it is not clear that data from such animal models can be generalized to full-term normal human infants. Premature infants in noisy environments (e.g. neonatal intensive care units), however, may be at risk

At the other extreme, increasing age has been hypothesized to be associated with decreasing susceptibility. This contention is based on the existence of presbycusis, hearing loss that increases with age and that is not known to be attributable to excessive noise exposure or other known etiology. The typical levels of presbycusis at various ages have recently been incorporated as Annex A in International Standards Organization Standard 1999.2 (1989). That standard may be used to estimate the portion of overall hearing loss that is attributable to exposure to excessive noise.

In summary, scientific knowledge is currently inadequate to predict that any individual will be safe in noise that exceeds established damage-risk criteria, nor that specific individuals will show greater-than-average loss following a given exposure. Among the many proposed explanations, the hypothesis that the resonant and transmission properties of the external and middle ear affect individual susceptibility deserves further attention. Empirical support for this hypothesis should not be difficult to obtain, but very few data have been collected on this question, both for TTS (experimentally) and PTS (retrospectively). Differences in susceptibility of the cochlear structures to NIHL may exist, but no practical approach to predicting them is yet available. Identification of susceptible humans will almost certainly be delayed until a successful animal model is available.

What Can Be Done to Prevent Noise-Induced Hearing Loss?

Noise-induced hearing loss occurs every day--in both occupational and nonoccupational settings. The crucial questions for prevention are as follows: (1) What can individuals do to protect themselves from NIHL? (2) What role should others, such as educators, employers, or the Government, play in preventing NIHL? (3) What general strategies should be employed to prevent NIHL? Answers to these questions have long been known, but solutions have not been effectively implemented in many cases. As a result, many people have needlessly suffered hearing loss.

Individual Protection Strategies

Hearing conservation must begin by providing each individual with basic information. NIHL is insidious, permanent, and irreparable, causing communication interference that can substantially affect the quality of life. Ringing in the ears and muffling of sounds after sound exposure are indicators of potential hazard. Dangerous sound exposures can cause significant damage without pain, and hearing aids do not restore normal hearing. Individuals should become aware of loud noise situations and avoid them if possible or properly use hearing protection. It is important to recognize that both the level of the noise and its duration (i.e., exposure) contribute to the overall risk. Certain noises, such as explosions, may cause immediate permanent damage.

Many sources, such as guns, power tools, chain saws, small airplanes, farm vehicles, firecrackers, some types of toys, and some medical and dental instruments may produce dangerous exposures. Music concerts, car and motorcycle races, and other spectator events often produce sound levels that warrant hearing protection. Similarly, some stereo headphones and loudspeakers are capable of producing hazardous exposures. Parents should exercise special care in supervising the use of personal headset listening devices, and adults and children alike should learn to operate them at safe volume settings.

Non-Occupational Strategies

Hearing loss from non-occupational noise is common, but public awareness of the hazard is low. Educational programs should be targeted toward children, parents, hobby groups, public role models, and professionals in influential positions such as teachers, physicians, audiologists and other health care professionals, engineers, architects, and legislators. In particular, primary health care physicians and educators who deal with young people should be targeted through their professional organizations. Consumers need guidance and product noise labeling to assist them in purchasing quieter devices and in implementing exposure reduction strategies. The public should be made aware of the availability of affordable, effective hearing protectors (ear plugs, ear muffs, and canal caps). Hearing protection manufacturers should supply comprehensive instructions concerning proper protector use and also be encouraged to increase device availability to the public sector. Newborn nurseries, including neonatal intensive care units, should be made quieter. Medical and dental personnel should be trained to educate their patients about NIHL.

Individuals with significant noise exposure need counseling. Basic audiometric evaluations should be widely available. The goal is to detect early noise-induced damage and interrupt its progression before hearing thresholds exceed the normal range.

Occupational Strategies

Hearing conservation programs for occupational settings must include the following interactive components: sound surveys to assess the degree of hazardous noise exposure, engineering and administrative noise controls to reduce exposures, education to inform at-risk individuals why and how to prevent hearing loss, hearing protection devices (earplugs, earmuffs, and canal caps) to reduce the sound reaching the ear, and audiometric evaluations to detect hearing changes. Governmental regulations that currently apply to most noisy industries should be revised to encompass all industries and all employees, strengthened in certain requirements, and strictly enforced with more inspections and more severe penalties for violations.

Many existing hearing conservation programs remain ineffective due to poor organization and inadequately trained program staff. Senior management must use available noise controls, purchase quieter equipment, and incorporate noise reduction in planning new facilities. Noise exposures must be measured accurately and the degree of hazard communicated to employees. Hearing protection devices must be available that are comfortable, practical for the demands of work tasks, and provide adequate attenuation. Labeled ratings of hearing protector attenuation must be more realistic so that the degree of protection achieved in the workplace can be properly estimated. Each employee must be individually fitted with protectors and trained in their correct use and care. Employees need feedback about their audiometric monitoring results annually.

Employers need to monitor program effectiveness by using appropriate techniques for analysis of group audiometric data. By detecting problem areas, managers can prioritize resource allocations and modify company policies to achieve effectiveness. Potential benefits include reduced costs for worker's compensation, enhanced worker morale, reduced absenteeism, fewer accidents, and greater productivity.

Enactment of uniform regulations for awarding worker's compensation for occupational hearing loss would stimulate employers' interest in achieving effective hearing conservation programs. Equitable criteria for compensability should be developed based on scientific investigations of the difficulties in communication and other aspects of auditory function encountered in everyday life by persons with differing degrees of NIHL.

General Strategies

Both non-occupational and occupational NIHL could be reduced by implementing broader preventive efforts. Labeling of consumer product noise emission levels should be enforced according to existing regulations. Incentives for manufacturers to design quieter industrial equipment and consumer goods are needed along with regulations governing the maximum emission levels of certain consumer products, such as power tools. Reestablishment of a Federal agency coordinating committee with central responsibility for practical solutions to noise issues is essential. Model community ordinances could promote local planning to control environmental noise and, where feasible, noise levels at certain spectator events. High-visibility media campaigns are needed to develop public awareness of the effects of noise on hearing and the means for self-protection. Prevention of NIHL should be part of the health curricula in elementary through high schools. Self-education materials for adults should be readily available.

What Are the Directions for Future Research?

The panel recommends that research be undertaken in two broad categories: (1) Studies that use existing knowledge to prevent NIHL in the immediate future, and (2) research on basic mechanisms to prevent NIHL in the long-term future.

- Development of rationale and collection of empirical data to evaluate systems for combining sound level and duration to predict NIHL.

- Longitudinal studies to further delineate responses of the ear to noise over time in different groups of people with varying levels of exposure.

- Continued investigation of engineering noise measurement and control techniques, such as acoustic intensity measurement, active noise-cancellation systems, and cost-benefit analyses of noise reduction.

- Development and investigation of hearing protector designs that provide improved wearer comfort, usability, and more natural audition.

- Development of repeatable laboratory procedures that incorporate behavioral tests to yield realistic estimates of hearing protector attenuation performance that are accepted for device labeling purposes.

- Empirical evaluation of the efficacy of hearing conservation programs and the field performance of hearing protection devices in industry.

- Development and validation of evaluation techniques for detection of the following: a) subtle changes in hearing resulting from noise exposure and b) early indicators of NIHL.

- Determination of the pathophysiological correlates of TTS and PTS.

- Investigation of the anatomic and physiologic bases of presbycusis and interactive effects with NIHL.

- Investigation of genetic bases for susceptibility to NIHL, using contemporary techniques, including molecular biology.

- Further studies of drugs (e.g., vasodilating agents) and other pre-exposure conditions (e.g., activation of efferent systems or exposure to "conditioning" noise) that have been suggested in preliminary reports to protect the inner ear from NIHL and elucidation of the underlying mechanisms.

- Investigation into the physiologic mechanisms underlying the synergistic effects of certain drugs and noise exposure in animal models.

Conclusions and Recommendations

- Sounds of sufficient intensity and duration will damage the ear and result in temporary or permanent hearing loss at any age.

- NIHL is characterized by specific anatomic and physiologic changes in the inner ear.

- Sounds with levels less than 75 dB(A), even after long exposures, are unlikely to cause permanent hearing loss.

- Sounds with levels above 85 dB(A) with exposures of 8 hours per day will produce permanent hearing loss after many years.

- There is a broad range of individual differences among people in the amount of hearing loss each suffers as a result of identical exposures.

- Current scientific knowledge is inadequate to predict that any particular individual will be safe when exposed to a hazardous noise.

- Because sources of potentially hazardous sound are present in both occupational and nonoccupational settings, personal hearing protection should be used when hazardous exposures are unavoidable.

- Vigorous enforcement of existing regulations, particularly for the workplace and consumer product labeling, would significantly reduce the risk of workplace NIHL. Regulations should be broadened to encompass all employees with hazardous noise exposures.

- Application of existing technologies for source noise control, especially in the manufacture of new equipment and construction of new facilities, would significantly reduce sound levels at the ear.

- In addition to existing hearing conservation programs, a comprehensive program of education regarding the causes and prevention of NIHL should be developed and disseminated, with specific attention directed toward educating school-age children.

APPENDIX E. MORE ON NOISE-INDUCED HEARING LOSS

Overview[50]

Every day we experience sound in our environment such as the television, radio, washing machine, automobiles, buses and trucks. But when an individual is exposed to harmful sounds—sounds that are too loud or loud sounds over a long time—sensitive structures of the inner ear can be damaged causing Noise-Induced Hearing Loss (NIHL).

How Do We Hear?

Hearing is a series of events in which sound waves in the air produce electrical signals and cause nerve impulses to be sent to the brain where they are interpreted as sound. The ear has three main parts: the outer, middle and inner ear. Sound waves enter through the outer ear and reach the middle ear where they cause the ear drum to vibrate.

The vibrations are transmitted through three tiny bones in the middle ear, called the ossicles. These three bones are named the malleus, incus and stapes (and are also known as the hammer, anvil and stirrup). The ear drum and ossicles amplify the vibrations and carry them to the inner ear. The stirrup transmits the amplified vibrations through the oval window and into the fluid that fills the inner ear. The vibrations move through fluid in the snail-shaped hearing part of the inner ear (cochlea) that contains the hair cells. The fluid in the cochlea moves the top portion of the hair cells, called the hair bundle, which initiates the changes that lead to the production of the

---

[50] Adapted from The National Institute on Deafness and Other Communication Disorders (NIDCD): http://www.nidcd.nih.gov/health/pubs_hb/noise.htm.

nerve impulses. These nerve impulses are carried to the brain where they are interpreted as sound. Different sounds move to the population of hair cells in different ways, thus allowing the brain to distinguish among various sounds, for example, different vowel and consonant sounds.

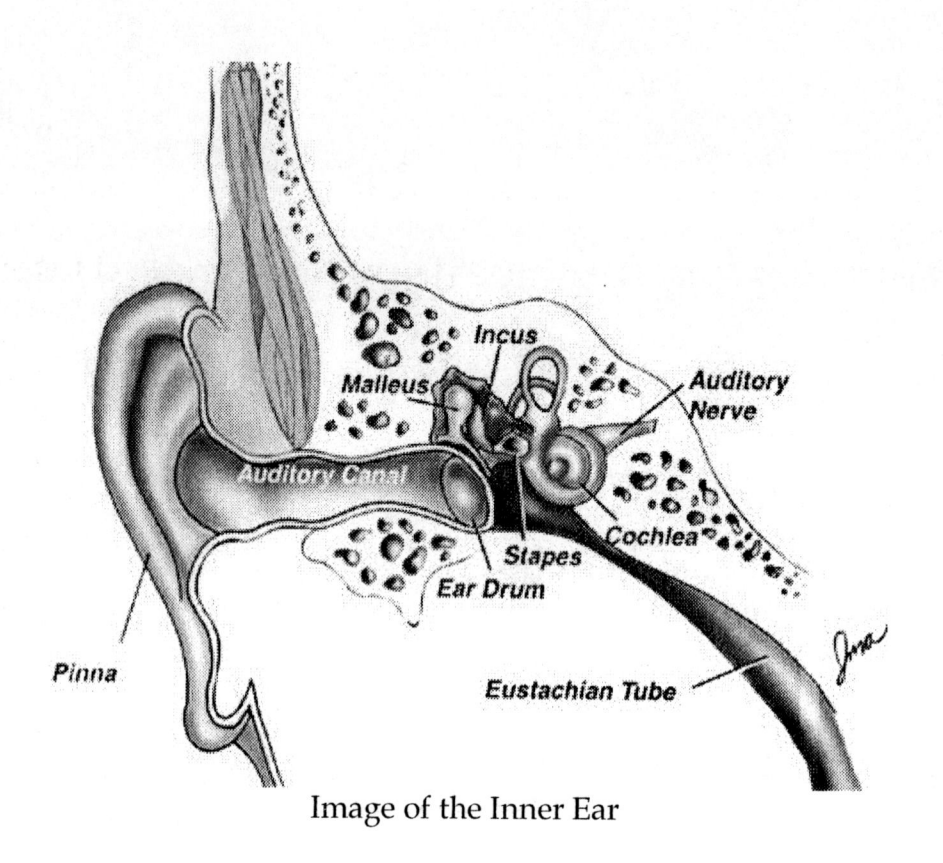

Image of the Inner Ear

What Sounds Cause NIHL?

NIHL can be caused by a one-time exposure to loud sound as well as by repeated exposure to sounds at various loudness levels over an extended period of time. The loudness of sound is measured in units called decibels. For example, usual conversation is approximately 60 decibels, the humming of a refrigerator is 40 decibels and city traffic noise can be 80 decibels. Examples of sources of loud noises that cause NIHL are motorcycles, firecrackers and small arms fire, all emitting sounds from 120 decibels to 140 decibels. Sounds of less than 75 decibels, even after long exposure, are unlikely to cause hearing loss.

Exposure to harmful sounds causes damage to the sensitive hair cells of the inner ear and to the nerve of hearing. These structures can be injured by noise in two different ways: from an intense brief impulse, such as an explosion, or from continuous exposure to noise, such as that in a woodworking shop.

What Are the Effects of NIHL?

The effect from impulse sound can be instantaneous and can result in an immediate hearing loss that may be permanent. The structures of the inner ear may be severely damaged. This kind of hearing loss may be accompanied by tinnitus, an experience of sound like ringing, buzzing or roaring in the ears or head, which may subside over time. Hearing loss and tinnitus may be experienced in one or both ears, and tinnitus may continue constantly or intermittently throughout a lifetime.

The damage that occurs slowly over years of continuous exposure to loud noise is accompanied by various changes in the structure of the hair cells. It also results in hearing loss and tinnitus. Exposure to impulse and continuous noise may cause only a temporary hearing loss. If the hearing recovers, the temporary hearing loss is called a temporary threshold shift. The temporary threshold shift largely disappears within 16 hours after exposure to loud noise.

Both forms of NIHL can be prevented by the regular use of hearing protectors such as ear plugs or ear muffs.

What Are the Symptoms of NIHL?

The symptoms of NIHL that occur over a period of continuous exposure increase gradually. Sounds may become distorted or muffled, and it may be difficult for the person to understand speech. The individual may not be aware of the loss, but it can be detected with a hearing test.

Who Is Affected by NIHL?

More than 30 million Americans are exposed to hazardous sound levels on a regular basis. Individuals of all ages including children, adolescents, young adults and older people can develop NIHL. Exposure occurs in the work place, in recreational settings and at home. There is an increasing awareness of the harmful noises in recreational activities, for example, target shooting or hunting, snowmobiles, go-carts, woodworking and other hobby equipment, power horns, cap guns and model airplanes. Harmful noises at home may come from vacuum cleaners, garbage disposals, lawn mowers, leaf blowers and shop tools. People who live in either urban or rural settings may be exposed to noisy devices on a daily basis. Of the 28 million Americans who have some degree of hearing loss, about one-third have been affected, at least in part, by noise.

Can NIHL Be Prevented?

Noise-induced hearing loss is preventable. All individuals should understand the hazards of noise and how to practice good health in everyday life.

- Know which noises can cause damage (those above 75 decibels)
- Wear ear plugs or other hearing protective devices when involved in a loud activity (special earplugs and ear muffs are available at hardware stores and sporting good stores)
- Be alert to hazardous noise in the environment
- Protect children who are too young to protect themselves
- Make family, friends and colleagues aware of the hazards of noise.
- Have a medical examination by an otolaryngologist, a physician who specializes in diseases of the ears, nose, throat, head and neck, and a hearing test by an audiologist, a health professional trained to identify and measure hearing loss and to rehabilitate persons with hearing impairments.

What Research Is Being Done for NIHL?

Scientists focusing their research on the mechanisms causing NIHL hope to understand more fully the internal workings of the ear, that will result in better prevention and treatment strategies. For example, scientists have discovered that damage to the structure of the hair bundle of the hair cell is related to temporary and permanent loss of hearing. They have found that when the hair bundle is exposed to prolonged periods of damaging sound, the basic structure of the hair bundle is destroyed and the important connections among hair cells are disrupted which directly lead to hearing loss.

Other studies are investigating potential drug therapies that may provide insight into the mechanisms of NIHL. For example, scientists studying altered blood flow in the cochlea are seeking the effect on the hair cells. They have shown reduced cochlear blood flow following exposure to noise. Further research has shown that a drug which promotes blood flow used for treatment of peripheral vascular disease (any abnormal condition in blood vessels outside the heart), maintains circulation in the cochlea during exposure to noise. These findings may lead to the development of treatment strategies to reduce NIHL.

Continuing efforts will provide opportunities that can aid research on noise-induced hearing loss as well as other diseases and disorders that cause hearing loss. Research is the way to develop new, more effective methods to prevent, diagnose, treat and eventually eliminate these diseases and disorders and improve the health and quality of life for all Americans.

Where Can I Get Additional Information?

For more information, contact:

American Academy of Audiology
8201 Greensboro Drive, Suite 300
McLean, VA 22102
Voice: (800) AAA-2336
Voice/TTY: (703) 610-9022
Internet: **www.audiology.org**

American Academy of Otolaryngology — Head and Neck Surgery
One Prince Street
Alexandria, VA 22314
Voice: (703) 519-1589
TTY: (703) 519-1585
E-mail: entinfo@aol.com
Internet: **www.entnet.org**

American Auditory Society
512 East Canterbury Lane
Phoenix, AZ 85022
Voice: (602) 789-0755
Fax: (603) 942-1486
E-mail: amaudsoc@aol.com

American Speech-Language-Hearing Association
10801 Rockville Pike
Rockville, MD 20852
Voice/TTY: (301) 897-5700
Voice: (800) 638-8255
Fax: (301) 571-0457
E-mail: actioncenter@asha.org
Internet: **www.asha.org**

American Tinnitus Association
P.O. Box 5
Portland, OR 97207
Voice: (800) 634-8978
E-mail: tinnitus@ata.org
Internet: **www.ata.org**

Self Help for Hard of Hearing People Inc. (SHHH)
7910 Woodmont Avenue, Suite 1200
Bethesda, MD 20814
Voice: (301) 657-2248
TTY: (301) 657-2249
E-mail: national@shhh.org
Internet: **www.shhh.org**

APPENDIX F. PROTECT YOURSELF AND YOUR FAMILY FROM NOISE-INDUCED HEARING LOSS

Overview[51]

Everyone should worry about noise. No matter how old or young you are, too much exposure to loud noise can permanently damage your hearing. Whether it's the screech of a chain saw, the sudden blast of a hunting rifle, or the roar of a lawn mower, exposure to loud sounds can cause Noise-Induced Hearing Loss (NIHL).

NIHL is serious. Some 30 million people are at risk in the workplace, in recreational settings, and at home. In fact, it is the most common work-related disease. Already, 10 million Americans have permanently damaged their hearing.

What Is the WISE EARS! Campaign?

To help prevent NIHL, the National Institute on Deafness and Other Communication Disorders (NIDCD) has teamed with the National Institute for Occupational Safety and Health (NIOSH) and more than 60 diverse national organizations to create the WISE EARS! health education campaign. WISE EARS! is spreading the word that:

- Hearing matters;
- NIHL is preventable; and
- WISE EARS! will last a lifetime.

---

[51] Adapted from the National Institute on Deafness and Other Communication Disorders (NIDCD): **http://www.nidcd.nih.gov/health/parents/wiseears.htm**.

How Can I Prevent NIHL and Have WISE EARS! for Life?

No matter what kinds of work and recreation are a part of your life, you can take steps to prevent NIHL.

- Know how much noise is too much
- Protect your hearing in noisy environments
- Tell others how to prevent NIHL
- Contact WISE EARS! coalition members for assistance

How Much Noise Is Too Much?

Sounds louder than 85 decibels (dB) can damage your ears. A decibel is a unit that measures the intensity of sound on a scale from zero to 140. A normal conversation is about 60 dB. Chainsaws, hammer drills, and bulldozers ring in at over 100 dB. So if you are a construction worker, harmful sounds may be a regular part of your job. The same goes for people working around lawn mowers and factory machinery every day. Airport workers and farmers are two more groups that are regularly exposed to loud noise. However, loud noise does not have to be an everyday happening to cause damage. One-time exposure, such as the sound of a gun firing at close range, can harm your ears permanently.

How Can I Protect My Hearing in Noisy Situations?

Wear ear plugs or special earmuffs when you are exposed to dangerous levels of noise; they can keep your hearing from being damaged. Hearing protection is important any time you're exposed to loud noise.

Where Can I Buy Hearing Protection Devices?

Several different types of protective plugs and muffs are available in most pharmacies, hardware stores, and sporting goods stores.

What Should I Tell Others about Hearing Protection?

You can share what you know about NIHL with your family, friends, classmates, and co-workers. If you have children, explain to them that hearing is delicate and important. Call their attention to sounds that are harmful. Encourage them to protect their ears by avoiding loud noises or using special ear muffs. If they are too young to protect themselves, do it for them. For your co-workers and other family members, make a copy of this flyer and share what you know about NIHL.

Additional Resources

Many organizations are committed to preventing NIHL. They can answer questions, offer suggestions, and provide printed or electronic (online) information. Contacting any of the following organizations can be very helpful:

WISE EARS!
(800) 241-1044
www.nidcd.nih.gov/health/wise/
Visit the Web site or call the toll free phone number at for additional coalition members' addresses and phone numbers.

The National Institute for Occupational Safety and Health (NIOSH)
1-800-35-NIOSH
www.cdc.gov/niosh
A Federal agency, offers publications and other information to anyone interested in work-related hearing loss. NIOSH publications focus on both general issues, such as practical guides to preventing hearing loss, and specific issues, such as noise levels in underground coal mines.

The National Hearing Conservation Association (NHCA)
(303) 224-9022
www.hearingconservation.org
An association of hearing conservation professionals, distributes and exchanges information on NIHL.

The American Tinnitus Association (ATA)
1-800-634-8978
www.ata.org
A nonprofit group offering services to people with tinnitus (ringing in the ears). Education, information, hearing-health referrals are available.

Hearing Education and Awareness for Rockers (HEAR)
(415) 431-3277
24-hour hotline: (415) 773-9590
www.hearnet.com
A nonprofit group dedicated to educating people about the dangers of exposure to loud music. HEAR provides many services, including custom hearing protection, hearing testing, and outreach to increase public awareness.

APPENDIX G. HOW LOUD IS TOO LOUD?

Loud noise can cause damage at the following levels and durations[52]:

- 110 Decibels: Regular exposure of more than 1 minute risks permanent hearing loss.

- 100 Decibels: No more than 15 minutes unprotected exposure recommended.

- 90 Decibels: Prolonged exposure to any noise above 90 decibels can cause gradual hearing loss.

Know which noises can cause damage and wear ear plugs when you are involved in a loud activity.

---

[52] Adapted from the National Institute on Deafness and Other Communication Disorders (NIDCD): **http://www.nidcd.nih.gov/health/pubs_hb/ruler.htm**.

How loud is too loud?

— 140 Rock concerts, Firecrackers

— 120 Boom cars, Snowmobile

— 110 Chainsaw

— 100 Wood shop

— 90   Lawn mower, Motorcycle

— 80   City traffic noise

— 60   Normal conversation

— 40   Refrigerator humming

— 20   Whispered voice

— 0   Threshold of normal hearing

DECIBELS

ONLINE GLOSSARIES

The Internet provides access to a number of free-to-use medical dictionaries and glossaries. The National Library of Medicine has compiled the following list of online dictionaries:

- ADAM Medical Encyclopedia (A.D.A.M., Inc.), comprehensive medical reference: **http://www.nlm.nih.gov/medlineplus/encyclopedia.html**
- MedicineNet.com Medical Dictionary (MedicineNet, Inc.): **http://www.medterms.com/Script/Main/hp.asp**
- Merriam-Webster Medical Dictionary (Inteli-Health, Inc.): **http://www.intelihealth.com/IH/**
- Multilingual Glossary of Technical and Popular Medical Terms in Eight European Languages (European Commission) - Danish, Dutch, English, French, German, Italian, Portuguese, and Spanish: **http://allserv.rug.ac.be/~rvdstich/eugloss/welcome.html**
- On-line Medical Dictionary (CancerWEB): **http://www.graylab.ac.uk/omd/**
- Technology Glossary (National Library of Medicine) - Health Care Technology: **http://www.nlm.nih.gov/nichsr/ta101/ta10108.htm**
- Terms and Definitions (Office of Rare Diseases): **http://rarediseases.info.nih.gov/ord/glossary_a-e.html**

Beyond these, MEDLINEplus contains a very user-friendly encyclopedia covering every aspect of medicine (licensed from A.D.A.M., Inc.). The ADAM Medical Encyclopedia can be accessed via the following Web site address: **http://www.nlm.nih.gov/medlineplus/encyclopedia.html**. ADAM is also available on commercial Web sites such as Web MD (**http://my.webmd.com/adam/asset/adam_disease_articles/a_to_z/a**) and drkoop.com (**http://www.drkoop.com/**). Topics of interest can be researched by using keywords before continuing elsewhere, as these basic definitions and concepts will be useful in more advanced areas of research. You may choose to print various pages specifically relating to tinnitus and keep them on file.

Online Dictionary Directories

The following are additional online directories compiled by the National Library of Medicine, including a number of specialized medical dictionaries and glossaries:

- Medical Dictionaries: Medical & Biological (World Health Organization):
  http://www.who.int/hlt/virtuallibrary/English/diction.htm#Medical

- MEL-Michigan Electronic Library List of Online Health and Medical Dictionaries (Michigan Electronic Library):
  http://mel.lib.mi.us/health/health-dictionaries.html

- Patient Education: Glossaries (DMOZ Open Directory Project):
  http://dmoz.org/Health/Education/Patient_Education/Glossaries/

- Web of Online Dictionaries (Bucknell University):
  http://www.yourdictionary.com/diction5.html#medicine

TINNITUS GLOSSARY

The following is a complete glossary of terms used in this sourcebook. The definitions are derived from official public sources including the National Institutes of Health [NIH] and the European Union [EU]. After this glossary, we list a number of additional hardbound and electronic glossaries and dictionaries that you may wish to consult.

Ablation: The removal of an organ by surgery. [NIH]

Adjustment: The dynamic process wherein the thoughts, feelings, behavior, and biophysiological mechanisms of the individual continually change to adjust to the environment. [NIH]

Afferent: Concerned with the transmission of neural impulse toward the central part of the nervous system. [NIH]

Ageing: A physiological or morphological change in the life of an organism or its parts, generally irreversible and typically associated with a decline in growth and reproductive vigor. [NIH]

Amplification: The production of additional copies of a chromosomal DNA sequence, found as either intrachromosomal or extrachromosomal DNA. [NIH]

Anchorage: In dentistry, points of retention of fillings and artificial restorations and appliances. [NIH]

Antibiotic: A substance usually produced by vegetal micro-organisms capable of inhibiting the growth of or killing bacteria. [NIH]

Aphasia: An inability, caused by cerebral dysfunction, to communicate in reading, writing or speaking or to receive meaning from spoken or written words. [NIH]

Apraxia: Loss of ability to perform purposeful movements, in the absence of paralysis or sensory disturbance, caused by lesions in the cortex. [NIH]

Attenuated: Strain with weakened or reduced virulence. [NIH]

Audiologist: Study of hearing including treatment of persons with hearing defects. [NIH]

Audition: The sense of hearing. [NIH]

Autoradiography: A process in which radioactive material within an object produces an image when it is in close proximity to a radiation sensitive emulsion. [NIH]

Axonal: Condition associated with metabolic derangement of the entire neuron and is manifest by degeneration of the distal portion of the nerve fiber. [NIH]

Basalis: Chiasmatic cistern. [NIH]

Binaural: Used of the two ears functioning together. [NIH]

Bioluminescence: The emission of light by living organisms such as the firefly, certain mollusks, beetles, fish, bacteria, fungi and protozoa. [NIH]

Broadband: A wide frequency range. Sound whose energy is distributed over a broad range of frequency (generally, more than one octave). [NIH]

Bruit: An abnormal sound heard over an artery, related to the cardiac cycle but unrelated to the respiratory cycle or to muscle, joint, or swallowing activity. [NIH]

Canonical: A particular nucleotide sequence in which each position represents the base more often found when many actual sequences of a given class of genetic elements are compared. [NIH]

CDNA: Synthetic DNA reverse transcribed from a specific RNA through the action of the enzyme reverse transcriptase. DNA synthesized by reverse transcriptase using RNA as a template. [NIH]

Circadian: Repeated more or less daily, i. e. on a 23- to 25-hour cycle. [NIH]

Clamp: A u-shaped steel rod used with a pin or wire for skeletal traction in the treatment of certain fractures. [NIH]

Clavicle: A long bone of the shoulder girdle. [NIH]

Consultation: A deliberation between two or more physicians concerning the diagnosis and the proper method of treatment in a case. [NIH]

Consumption: Pulmonary tuberculosis. [NIH]

Contraindications: Any factor or sign that it is unwise to pursue a certain kind of action or treatment, e. g. giving a general anesthetic to a person with pneumonia. [NIH]

Deletion: A genetic rearrangement through loss of segments of DNA (chromosomes), bringing sequences, which are normally separated, into close proximity. [NIH]

Density: The logarithm to the base 10 of the opacity of an exposed and processed film. [NIH]

Dermatitis: Inflammation of the skin. [NIH]

Dimethyl: A volatile metabolite of the amino acid methionine. [NIH]

Discrimination: The act of qualitative and/or quantitative differentiation between two or more stimuli. [NIH]

Dissection: Cutting up of an organism for study. [NIH]

Disulphide: A covalent bridge formed by the oxidation of two cysteine residues to a cystine residue. The-S-S-bond is very strong and its presence confers additional stability. [NIH]

Dyslexia: Partial alexia in which letters but not words may be read, or in which words may be read but not understood. [NIH]

Dysphonia: Difficulty or pain in speaking; impairment of the voice. [NIH]

Eardrum: A thin, tense membrane forming the greater part of the outer wall of the tympanic cavity and separating it from the external auditory meatus; it constitutes the boundary between the external and middle ear. [NIH]

EEG: A graphic recording of the changes in electrical potential associated with the activity of the cerebral cortex made with the electroencephalogram. [NIH]

Efferent: Nerve fibers which conduct impulses from the central nervous system to muscles and glands. [NIH]

Electrode: Component of the pacing system which is at the distal end of the lead. It is the interface with living cardiac tissue across which the stimulus is transmitted. [NIH]

EMG: Recording of electrical activity or currents in a muscle. [NIH]

Empirical: A treatment based on an assumed diagnosis, prior to receiving confirmatory laboratory test results. [NIH]

Enhancer: Transcriptional element in the virus genome. [NIH]

Enzymatic: Phase where enzyme cuts the precursor protein. [NIH]

Epilepticus: Repeated and prolonged epileptic seizures without recovery of consciousness between attacks. [NIH]

Equalization: The reduction of frequency and/or phase distortion, or modification of gain and or phase versus frequency characteristics of a transducer, by the use of attenuation circuits whose loss or delay is a function of frequency. [NIH]

Excitatory: When cortical neurons are excited, their output increases and each new input they receive while they are still excited raises their output markedly. [NIH]

Exhaustion: The feeling of weariness of mind and body. [NIH]

Fatigue: The feeling of weariness of mind and body. [NIH]

Fold: A plication or doubling of various parts of the body. [NIH]

Formulary: A book containing a list of pharmaceutical products with their formulas and means of preparation. [NIH]

Fossa: A cavity, depression, or pit. [NIH]

Generator: Any system incorporating a fixed parent radionuclide from which is produced a daughter radionuclide which is to be removed by elution or by any other method and used in a radiopharmaceutical. [NIH]

Genetics: The biological science that deals with the phenomena and mechanisms of heredity. [NIH]

Glutamate: Excitatory neurotransmitter of the brain. [NIH]

Gould: Turning of the head downward in walking to bring the image of the ground on the functioning position of the retina, in destructive disease of the peripheral retina. [NIH]

Gravis: Eruption of watery blisters on the skin among those handling animals and animal products. [NIH]

Growth: The progressive development of a living being or part of an organism from its earliest stage to maturity. [NIH]

Habituate: Eventual cessation of response to a repeated sound. [NIH]

Habituation: Decline in response of an organism to environmental or other stimuli with repeated or maintained exposure. [NIH]

Handicap: A handicap occurs as a result of disability, but disability does not always constitute a handicap. A handicap may be said to exist when a disability causes a substantial and continuing reduction in a person's capacity to function socially and vocationally. [NIH]

Harmony: Attribute of a product which gives rise to an overall pleasant sensation. This sensation is produced by the perception of the product components as olfactory, gustatory, tactile and kinaesthetic stimuli because they are present in suitable concentration ratios. [NIH]

Hereditary: Of, relating to, or denoting factors that can be transmitted genetically from one generation to another. [NIH]

Homozygotes: An individual having a homozygous gene pair. [NIH]

Host: Any animal that receives a transplanted graft. [NIH]

Hybrid: Cross fertilization between two varieties or, more usually, two species of vines, see also crossing. [NIH]

Hypnotherapy: Sleeping-cure. [NIH]

Immunologic: The ability of the antibody-forming system to recall a previous experience with an antigen and to respond to a second exposure with the prompt production of large amounts of antibody. [NIH]

Impairment: In the context of health experience, an impairment is any loss or abnormality of psychological, physiological, or anatomical structure or function. [NIH]

Infancy: The period of complete dependency prior to the acquisition of competence in walking, talking, and self-feeding. [NIH]

Infections: The illnesses caused by an organism that usually does not cause disease in a person with a normal immune system. [NIH]

Initiation: Mutation induced by a chemical reactive substance causing cell changes; being a step in a carcinogenic process. [NIH]

Insight: The capacity to understand one's own motives, to be aware of one's own psychodynamics, to appreciate the meaning of symbolic behavior. [NIH]

Involuntary: Reaction occurring without intention or volition. [NIH]

Jefferson: A fracture produced by a compressive downward force that is transmitted evenly through occipital condyles to superior articular surfaces of the lateral masses of C1. [NIH]

Joint: The point of contact between elements of an animal skeleton with the parts that surround and support it. [NIH]

Kb: A measure of the length of DNA fragments, 1 Kb = 1000 base pairs. The largest DNA fragments are up to 50 kilobases long. [NIH]

Koch: It was an early form of tuberculin of low specificity, devised by Robert Koch and made by heat concentration of a broth culture of Mycobacterium tuberculosis. [NIH]

Labyrinthine: A vestibular nystagmus resulting from stimulation, injury, or disease of the labyrinth. [NIH]

Loop: A wire usually of platinum bent at one end into a small loop (usually 4 mm inside diameter) and used in transferring microorganisms. [NIH]

Meatus: A canal running from the internal auditory foramen through the petrous portion of the temporal bone. It gives passage to the facial and auditory nerves together with the auditory branch of the basilar artery and the internal auditory veins. [NIH]

Medial: Lying near the midsaggital plane of the body; opposed to lateral. [NIH]

Metabotropic: A glutamate receptor which triggers an increase in production of 2 intracellular messengers: diacylglycerol and inositol 1, 4, 5-triphosphate. [NIH]

Modeling: A treatment procedure whereby the therapist presents the target behavior which the learner is to imitate and make part of his repertoire. [NIH]

Modification: A change in an organism, or in a process in an organism, that is acquired from its own activity or environment. [NIH]

Monoamine: Enzyme that breaks down dopamine in the astrocytes and microglia. [NIH]

Morphological: Relating to the configuration or the structure of live organs. [NIH]

MRNA: The RNA molecule that conveys from the DNA the information that is to be translated into the structure of a particular polypeptide molecule. [NIH]

Naive: Used to describe an individual who has never taken a certain drug or class of drugs (e. g., AZT-naive, antiretroviral-naive), or to refer to an undifferentiated immune system cell. [NIH]

Narcolepsy: A condition of unknown cause characterized by a periodic uncontrollable tendency to fall asleep. [NIH]

Need: A state of tension or dissatisfaction felt by an individual that impels him to action toward a goal he believes will satisfy the impulse. [NIH]

Nerve: A cordlike structure of nervous tissue that connects parts of the nervous system with other tissues of the body and conveys nervous impulses to, or away from, these tissues. [NIH]

Networks: Pertaining to a nerve or to the nerves, a meshlike structure of interlocking fibers or strands. [NIH]

Neurosyphilis: A late form of syphilis that affects the brain and may lead to dementia and death. [NIH]

Niche: The ultimate unit of the habitat, i. e. the specific spot occupied by an individual organism; by extension, the more or less specialized relationships existing between an organism, individual or synusia(e), and its environment. [NIH]

Nuclei: A body of specialized protoplasm found in nearly all cells and containing the chromosomes. [NIH]

Nucleus: A body of specialized protoplasm found in nearly all cells and containing the chromosomes. [NIH]

Nystagmus: Rhythmical oscillation of the eyeballs, either pendular or jerky. [NIH]

Orderly: A male hospital attendant. [NIH]

Ossicles: The hammer, anvil and stirrup, the small bones of the middle ear, which transmit the vibrations from the tympanic membrane to the oval window. [NIH]

Otology: The branch of medicine which deals with the diagnosis and treatment of the disorders and diseases of the ear. [NIH]

Outpatient: A patient who is not an inmate of a hospital but receives diagnosis or treatment in a clinic or dispensary connected with the hospital. [NIH]

Palsy: Disease of the peripheral nervous system occurring usually after many years of increased lead absorption. [NIH]

Paralysis: Loss or impairment of muscle function or sensation. [NIH]

Pathologies: The study of abnormality, especially the study of diseases. [NIH]

Pediatrics: The branch of medical science concerned with children and their diseases. [NIH]

Perilymph: The fluid contained within the space separating the membranous from the osseous labyrinth of the ear. [NIH]

Phantom: Used to absorb and/or scatter radiation equivalently to a patient, and hence to estimate radiation doses and test imaging systems without actually exposing a patient. It may be an anthropomorphic or a physical test object. [NIH]

Physiology: The science that deals with the life processes and functions of organismus, their cells, tissues, and organs. [NIH]

Plasticity: In an individual or a population, the capacity for adaptation: a) through gene changes (genetic plasticity) or b) through internal physiological modifications in response to changes of environment (physiological plasticity). [NIH]

Polymerase: An enzyme which catalyses the synthesis of DNA using a single DNA strand as a template. The polymerase copies the template in the 5'-3'direction provided that sufficient quantities of free nucleotides, dATP and dTTP are present. [NIH]

Postsynaptic: Nerve potential generated by an inhibitory hyperpolarizing stimulation. [NIH]

Potassium: It is essential to the ability of muscle cells to contract. [NIH]

Presumptive: A treatment based on an assumed diagnosis, prior to receiving confirmatory laboratory test results. [NIH]

Probe: An instrument used in exploring cavities, or in the detection and dilatation of strictures, or in demonstrating the potency of channels; an elongated instrument for exploring or sounding body cavities. [NIH]

Promoter: A chemical substance that increases the activity of a carcinogenic process. [NIH]

Protocol: The detailed plan for a clinical trial that states the trial's rationale, purpose, drug or vaccine dosages, length of study, routes of administration, who may participate, and other aspects of trial design. [NIH]

Pterygoid: A canal in the sphenoid bone for the vidian nerve. [NIH]

Race: A population within a species which exhibits general similarities within itself, but is both discontinuous and distinct from other populations of that species, though not sufficiently so as to achieve the status of a taxon. [NIH]

Racemic: Optically inactive but resolvable in the way of all racemic compounds. [NIH]

Radiological: Pertaining to radiodiagnostic and radiotherapeutic procedures, and interventional radiology or other planning and guiding medical radiology. [NIH]

Reassurance: A procedure in psychotherapy that seeks to give the client confidence in a favorable outcome. It makes use of suggestion, of the prestige of the therapist. [NIH]

Recombination: The formation of new combinations of genes as a result of segregation in crosses between genetically different parents; also the rearrangement of linked genes due to crossing-over. [NIH]

Refer: To send or direct for treatment, aid, information, de decision. [NIH]

Rehabilitative: Instruction of incapacitated individuals or of those affected with some mental disorder, so that some or all of their lost ability may be regained. [NIH]

Reliability: Used technically, in a statistical sense, of consistency of a test with itself, i. e. the extent to which we can assume that it will yield the same result if repeated a second time. [NIH]

Restoration: Broad term applied to any inlay, crown, bridge or complete denture which restores or replaces loss of teeth or oral tissues. [NIH]

Retrogression: A reversion to some earlier stage of succession consequent on the introduction of an adverse factor, commonly soil degradation. [NIH]

Salicylate: Non-steroidal anti-inflammatory drugs. [NIH]

Schizophrenia: A mental disorder characterized by a special type of disintegration of the personality. [NIH]

Secretory: Secreting; relating to or influencing secretion or the secretions. [NIH]

Senile: Relating or belonging to old age; characteristic of old age; resulting from infirmity of old age. [NIH]

Specialist: In medicine, one who concentrates on 1 special branch of medical science. [NIH]

Specificity: Degree of selectivity shown by an antibody with respect to the number and types of antigens with which the antibody combines, as well as with respect to the rates and the extents of these reactions. [NIH]

Sperm: The fecundating fluid of the male. [NIH]

Spike: The activation of synapses causes changes in the permeability of the dendritic membrane leading to changes in the membrane potential. This difference of the potential travels along the axon of the neuron and is called spike. [NIH]

Splint: A rigid appliance used for the immobilization of a part or for the correction of deformity. [NIH]

Stereotactic: Radiotherapy that treats brain tumors by using a special frame affixed directly to the patient's cranium. By aiming the X-ray source with respect to the rigid frame, technicians can position the beam extremely precisely during each treatment. [NIH]

Stethoscope: An instrument used for the detection and study of sounds within the body that conveyed to the ears of the observer through rubber tubing. [NIH]

Stimulants: Any drug or agent which causes stimulation. [NIH]

Stimulus: That which can elicit or evoke action (response) in a muscle, nerve, gland or other excitable issue, or cause an augmenting action upon any function or metabolic process. [NIH]

Suppression: A conscious exclusion of disapproved desire contrary with repression, in which the process of exclusion is not conscious. [NIH]

Synapse: The region where the processes of two neurons come into close contiguity, and the nervous impulse passes from one to the other; the fibers of the two are intermeshed, but, according to the general view, there is no direct contiguity. [NIH]

Synchrony: The normal physiologic sequencing of atrial and ventricular activation and contraction. [NIH]

Temporal: One of the two irregular bones forming part of the lateral surfaces and base of the skull, and containing the organs of hearing. [NIH]

Tetanic: Having the characteristics of, or relating to tetanus. [NIH]

Therapeutics: The branch of medicine which is concerned with the treatment of diseases, palliative or curative. [NIH]

Threshold: For a specified sensory modality (e. g. light, sound, vibration), the lowest level (absolute threshold) or smallest difference (difference threshold, difference limen) or intensity of the stimulus discernible in prescribed conditions of stimulation. [NIH]

Tonal: Based on special tests used for a topographic diagnosis of perceptive deafness (damage of the Corti organ, peripheral or central damage, i. e. the auditive cortex). [NIH]

Transduction: The transfer of genes from one cell to another by means of a viral (in the case of bacteria, a bacteriophage) vector or a vector which is similar to a virus particle (pseudovirion). [NIH]

Translational: The cleavage of signal sequence that directs the passage of the protein through a cell or organelle membrane. [NIH]

Transmitter: A chemical substance which effects the passage of nerve impulses from one cell to the other at the synapse. [NIH]

Trigeminal: Cranial nerve V. It is sensory for the eyeball, the conjunctiva, the eyebrow, the skin of face and scalp, the teeth, the mucous membranes in the mouth and nose, and is motor to the muscles of mastication. [NIH]

Ulcer: A localized necrotic lesion of the skin or a mucous surface. [NIH]

Vasodilators: Any nerve or agent which induces dilatation of the blood vessels. [NIH]

Vitro: Descriptive of an event or enzyme reaction under experimental investigation occurring outside a living organism. Parts of an organism or microorganism are used together with artificial substrates and/or conditions. [NIH]

Wound: Any interruption, by violence or by surgery, in the continuity of the external surface of the body or of the surface of any internal organ. [NIH]

Zoster: A virus infection of the Gasserian ganglion and its nerve branches, characterized by discrete areas of vesiculation of the epithelium of the forehead, the nose, the eyelids, and the cornea together with subepithelial infiltration. [NIH]

General Dictionaries and Glossaries

While the above glossary is essentially complete, the dictionaries listed here cover virtually all aspects of medicine, from basic words and phrases to more advanced terms (sorted alphabetically by title; hyperlinks provide rankings, information and reviews at Amazon.com):

- **Dictionary of Medical Acronymns & Abbreviations** by Stanley Jablonski (Editor), Paperback, 4th edition (2001), Lippincott Williams & Wilkins Publishers, ISBN: 1560534605,
  http://www.amazon.com/exec/obidos/ASIN/1560534605/icongroupinterna

- **Dictionary of Medical Terms : For the Nonmedical Person (Dictionary of Medical Terms for the Nonmedical Person, Ed 4)** by Mikel A. Rothenberg, M.D, et al, Paperback - 544 pages, 4th edition (2000), Barrons Educational Series, ISBN: 0764112015,
  http://www.amazon.com/exec/obidos/ASIN/0764112015/icongroupinterna

- **A Dictionary of the History of Medicine** by A. Sebastian, CD-Rom edition (2001), CRC Press-Parthenon Publishers, ISBN: 185070368X,
  http://www.amazon.com/exec/obidos/ASIN/185070368X/icongroupinterna

- **Dorland's Illustrated Medical Dictionary (Standard Version)** by Dorland, et al, Hardcover - 2088 pages, 29th edition (2000), W B Saunders Co, ISBN: 0721662544,
  http://www.amazon.com/exec/obidos/ASIN/0721662544/icongroupinterna

- **Dorland's Electronic Medical Dictionary** by Dorland, et al, Software, 29th Book & CD-Rom edition (2000), Harcourt Health Sciences, ISBN:

0721694934,
http://www.amazon.com/exec/obidos/ASIN/0721694934/icongroupinterna

- **Dorland's Pocket Medical Dictionary (Dorland's Pocket Medical Dictionary, 26th Ed)** Hardcover - 912 pages, 26th edition (2001), W B Saunders Co, ISBN: 0721682812,
http://www.amazon.com/exec/obidos/ASIN/0721682812/icongroupinterna/103-4193558-7304618

- **Melloni's Illustrated Medical Dictionary (Melloni's Illustrated Medical Dictionary, 4th Ed)** by Melloni, Hardcover, 4th edition (2001), CRC Press-Parthenon Publishers, ISBN: 85070094X,
http://www.amazon.com/exec/obidos/ASIN/85070094X/icongroupinterna

- **Stedman's Electronic Medical Dictionary Version 5.0 (CD-ROM for Windows and Macintosh, Individual)** by Stedmans, CD-ROM edition (2000), Lippincott Williams & Wilkins Publishers, ISBN: 0781726328,
http://www.amazon.com/exec/obidos/ASIN/0781726328/icongroupinterna

- **Stedman's Medical Dictionary** by Thomas Lathrop Stedman, Hardcover - 2098 pages, 27th edition (2000), Lippincott, Williams & Wilkins, ISBN: 068340007X,
http://www.amazon.com/exec/obidos/ASIN/068340007X/icongroupinterna

- **Tabers Cyclopedic Medical Dictionary (Thumb Index)** by Donald Venes (Editor), et al, Hardcover - 2439 pages, 19th edition (2001), F A Davis Co, ISBN: 0803606540,
http://www.amazon.com/exec/obidos/ASIN/0803606540/icongroupinterna

INDEX

A
Ablation 108, 111
Adjustment 66, 379
Afferent 85, 111, 114, 138, 196, 216
Amplification .73, 83, 84, 190, 194, 206, 285, 287, 288
Aphasia 266, 287
Apraxia 287
Attenuated 240
Audiologist 11, 28, 33, 65, 66, 77, 82, 244, 287, 394
Audition 388
Autoradiography 88
Axonal 108

B
Basalis 92
Binaural 113, 290
Bioluminescence 108
Broadband 60, 189, 258, 378
Bruit 240

C
Canonical 257
Circadian 224
Clamp 102
Clavicle 80
Consultation .... ii, iii, 3, 57, 244, 259
Consumption 354
Contraindications ii

D
Density 91, 106
Dermatitis 185
Dimethyl 225
Discrimination 288
Dissection 80, 162, 163
Disulphide 208
Dyslexia 92, 184, 266
Dysphonia 266

E
Eardrum 26, 78, 186, 187, 196, 212, 216
Electrode 188, 207, 265, 328
Empirical 382, 383, 387
Enzymatic 85
Epilepticus 218
Equalization 78
Excitatory 86, 95, 111
Exhaustion 377

F
Fatigue 215, 283, 284, 379
Fold 33
Fossa 121, 286

G
Generator 60, 69, 178, 198
Genetics 106
Glutamate 85, 86, 101, 111, 172, 243, 409
Gravis 89
Growth .36, 86, 108, 240, 241, 268, 282, 352, 353, 354, 405

H
Habituate 256
Habituation 29, 32, 64, 67, 69, 73, 75, 76, 83, 90, 113, 136, 178, 205, 230, 231, 246, 259, 263
Handicap 63, 110, 113, 128, 137, 158, 160, 172, 261, 408
Harmony 301
Hereditary 104
Homozygotes 104
Host 218
Hybrid 84
Hypnotherapy 127, 305, 308, 312, 315

I
Immunologic 141, 320
Infancy 374
Infections 22, 182, 195, 264, 287
Initiation 64, 208
Insight 112, 395
Involuntary 184, 240

J
Joint 83, 110, 118, 179, 225, 232, 240, 268, 277, 283, 328, 406

L
Labyrinthine 192
Loop 75, 103, 172, 409

M
Meatus 36, 196, 216, 407
Medial ... 87, 94, 103, 108, 114, 143, 196, 217, 241
Metabotropic 85
Modeling 84
Modification 69, 171, 183, 230, 407
Morphological 101, 111, 268, 405

N
Naive 76, 92, 173, 410
Narcolepsy 219, 224
Networks 3, 129
Neurosyphilis 240

Niche 243
Nuclei 88, 97, 108, 112
Nucleus...86, 87, 88, 92, 94, 95, 97, 109, 111, 112, 114, 142, 161, 317, 319
Nystagmus 192, 228, 409

O
Orderly 99
Ossicles 391
Outpatient 164

P
Palsy 123, 182
Paralysis...125, 182, 283, 286, 296, 333, 357, 405
Pathologies 103, 104, 178
Perilymph 101, 240, 377
Phantom 111, 126, 195, 222
Physiology .. 24, 212, 232, 233, 285, 290, 382
Plasticity 92, 96, 105, 108, 112, 114, 138, 174, 330, 411
Polymerase 101, 174, 411
Postsynaptic 94
Potassium 87, 94, 102, 226, 354
Presumptive 101
Promoter 99
Protocol 48, 66, 68, 69, 113, 117, 255
Pterygoid 196, 217

R
Race 49, 228, 411
Racemic 228, 411
Radiological 182
Reassurance 61, 73, 83, 251, 330
Recombination 94
Refer 3, 4, 11, 42, 173, 249, 279, 410
Reliability 71, 117, 248
Restoration 301, 302

Retrogression 208

S
Salicylate 28, 304, 307, 309
Schizophrenia 89, 123, 218, 219, 224, 227
Secretory 219
Senile 225
Specialist 41, 42, 45, 163, 182, 253
Specificity 112, 172, 409
Sperm 354
Spike 200, 221, 228, 412
Splint 284
Stethoscope 223
Stimulants 26
Stimulus .73, 81, 93, 114, 175, 178, 188, 193, 201, 221, 227, 245, 407, 413
Suppression 127, 133, 134, 167, 222, 262, 313, 316, 318, 334, 335, 337
Synapse 175, 413
Synchrony 201, 221

T
Temporal.....70, 78, 79, 90, 92, 110, 156, 163, 228, 381, 409
Tetanic 112
Therapeutics 357
Threshold. 103, 107, 115, 175, 183, 189, 256, 265, 287, 317, 377, 378, 381, 382, 393, 413
Tonal 63, 183, 306, 317
Transduction 85, 104, 109, 115, 127, 254
Translational 106
Transmitter 86, 94, 101, 111, 115

V
Vasodilators 64
Vitro 101, 102, 103, 104, 108

Z
Zoster 106